T0356084

PRESCRIPTION FOR PAIN

How a Once-Promising Doctor Became the "PILL MILL KILLER"

PHILIP EIL

STEERFORTH PRESS
LEBANON, NEW HAMPSHIRE

For information about permission to reproduce
selections from this book, write to:
Steerforth Press, 31 Hanover Street, Suite 1
Lebanon, New Hampshire 03766

Cataloging-in-Publication Data is available from the Library of Congress

ISBN 978-1-58642-405-3 (paperback)
Printed in the United States of America

1 3 5 7 9 10 8 6 4 2

For my parents, Adele and Charles.

The ability of human beings to find pleasing explanations for the most grotesque kinds of things that they do is, of course, one of our saving characteristics. Self-deception allows us to act indecently and transmute such actions, in our minds, into more palatable fare. It is the extraordinarily rare murderer or thief who tells us that he did what he did because he is a mean, ugly, and vicious human being.

For the physicians in our sample, the intensity of their defense of what they had done, and their skill and resourcefulness in locating villains who, out of malevolence or ineptness, had gotten them into trouble with the authorities, were particularly pronounced.

— *Journal of the American Medical Association (JAMA)*, "Fraud by Physicians Against Medicaid," Paul Jesilow, Gilbert Geis, and Henry Pontell, December 1991

CONTENTS

ACKNOWLEDGMENTS

I began working on this project in the spring of 2009, a few weeks before I turned twenty-four. The book will be released in April 2024, a few days before my thirty-ninth birthday. During the intervening years, I received help from so many people.

First and foremost, my gratitude goes to the family members of deceased Volkman patients who spoke with me. I was a stranger contacting them about a deeply painful subject, and yet they placed their trust in me. This book would not have been possible without their cooperation, and telling their stories has been an honor and a privilege. In particular, I want to thank Melissa Flaugher-Ratcliff, Brad Nolan, Jakkie Layne, and Megan Rose Estep, who spoke with me multiple times. I am also indebted to many other folks in southern Ohio, especially Lisa Roberts, Andrew Feight, Diana Colley, Lisa Carver, and Ed Hughes.

This book would also not have been possible without interviews with more than a dozen experts on pain and addiction. None were more generous with their time and expertise than Steven Passik, whom I now consider a friend.

I also want to thank Adam and Elizabeth Volkman, Jane Volkman, and David Volkman for our many conversations over the years.

Another thank-you goes to the folks who helped me to understand Paul Volkman's malpractice cases, including Joanne and Nicole De Masi, Margaret O'Leary, Dale Ryder, Steve Jambois, and Sarah Olson.

Thank you, also, to Sara Martinez and William Hurwitz. And thank you to the many clerks, court reporters, and librarians who helped me along the way, in particular, the staff in the local history room at the Portsmouth Public Library.

Over the course of this project, I received extraordinary hospitality. Thank you to Adam Kistler in Chicago; Evan McGarvey in State College, Pennsylvania; Marty Austin in Louisville; Oliver and Susan Cameron in Ann Arbor; Jessica Fornari and her parents, Barbara and Ralph, in Chicago; Michael and China Hoffman in Pittsburgh; Jeremy Katzen and Sarah Folit-Weinberg in Rochester, New York; Jane Holding in Chapel Hill; Ryan Scanlon in Boston and Woodstock, Vermont; Lucas Owens in Cumberland, Maryland; Maria Clark in New Orleans; Andrew Eil and Hannah Seligson in Washington, DC; Mark Cohen and Jerry Hyman in

New York; Tanya Paperny in Washington, DC; and Sean Kostamo and Jessica Hill in Alexandria, Virginia. Thank you, also, to Katy Mathuews, who helped me to feel welcome in southern Ohio.

This book began to take shape at the Columbia University School of the Arts MFA Writing Program from 2009 to 2011 and in Sam Freedman's book-writing seminar at the Columbia School of Journalism in 2011. I am indebted to my teachers Stephen O'Connor, Richard Locke, Paul Elie, Patricia O'Toole, Leslie Sharpe, and Sam Freedman. Thank you, also, to MFA classmates Dax Proctor, Brian Spitulnick, Suzanne Mozes, Sophia Efthimiatou, Casey Plett, Sarah Perry, Raina Lipsitz, Abigail Rasminsky, Channing Kehoe, and Ray Dademo, and book-seminar classmates Jaime Joyce and Joe Alexiou.

Thank you to the Norman Mailer Center and to my friend from the 2012 Nonfiction Fellowship (and fellow Steerforth Press author), Steve Jimenez.

Thank you to my colleagues in the Rhode Island press corps: Ian Donnis, Ted Nesi, Dan McGowan, Tim White, Amanda Milkovits, Ed Fitzpatrick, G. Wayne Miller, Sarah Francis, Ethan Shorey, Lou Papineau, Steve Ahlquist, Katie Mulvaney, Mike Stanton, Jamie Coelho, Janine Weisman, and Antonia Noori Farzan. Thank you to other Rhode Island writer/editor-friends: Mary-Kim Arnold, Vanessa Lillie, Josie Riesman, SI Rosenbaum (who read an early draft of this book), Tom Stackpole, Nora Caplan-Bricker, and Bill Clements (another early reader). Thank you to my friends, mentors, editors, and colleagues from my years in journalism: David Scharfenberg, Rajul Punjabi, Peter Kadzis, Dan Kennedy, Adam Flango, Adam Langer, Cory Schouten, Dan Bloom, Robin Amer, and Felice Freyer.

A very special thank-you goes to the folks who helped me in my multi-year Freedom of Information Act battle, which ultimately prompted the release of tens of thousands of pages of evidence from the Volkman trial. Thank you to Rhode Island ACLU Executive Director Steve Brown; my pro bono attorneys, Jessica Schacter Jewell and Neal McNamara, from Nixon Peabody; and US District Court Judge John McConnell, who gave my case a thorough hearing and a fair ruling. Thank you, also, to the journalists, organizations, and news outlets who helped me during this odyssey: Luke O'Neil; John Marion; Mark Schieldrop; Bob Plain; Nick Inglis; Dan Yorke; Justin Silverman at the New England First Amendment Coalition; Trevor Timm at the Freedom of the Press Foundation; Michael Morisy, JPat Brown, and Beryl Lipton at MuckRock; the opinion pages at the *Columbus*

Dispatch and *Portsmouth Daily Times*; the Electronic Frontier Foundation; and the Investigative Reporters and Editors podcast.

Thank you to the many authors who were supportive of this project: Leah Carroll, John Temple, Charlotte Bismuth, Harold Schechter, Joanna Connors, Brad Balukjian, Laura Jean Moore, Elon Green, and Sarah Weinman.

Thank you to my therapist, Deborah, without whom I would have never finished this project.

Thank you to my dear friends Ryan and Emily Scanlon, John and Samantha Kokolski, Greg Katzen, Sam Miner, Ben Horowitz, Becca Bender and Seth Mulliken, Joe Manok and Kate Jennings, Howard Voss-Altman, Jesus Hernandez, Jarvis Green, Jose Itzigsohn, Mark Douglas (another early manuscript reader), and Nadje Al-Ali. A special thank-you to my wonderful longtime friends Tanya Paperny, Liz Greenwood, and Jean Murley, each of whom helped this project in innumerable ways.

Thank you to my grandmother Dr. Lois Eil, who was a steadfast supporter of this book project until her passing in 2017.

Thank you to my parents, Adele and Charles, who had front-row seats to this project's many delays, detours, and obstacles and remained unwavering supporters. Thank you to my brothers, Matt and Andrew; my sisters-in-law, Ariella and Hannah; and my beautiful nieces and nephews: Ellie, Ollie, Leah, and Gabriel. Thank you, also, to my cousin (and early reader), David Eil, and to my aunt, Phyllis Zavatsky.

Thank you to Chip Fleischer and the entire team at Steerforth Press. Their team has been incredibly warm and supportive, and I have always felt seen, heard, and valued, which I know is not always the case for authors in the publishing world. To Chip, in particular: I will never forget the faith you placed in me as an unknown first-time author. Over the course of this project, I treasured your patience, professionalism, and wisdom.

Finally, I want to thank my partner, Georgina, who was my co-pilot for the last four years of this journey. Georgina supported this project in too many ways to count. She helped to keep me sane and steady in difficult moments. She was a reliable source of encouragement and a sensitive listener to my book-related thoughts, plans, questions, and fears. She saw me spend mornings, nights, weekends, and portions of "vacations" working on the book and did not protest. She read drafts and offered incisive feedback. During particularly demanding stretches, she kept me well-fed. And when I was too mired in self-criticism or pessimism, she helped me to see the project, and what I had accomplished, more clearly.

She is a brilliant, beautiful, sensitive, and generous person. And I am so lucky to have her — and our two precious kitties, Jack and Jill — in my life.

PROLOGUE: THE ARREST

Lake Shore Drive runs along the eastern edge of the city of Chicago, separating the skyscrapers of downtown from the shores of Lake Michigan. The roadway begins in the South Side and continues north to the city's upper outskirts. Along the way, travelers pass an array of dazzling sights: beaches, parks, museums, a football stadium, a Ferris wheel. With four lanes in each direction, the road carries more than a hundred thousand vehicles every day, while countless additional bikers, walkers, joggers, and in-line skaters use the abutting paths.

But Lake Shore Drive is more than just a means of transportation; it's also a status symbol. The highway has been the address of movie stars, professional athletes, and other celebrities. In this way, Lake Shore Drive is a bit like Park Avenue in New York or Ocean Drive in Miami: It's both a mark of prestige and an instantly recognizable landmark. The road makes appearances in famous Chicago-set films like *Risky Business, Ferris Bueller's Day Off*, and *The Blues Brothers*. In 1998, a *Chicago Tribune* architecture critic wrote that "the lakefront is Chicago's undisputed crown jewel . . . the face Chicago presents to the world."

And, of course, if you live in Chicago, Lake Shore Drive needs no introduction at all. I recently spoke with someone from the city who described it in blunt and memorable terms. "When you are from Chicago and you say or hear 'Lake Shore Drive,' you immediately think of money," she said.

The apartment building at 3240 North Lake Shore Drive was completed in 1929, just months before the stock market crashed. And the twenty-story brick building is a reflection of the high-flying era that preceded the Depression. The entrance features stone archways, gas-lamp-style light fixtures, wrought-iron railings, and carefully maintained beds of flowers. The lobby has crystal chandeliers, gilded ceilings, and black and white marble floor tiles installed in a chessboard pattern. Some apartments in the building have wood-burning fireplaces. The building is staffed by a small army of employees, including doormen, maintenance workers, car valets, and elevator operators.

In May 2007, Dr. Paul Volkman lived with his wife, Nancy, on the ninth floor, in a spacious apartment with three bedrooms. Six windows looked out over the bright-blue waters of Lake Michigan. The apartment had a grand piano, and Nancy had worked with an interior decorator to outfit the place with artwork and furniture. Rent was $4,500 per month. It was, in the words of Volkman's daughter, Jane, a "rich man's apartment."

It was in this apartment, at around seven thirty on Monday morning, May 21, when Volkman heard a loud banging on the door. This was unusual. If the Volkmans had visitors, they would usually receive a phone call from the building's front desk. Behind the door was a group of law enforcement agents with guns drawn. They were there to arrest him.

Volkman had just gotten out of bed, and the agents allowed him to get dressed. After he was handcuffed and his legs were shackled, he was led to the elevator, walked through the lobby, and ushered into an SUV that waited outside. The indignity of that moment, in which he was marched through the lobby in shackles, was something he described repeatedly in the years that followed. It was as if the scene were playing on a loop in his mind.

The reason for Volkman's arrest was a thirty-five-page federal indictment that had been filed three hundred miles away in Cincinnati, Ohio. That document alleged that he was one of three players in a massive scheme to illegally distribute prescription drugs. Prosecutors said that his criminal activity had taken place over a span of nearly three years, from April 2003 to February 2006, in towns in the Appalachian foothills of southern Ohio.

According to the indictment, Volkman had worked as a physician in a series of cash-only pain clinics that prescribed high doses of narcotics and other controlled substances. Some clinics were patrolled by armed guards. And when local pharmacies refused to fill Volkman's prescriptions, one clinic opened its own on-site dispensary. Prosecutors alleged that Volkman continued to prescribe medications despite obvious indicators that patients were addicted to the medications, reselling their pills, or both.

Volkman's partners in this scheme — and his codefendants in the indictment — were a mother-daughter duo, Denise and Alice Huffman, who owned and operated the clinic. The indictment noted that neither woman had any medical education. And during the course of the Volkman-Huffman partnership, the document said, more than a million pills had gone missing from the clinic, in addition to the hundreds of thousands that were prescribed and dispensed.

Prosecutors claimed that the consequences of this operation were catastrophic. Though Volkman wasn't formally charged with murder or manslaughter, the indictment described a disturbing pattern where people traveled to the clinic, met with the doctor, received a prescription, and, within a few days, died from an apparent overdose. Included in the indictment were names of fourteen patients whom prosecutors claimed to have died as a direct result of medication Volkman prescribed.

The indictment ended with an estimate of how much Volkman and the Huffmans had made from this operation, which the government was now seeking to recoup: $3,087,500 from each of the Huffmans, and $3,787,500 from the doctor himself.

Following his arrest, Volkman was driven to a building downtown where he said he was strip-searched, given an orange uniform, and placed in a holding room for hours with what he later described as "a bunch of gang members that were awaiting arraignment." After his bond was denied, he was transferred to the Metropolitan Correctional Center, a mustard-colored skyscraper with thin window slats in downtown Chicago.

The sixty-year-old physician remained in custody there for the next few weeks while word of his indictment spread. Wire reports about the case appeared in newspapers in Maine, Florida, Pennsylvania, and Texas. The Drug Enforcement Administration — the federal agency that had led the investigation — issued a press release with a quote from a high-ranking agent who said, "This indictment serves as a warning to all medical professionals that if you illegally prescribe medication for personal gain you will be prosecuted to the fullest extent of the law." An article in the *Chicago Tribune* mentioned that, at an early stage in his career, Volkman had run a pediatrics office in Chicago. The piece included a quote from Volkman's daughter, Jane, who said that her father was "completely innocent." Meanwhile, Ohio's capital-city newspaper, the *Columbus Dispatch*, ran a story noting that, in 2004, Volkman was the largest single purchaser of oxycodone in the United States.

It was more than two weeks into his stay at the Metropolitan Correctional Center that Volkman handwrote a letter to the magistrate overseeing his detention. His immediate purpose was to refute the idea that he was a flight risk, which prosecutors had used to justify his ongoing imprisonment. (An agent present at his arrest would later testify that Volkman told agents that "he had money in the Bahamas, and that as soon as he got out, he was going to go there.")

But over the course of six pages, Volkman took aim at the entire case against him. He argued that he was fully innocent of the charges and that he was a "law abiding, responsible physician and family man with no previous history of violations of law and no history of any actions against him by any state medical board." And he vowed that he had every intention of appearing for any scheduled court date to "vigorously contest the vicious, fabricated allegations with which the gov't has attacked me and my family."

Years later, I would interview various people from Volkman's life, including med school classmates, his two children, and people who knew him in Chicago. And among these people, the most frequent reaction was shock. One person who had known him in college and graduate school told me, "I honestly thought that one day I would pick up the newspaper and I would see that Paul had been given the Nobel Prize in Medicine."

I understand their confusion.

The facts of Paul Volkman's story were like puzzle pieces that didn't seem to fit together.

How had a man who lived in Chicago committed a multiyear crime spree hundreds of miles from where he lived?

How had this former high school valedictorian wound up working in a cash-only pain clinic with armed guards and an on-site pharmacy?

Why was Volkman working in a clinic owned by a woman with no medical training and who had previously worked in factories and fast-food restaurants?

And how could prosecutors claim that he had caused so much damage while Volkman claimed to be completely innocent?

Some of that factual dissonance would have been visible during his early-morning arrest on Lake Shore Drive, as he shuffled across the lobby's marble floors with shackled feet. And some of it was captured in Volkman's signature at the bottom of his letter from jail, written on June 4, 2007. In a sense, that signature captured the entirety of his life and career:

Respectfully
Paul H Volkman, M.D., Ph.D.
Inmate 22435–424

Over the course of the American opiate epidemic, more than a hundred doctors have been convicted of illegally dispensing prescription drugs. The long list includes Kevin Clemmer in Colorado, Sanjay Kumar in North Carolina, David Webb in Florida, Philip Dean in Missouri, Howard

Diamond in Texas, Shannon Caesar in Louisiana, and Jerrold Rosenberg in my home state of Rhode Island. There have been prosecutions of doctors in New York City, Los Angeles, Dallas, Detroit, Las Vegas, Louisville, Richmond, Honolulu, Savannah, Tulsa, and Wichita, among other cities. In 2020, the journal *Injury Epidemiology* published an article based on a review of media coverage between 1995 and 2019. The authors found 372 instances of physicians "involved in opioid-related criminal cases," including cases of alleged fraud, money laundering, and manslaughter.

And yet, even in this era of widespread medical corruption, the case of Paul Volkman stands out.

It stands out, first, for the sheer number of pills that moved through his clinics. By Volkman's own admission, many of his patients were being prescribed between six hundred and eight hundred pills per month. And when authorities executed a raid of his clinic in 2005, they found stacks of prefilled, prelabeled bottles of pills in the dispensary, waiting to go into the hands of patients. At one point, a medical supply company notified the DEA that Volkman had placed the largest order for the opioid hydrocodone the company had ever seen.

Second is the fact that, training-wise, Volkman had obtained not just a medical degree but also a doctorate in pharmacology and toxicology. And as he explained under oath at one point in his career, "Pharmacology involves the study of drugs, pharmaceutical agents, and the way they act. And toxicology involves the study of overdoses, poisons, and the treatment thereof." If anyone should have known the consequences of overprescribing dangerous medications, it was Paul Volkman, MD, PhD.

And then there was the sentence. On February 14, 2012, Paul Volkman was sentenced to four *consecutive* life terms in federal prison. This appears to be the longest sentence imposed on any convicted doctor during the country's opiate epidemic. To find a comparable sentence, you have to step out of the world of medical crimes and into the realms of mob activity, terrorism, murder, and rape. Perhaps the closest match to Volkman's sentence is the punishment given to the Unabomber, Theodore Kaczynski, who also received four life sentences for a campaign of mail bombing that left three people dead and more than twenty injured.

But there is one more thing that, for me specifically, makes the Volkman case stick out: He and my dad were classmates and friends for ten years.

My father, Dr. Charles Eil, first met Volkman when they were freshmen at the University of Rochester, in 1964. And then, by coincidence, after college, they attended the same MD/PhD program at the University of Chicago, from 1968 to 1974. During those years their lives ran on close parallel tracks. They took classes, played bridge, and sang in the glee club together. On graduation day at the University of Chicago, their families ate at the same restaurant.

Photos from the 1968 University of Rochester yearbook even show a visual resemblance between the two young men. In his photograph, Volkman is wearing a jacket, a white shirt, a necktie, and dark-framed glasses, with his hair neatly combed to the side. In the other image, my dad is dressed similarly. There are certainly some differences between the photos, but a viewer's immediate impression is that these two guys could pass for brothers.

I first learned about Volkman in 2009, when I was twenty-three years old. I had just embarked on a career in journalism, and the news of my dad's indicted former classmate hit me like a lightning bolt.

Much of that reaction was sheer surprise. My dad is a quiet, mild-mannered guy who spends his free time singing in civic chorale groups, reading books, and playing golf. I don't think he's ever even gotten a speeding ticket. And now, I had just learned, he knows a guy charged with prescription drug dealing? It was astonishing.

My lack of any prior knowledge about Volkman further fueled my interest. Unlike some of my dad's other friends and colleagues, Volkman had not been to dinner parties at our house. The Eil and Volkman families had not gone on vacations together. When I first learned about his case, I knew little more than two basic facts:

> FACT #1: From the late 1960s to the mid-1970s, Paul Volkman had, like my dad, earned two degrees from the University of Chicago: an MD and a PhD. The federal government had paid for this education through a scholarship program known as the Medical Scientist Training Program (MSTP).
>
> FACT #2: In 2007, Volkman was charged with a massive prescription drug-dealing scheme that, according to prosecutors, involved guns, cash, pills, and the overdose deaths of more than a dozen patients.

What on earth had happened in the thirty-some-odd years between these two facts? I found the mystery irresistible.

A few months after I learned about Volkman's case, I sent him a letter. By this point — September 2009 — he was out of jail, living in Chicago, and awaiting trial. And to my surprise (and surely against what his lawyers would have advised, if he had asked them), he was willing to speak with me. A few months later, I drove to Chicago for a series of in-person interviews. And we continued to speak and correspond for more than a decade.*

By now, as I write this, I am extremely well versed in Volkman's version of what happened in his life and career. I have read and re-read the transcripts of our seventeen hours of in-person interviews, plus the hundreds of pages of letters and emails he sent to me after his trial. I have also assembled a trove of his other letters, emails, interviews, essays, comments on news websites, legal filings, and sworn testimony in various court proceedings. You will see excerpts and quotes from these materials throughout this book.

In his telling, it is a story in which Volkman is mistreated by various people and institutions. During his brief time as a medical researcher, a lab director refused to allow Volkman to publish his "major paper with major implications," which prompted him to leave the field in disgust. Later, during his decades as a pediatrician and emergency room physician, he was sued several times for malpractice. Those lawsuits were, in his telling, "all cases without any remotely cognizable negligence" filed by unscrupulous lawyers. But because of the verdicts and settlements they produced, he found himself unable to obtain malpractice insurance. At this point, in the early 2000s, he pivoted to pain management, where he was victimized yet again.

To hear Volkman tell it, his criminal case was the crowning injustice of a career defined by bad luck and the corruption of others. According to one of his legal filings, in southern Ohio, he was "an accomplished, experienced, competent physician working in a rural under-served area trying to help manage the pain of his patients." But because of his willingness to prescribe medications that the government overzealously regulated, he became, in his words, "just another doctor the government decided to put out of business and into jail, absent any evidence at all of wrongdoing."

In Volkman's telling, he is an honest man and a good doctor who was robbed of his livelihood, his medical license, his reputation, and ultimately his freedom for performing the physician's most basic duty: relieving pain.

---

* Yet another unique aspect of this case is how eager Volkman is to speak on the record. He is certainly not the only convicted doctor who maintains his innocence, but few, if any, have gone to such lengths to try to explain themselves.

But I have no intention of merely publishing the lightly edited commentary of a disgraced doctor who believes unequivocally in his own innocence. This was never my goal, as a journalist. Nor do I think, after fact-checking Volkman's account of his career, that his version of events is particularly trustworthy or accurate.

And so, to obtain a truthful and properly contextualized account of this man's life, I have spent years independently piecing together his story. I have traveled to southern Ohio repeatedly to speak with people there. I have attended key moments during Volkman's legal proceedings, including pretrial hearings, opening arguments of the trial, and his sentencing. I have collected and combed through thousands of pages of documents from nearly every stage of his career, including lawsuits, depositions, news clippings, disciplinary records from state medical boards, and other documents. I have read all forty-three hundred pages of the transcript of Volkman's two-month criminal trial. I have also spoken with more than 150 people who helped me to better understand Volkman's life, career, and crimes. This includes more than twenty family members of his deceased patients.

I have, year by year, interview by interview, document by document, answered the question that first drew me to this story: "What the hell happened to Paul Volkman?"

It took quite a while to complete all that reporting. As I write this, more than fourteen years have passed since I first heard my dad mention Volkman. During that time I went to graduate school in New York, moved back home to Rhode Island, and made a name for myself as a journalist. My professional experience, which was so scant when I first heard Volkman's name, now includes bylines in nationally known magazines, websites, and newspapers. I have worked as the news editor of my hometown's alt-weekly newspaper, the *Providence Phoenix*. I have published stories on authors, artists, journalists, activists, academics, and politicians. I have been a guest on TV shows, radio programs, and podcasts. I have flown to Brazil to appear on a panel about access to public records. I have won journalism awards.

This book represents the application of those journalistic skills to the mystery of my dad's old classmate. Even with my added years of journalism experience, it remains the biggest, strangest, and saddest story I have ever told.

— PART ONE —
MALPRACTICE

THE VALEDICTORIAN

Paul Volkman is the grandson of Jewish immigrants.

His maternal grandfather, Simon, was a rabbi who arrived in New York from Russia in 1903 and eventually settled in Denver, Colorado. His paternal grandfather, Edward, was born in Austria and emigrated to the United States in 1901, where he worked in the grocery business in New York City.[*] Both of Paul's grandmothers, Ida and Bessie, were born in Russia.

Details of Volkman's parents' lives are a bit scant. His mother, Rebecca, grew up in Denver before moving to Washington, DC, where she worked as a clerk in the US Treasury Department. Volkman's father, Murray, grew up in New York City before he, too, moved to DC, where he worked as a pharmacist. A World War II draft registration card from 1940 offers a sketch of his physical appearance. He was 5'6½" and 186 pounds, with brown eyes, brown hair, and eyeglasses.

Murray and Rebecca were married in October 1941. Two years later, in 1943, their first son, Seymour Alan, was born. On October 27, 1946, they had a second son, whom they named Paul.

Census records from 1950 indicate that the Volkmans lived in a three-story brick apartment building in the northern part of Washington. In a black-and-white photo from a few years later, Paul's mother, Rebecca, stands on a grassy hill with her two sons on either side. Alan is wearing what appears to be a Boy Scout uniform. And young Paul, who appears to be about six or seven, is wearing crisply ironed slacks, a buttoned-up blazer, and a bow tie.

The rest of what I know about Paul's early years comes mostly from Volkman himself. And it is, like much of the story he tells about his life, strikingly bleak.

He has described his father as a "very angry, depressed kind of guy" who once aspired to pursue medicine but never achieved the dream. After this, in Paul's telling, his dad harbored a simmering loathing for doctors, whom he felt were "absolutely stupid compared to him."

For a time, Murray Volkman ran his own small, independent pharmacy, where he worked long hours. According to Paul, Murray complained

---

[*] Volkman has rabbinical lineage on his father's side as well. His great-uncle Aaron — Edward's brother — was a renowned rabbi who founded the Beth El Congregation in Washington, DC, in 1936. When Aaron died in 1950, a *Washington Post* obituary described him as a "Senior Rabbi of [the] District" and noted that he was the "descendant of 12 generations of spiritual leaders."

frequently about the big drugstore chains, which were able to undercut his prices. His venture into small business ownership eventually failed. Afterward, Murray took a job as a pharmacist at a pharmacy chain, but in Paul's words, he "never stopped his grumbling."

Paul's overall assessment of his father is similarly unflattering. He described his dad to me as an immature, narcissistic man who was uninterested in spending time with kids. And he felt that his dad's punishing work schedule was designed, at least in part, to avoid being at home with his family.

In Volkman's telling, his mother was also an immature and narcissistic person who had little idea about being a mother and not much inclination to learn. He once told me an anecdote from when he was around twelve years old that seemed to represent, to him, the emotional experience of his upbringing. In that story, his mother came home from work, flopped down on the couch, wrung her hands, and complained about her day, while young Paul was tasked with shopping for groceries and preparing dinner. In Volkman's telling, it never occurred to his mother to ask her son how his day had gone.

At one point, Volkman used the word "awful" to describe his parents. He has also said they had little to offer beyond providing two negative role models for him to avoid emulating. His comments about his brother, Alan, are even bleaker. "Hopefully, he's dead," he once told me. "I can't stand the son of a bitch."

Paul's daughter, Jane, meanwhile, has told me that her dad described his childhood home as notably silent, without much talking. She also believed that academic achievement was one of the few sources of affirmation he received from his parents.

"I don't think he felt very loved," she said.

Aside from his diatribes about his parents and his brother, Paul's references to early life are strikingly few. He once described his upbringing to me as "lower middle class." He also once briefly described the pharmacy his father owned, which he said had little red stools that spun around and a distinct "sort of a spicy" smell, perhaps from cough syrup. It was your typical "old ma-and-pa pharmacy," he said.

Additionally, in a letter he wrote from prison, he briefly mentioned family trips that he had taken as a child with his parents to Hershey, Pennsylvania, and the Corning Glass factory in western New York. He described such trips as "interesting, low budget vacations during hard times."

He did speak in some detail about the religious nature of his upbringing. He has explained that he was brought up culturally Jewish, which involved attending Hebrew school twice per week and completing a bar mitzvah. He felt his family's involvement in Judaism stemmed from his parents' sense of duty to raise him and his brother as Jews. But his parents were not particularly observant, and he said that he never heard either of them discuss a belief in God.

My picture of Volkman's life comes into clearer focus in high school. Photos from his sophomore yearbook show a clean-cut, bespectacled kid who participated in an array of bookish pursuits, including the Latin club, chess club, science club, the stamp and coin club, and a classical music ensemble, in which he played the flute. He once told me that during his free time in his early teens, he also enjoyed bowling and playing golf. In 1964, he graduated as valedictorian of his class.

Volkman scored well on his SATs and secured a partial scholarship to attend the University of Rochester, in western New York. He was apparently more than eager to leave Washington because, as he once told me, "I hate the place."

In 1964, when Volkman arrived in Rochester, Lyndon B. Johnson was the president, the Beatles had six Number 1 singles on *Billboard*'s Pop Singles chart, and the civil rights leader Martin Luther King Jr. was awarded a Nobel Peace Prize. Paul majored in chemistry and, in his free time, played chess and bridge and sang in the glee club. A friend who knew him at the time told me that Paul was "painfully shy" around women. "I would bet that he had not been on six dates in his life" before graduating from college, the friend said. Many years later, during the opening statement of his criminal trial in Cincinnati, in 2011, one of his defense attorneys described him as "a self-proclaimed nerd."

Volkman would later reflect on college and — with characteristic immodesty — describe it as "perhaps my happiest years, as I was developing my intellectual skills, which I found were quite considerable." He graduated with honors in the spring of 1968 and, after just a few weeks of summer vacation, headed to Chicago to begin the government-funded MD/PhD program at the University of Chicago. By coincidence, one of his classmates there was his friend from his previous four years in Rochester: my dad, Charles Eil.

———

Volkman once referred to my dad as his "best friend from Rochester." I never heard my dad describe that level of closeness, though he did at least attest that he and Paul became friends shortly after arriving on campus in Rochester in 1964.

The reasons they hit it off are easy to understand. They were bright Jewish guys from the East Coast who excelled in math and science. They both liked to play bridge. They both liked classical music. And they sang together in the glee club.

My dad had arrived in Rochester from the New York City suburb of Yonkers. He was the son of two physicians: Harry, a dermatologist; and Lois, a rare-for-the-era female doctor who worked for the New York City public school system and, later, for the New York State Health Department.

Like Paul, my dad's life at the U of Rochester tended toward nerdier pastimes. He attended concerts of the Rochester Philharmonic Orchestra and spent one summer working in the U of R medical school's biochemistry department.

When I asked what he remembered about Paul from that time, he described him as a smart guy who was not particularly outgoing, socially skilled, or interested in dating, and he specifically remembered Paul's glaring lack of any kind of fashion sense. One word he used to describe his old classmate was *nebbish*, which is a Yiddish word, defined by Oxford Dictionaries as "a person, especially a man, who is regarded as pitifully ineffectual, timid, or submissive."

The other thing that stuck out in my dad's memory was Paul's temperament. He was, in my dad's telling, a frequent complainer who "always thought that things weren't as good as they could have been." This gloominess, along with Paul's general reservedness, were two factors that my dad said kept him at a distance.

Paul "really never opened up like you would to a real close friend," my dad told me. He described him as "kind of a downer."

MSTP

Founded in 1890, the University of Chicago is a sapling compared with legendary East Coast institutions like Harvard (1636), Yale (1701), and Princeton (1746).

But by the time Paul and my father applied there in the late 1960s, the school had established itself as a place of intellectual rigor. These ambitions were reflected in its imposing stone, Gothic-style buildings, modeled after buildings at the Universities of Oxford and Cambridge. And the school's prestige was also visible in its roster of alumni, which, when Paul and Chas arrived in 1968, included several Nobel Prize winners, the National Book Award–winning author Philip Roth, and a recipient of the Fields Medal for mathematics. Other alumni, like astronomer and astrophysicist Carl Sagan, future Supreme Court justice John Paul Stevens, writer and cultural critic Susan Sontag, and economist Milton Friedman, were either well on their way to fame or established intellectual superstars.

Nowadays, the tongue-in-cheek motto that students and alumni have given the school — "Where Fun Goes to Die" — is so ingrained that T-shirts with the slogan are available for purchase online. And one of Volkman's classmates confirmed that this culture existed at the time of their arrival. He recalled studying in the biology library on a Friday night and asking a young woman what she was also doing there at that time. Her response was, "I just don't have anything else to do."

The first MD/PhD program in the United States was established at Case Western Reserve University in Cleveland, Ohio, in 1956. Around the same time, the National Institutes of Health began tinkering with publicly funded programs that combined research with traditional medical training. Then, in 1964, the NIH launched a fully funded dual-degree training program like the one at Case Western. It was called the Medical Scientist Training Program.

The federally funded MSTP debuted at three institutions: Albert Einstein College of Medicine in New York City, New York University, and Northwestern University. Soon, a fourth site was established at Duke University.

A *Chicago Tribune* article from this time offers a glimpse at the hopes behind the taxpayer-backed program. In the article, an official from the NIH said that, previously, medical scientists had pursued either clinical medicine or medical research, and then gradually "backed into" their second field. But this new program would allow students to plant feet in both realms from the start of their training, and in doing so become a "new type of scientist" who "will develop new ways to approach problems of disease." Soon after, three more schools joined the initial quartet of MSTP locations, including the University of Chicago.

But what exactly is medical research?

If you're like me when I first began this project, you won't find the term self-explanatory. And there are few good reasons for this.

First, according to the US Bureau of Labor Statistics, clinical doctors — that is, doctors who primarily see patients — outnumber researchers by a factor of more than five to one. Second, due to the nature of their work, medical researchers interact with the public far less than their clinical counterparts, and their research is primarily read by other members of the medical field, rather than a general audience. (Medical researchers are also the basis for far fewer films and network-TV dramas.)

The Bureau of Labor Statistics defines *medical research* as "dealing with the understanding of human diseases and the improvement of human health" and "engag[ing] in clinical investigation, research and development, or other related activities." The journal *Nature* describes it as "research in a wide range of fields, such as biology, chemistry, pharmacology and toxicology with the goal of developing new medicines or medical procedures or improving the application of those already available."

Much of this research takes place at universities, where those conducting it are employed as professors. This research, once completed and reviewed by peers, is submitted for publication to journals like the *New England Journal of Medicine*, the *American Journal of Medicine*, the *Journal of the American Medical Association* (*JAMA*), and various specialty-specific outlets, such as *Pediatrics*, the *American Journal of Cardiology*, and the *Journal of Clinical Oncology*.

It is through such research and publishing — much of it funded by the federal government — that the medical field slowly presses forward. In turn, this knowledge eventually trickles down into the lives of regular folks like you and me, in the form of the vaccines we receive, the medications we take, the procedures we undergo, and the advice we receive for the treatment of a particular ailment or injury.

This is what both Paul Volkman and my dad wanted to do as a career.

Due to the accelerated nature of U of C's dual-degree program, entrants would not wait until September to begin classes. The program started in the summer, just a few weeks after Chas, Paul, and their six classmates graduated from college. And it began with an age-old rite of passage for medical students: the weeks-long dissection of a cadaver as part of a course on human anatomy.

Their teacher was a colorful, charismatic, British professor named Charles Oxnard, who had previously studied and taught at the University of Birmingham in England. The course took place in the Anatomy Building, an imposing stone structure built in the late 1800s in the school's signature Gothic style. Within a few weeks, the building's air-conditioning gave out, but the course plodded on in what one participant described to me as "incredibly hot conditions."

One classmate of Paul's told me that prior to this course, most of the students had never seen a dead body, and they faced the experience in varying ways. Some students felt faint and barely made it through the dissections. Others steeled themselves and attempted to remain stoic. Volkman told me that he didn't care for it at all. "It was smelly and it was disgusting and it was nauseating," he said.

When researching this part of Volkman and my dad's story, I was fascinated by the fact that this hands-on entry to medical education took place during the summer of 1968, in the midst of what *Smithsonian* magazine has dubbed "The Year That Shattered America."

In the months prior to their arrival in Chicago, protests against the Vietnam War had taken place on college campuses and at recruitment offices. The assassination of Martin Luther King Jr. had sparked riots in dozens of cities across the country. President Lyndon B. Johnson's National Advisory Commission on Civil Disorders (known as the Kerner Commission) released a report warning that the country was "moving toward two societies, one black, one white — separate and unequal." Describing the year in his memoir, music critic Richard Goldstein wrote, "The whole country was inflamed, raw with anxiety and resentment, a land charred by fires of rage."

This tension would rise even higher during the Democratic National Convention in August in downtown Chicago, just a few miles from the MSTP anatomy classes. When antiwar protestors gathered outside the proceedings, Chicago police responded by bashing and brawling and punching through the crowd, leaving a trail of blood and broken glass. The melee, dubbed the Battle of Michigan Avenue, was a vivid manifestation of the country's turmoil. Much of it was broadcast on live television.

And yet, despite the chaos unfolding outside of the classroom, Volkman claims to have been largely detached from politics. He has acknowledged that the draft for the Vietnam War partly motivated his interest in a lengthy training program, stating, "Six years of medical school was more appealing than being drafted to fight in the jungle!"

But when I asked him about any direct involvement in the politics of the time, he said that he was much too busy with school. And when I asked specifically about the much-romanticized counterculture of the late 1960s — hippies, tie-dye, long hair, Woodstock, dancing, drugs, rock 'n' roll, "free love" — he told me that it didn't appeal to him. "It basically seemed like a bunch of unwashed, dirty people just sort of sitting around all day, smoking pot, [and] having sex," he said. "Kinda stupid."

Volkman's comments about his med school experience itself are contradictory. In one essay he wrote in 2019, he said that he "loved" his years at the U of C. But over the years that I spoke to him, he described the place in almost exclusively negative terms.

Volkman told me that the U of C MD/PhD cirriculum was a lofty, impractical program that, in its eagerness to produce what he described as "hotsy totsy researchers," left students clueless about the practical aspects of life as a doctor. He said he left there with no clue how to manage an office, how to bill Medicare and insurance companies, or which areas of medicine paid well compared with others. And over the years I interviewed him, he returned to these gripes. At the U of C, he once said, "clinical medicine and medical practice were options that were considered almost dishonorable, shameful options for those not good enough to be professors."

Although Volkman's classmates didn't seem to share his bitterness, some did, to an extent, affirm his assessment of the culture. One alum of the medical school described it to me as a "very cultured and very theoretical" place with a "rarified atmosphere." He said the joke used to be that if you were sick with some kind of common illness, you'd want to avoid the U of C hospital because you might receive a treatment in search of an exotic illness. It was a place that practiced medicine "based on the most unlikely zebras to occur in the field of pathology," he said.

And other MSTP classmates agree that there was indeed a palpable hierarchy between research and clinical medicine, as Volkman had recalled, although one told me this was simply a fact of academic medicine and not unique to the U of C. He told me that the currency of academic medicine was not necessarily treating patients or teaching; it was securing NIH funding, conducting research, and bringing distinction to your institution through published scholarship.

Generally, when speaking to Volkman's MSTP classmates decades after medical school, I found nobody who shared Volkman's enduring resentment about his training. My dad spoke of his experiences in Chicago in glowing terms. He recalled how he was "euphoric" to learn that he had been accepted and, later, how grateful he was for the program's intellectually stimulating environment. In particular, he described working under the tutelage of a professor of biochemistry whom he loved. And he told me that, overall, he looked back on his time there "very affectionately."

Another UC MSTP classmate, Richard Pauli, who went on to a distinguished career at the University of Wisconsin, also looked back on the program fondly. He explained to me that he had grown up as the son of a stay-at-home mother and a maintenance foreman for an asphalt manufacturer. Before the University of Chicago, he had never traveled outside of New Jersey and New York City.

Not only was the financial support of the scholarship crucial to Pauli's experience, but he told me that the culture of the U of C was important as well. He had applied to the university because he had heard that it was a "place of the mind." And he had found that to be true. Some thirty-five years later, when I interviewed him at his home in Madison, he remembered the ceremony celebrating the completion of his PhD, when his adviser told him, "Welcome to the community of scholars." He admitted that he still got emotional thinking about it decades later.

All told, I spoke to about half a dozen people who knew Volkman during his time at the University of Chicago, including classmates, colleagues, roommates, friends, and acquaintances. For the most part, Volkman seems not to have made a particularly strong impression. One classmate said that he found it interesting that when he thought back on those years, Paul was the classmate about whom he remembered the least. He's the "foggiest, shadiest" recollection, he said. "I really don't remember much about him at all."

But among those who did remember him, a few points of overlap emerged.

More than one person mentioned Volkman's obliviousness to his physical appearance. One remembered how he wore clothes with clashing patterns; another described how he had a "wispy beard and goatee" and unkempt hair.

Others recalled the same gloomy temperament that my dad had noticed at the University of Rochester. "No one would ever describe Paul as 'warm and fuzzy,'" one former roommate told me. Another acquaintance described him as a bit of a loner. "He wouldn't be someone I think you'd have a lot of fun going out and having a drink with," he said.

Many of the people I spoke to remembered him for his intelligence. His former roommate recalled that he was "amazingly bright and hardworking." A pharmacology lab mate told me that Volkman was clearly proud of his intelligence. She remembered that he talked about how he liked to crush his chess opponents.

And this aligned with an anecdote I heard from Richard Pauli. Pauli recalled that, during his years as a med student, there were times when he was awestruck by the responsibilities that came with being a doctor, and he channeled this fear into a determination to learn everything he could. But Volkman seemed to take a different approach. Pauli remembered one incident during a surgery lesson, where Volkman expressed a skepticism about the necessity of what he was learning and was kicked out of the classroom as a result.

When he told me this story, Pauli said that Volkman's remarks about the day's lesson weren't necessarily wrong. It was possible that the students did not, in fact, need to know the exact thing being taught that day for their eventual careers.

But Pauli told me that he would have never dreamed of speaking or acting in that kind of flippant way, out of a fear that perhaps one day, in some unexpected situation, he would need to know what they were being taught. But this mix of apprehension and humility "seemed not to be at all intrinsic to the way Paul felt."

NANCY

In the summer of 1973, Susan Cameron, the wife of one of Paul's med school classmates, introduced Paul to a friend of hers who was studying at U of C's graduate library school. Her name was Nancy Krinn. Susan thought that Nancy and Paul might make a good match, because "they were both single, they were both Jewish, [and] they were both smart."

Nancy had grown up in the Chicago area. People who knew her describe her as peppy and sociable. In high school, she had been a cheerleader, and in college at the University of Illinois, she was the treasurer of her sorority, Sigma Delta Tau. She dressed well and cared about her appearance. "She put herself together," Susan Cameron told me. "She looked very nice."

Despite the rather obvious differences between Paul and Nancy — he was glum, she was cheery; he was oblivious to fashion, she was excited by it — the pair did, in fact, hit it off. Paul would later write that he was "instantly" drawn to Nancy, whom he found "smart, energetic, bubbly, and attractive." They married the following year.

Nancy had passed away by the time I began working on this project, and her family members did not respond to my queries. So, much to my regret, I never heard her thoughts on many aspects of this story, including what drew her to Paul. But Paul's son Adam,* who said that his parents fought like "cats and dogs" during his upbringing, had a decidedly unromantic take.

Adam thought that at the time his parents first met, his mother, who was a few months shy of her thirtieth birthday, was feeling pressure to get married and start a family. And then along came this young Jewish doctor, in whom she saw the promise of stability, financial support, and prestige. In Adam's telling, he believed Nancy's reaction upon meeting Paul was to think: "Bingo. Jackpot. I'll take it."

Paul's marriage to Nancy took place around the time he was making another major life decision: choosing a medical specialty. For the MSTP students nearing the end of their six-year graduate studies, the decision had both short- and long-term implications. On one level, their chosen field would guide the focus of their post-med-school internship, residency, and fellowship. But the specialty was also a chance to set a course that, if things went well, they could pursue for their entire careers.

The choices varied among the cohort. One student chose pathology, the study of diseases. Another — my dad — pursued endocrinology, the study of hormones and their effect on the body. Paul decided to focus on pediatrics, the branch of medicine involving newborns, children, and adolescents.

For people who knew Paul at the time, it was a mystifying choice. Pediatrics was widely recognized as one of the lowest-paying medical specialties, which made it hard to discern an economic motive. More importantly, it just didn't seem to match with Paul's personality. One U of C classmate, who himself became a pediatrician, told me that Paul "hadn't struck [him] as being somebody who had that feel with kids."

My father said that Volkman's choice of career always puzzled him. Pediatrics was particularly demanding of soft skills, because children are

---

* Not his real name.

often fearful of doctors, and their parents can be demanding. Paul wasn't someone whom he thought to be particularly adept in these areas. My dad said, "I never thought of him as a good humanist, as a compassionate person."

Yet another former acquaintance from the U of C, Dr. Oliver Cameron (Susan Cameron's husband), who went on teach psychiatry at the University of Michigan, said that Volkman's career choice surprised him for two reasons. First was his lack of people skills. If Paul had asked him for career advice at the time, he would have advised him not to pursue a specialty with a lot of hands-on patient care.

But Cameron's second reason for surprise was due to how sharply pediatrics diverged from Paul's previous areas of focus. "He got a PhD in pharmacology. Why the hell didn't this guy become a clinical pharmacologist?" He couldn't understand it. "That's like being a world-class downhill skier and decid[ing] that you're going to do figure skating," he said.

Volkman's explanations for this decision tended to be clipped and terse.* During one in-person interview, he told me, "I like interacting with kids." Another time he told me that during med school rotations through various specialties, he found pediatrics the most appealing. He added that he thought kids were cute and "relatively easy to deal with." Elsewhere, in a written account of his career, he described pediatrics as "the area of medicine which most appealed to me, because I loved dealing with kids."

In a couple of instances, he offered slightly more detail. In one case, he seemed to acknowledge that choosing pediatrics was an extension of his distaste for dealing with adults. "I went into pediatrics because I always (and still do) like animals and kids far better than anybody I have ever met over the age of 4," he wrote. At another point, he explained that pediatrics was a specialty in which success was, comparatively speaking, more visible and common. "Mostly, kids get better," he explained. "Some don't. But most of the kids recover from whatever illnesses they have."

Paul graduated from the University of Chicago with his medical degree in 1974. (He had received his PhD two years prior.) And after one year of pediatrics residency at Duke University in North Carolina, he and Nancy returned to Chicago.

---

* This was often the case when I asked him to describe things that he liked or viewed favorably; whereas, when discussing the many subjects of his disdain, his language grew varied and animated.

In August 1975, Nancy gave birth to the couple's first child, their son, Adam. Three years later, in the spring of 1978, their daughter, Jane, was born. A photo from this era shows Nancy, beaming, and holding her two children close. A young Adam, who is also smiling, clutches his baby sister in his arms.

In these early years of fatherhood, Volkman continued to lay the groundwork for a career in academic medicine. Between 1975 and 1977, he completed a fellowship in pharmacology at the U of Chicago, and then spent the two years in a pediatrics residency program at Loyola Medical Center, outside Chicago. During the opening statements of his criminal trial in 2011, one of his defense attorneys, who was keen to cite her client's academic credentials, noted that "during his time at Loyola, he actually taught pharmacology to medical students, he did research, and he published a paper based on that research." After Loyola he moved to a research position in the anesthesiology department at Michael Reese Hospital in Chicago.

And it was here that he ran into a spell of professional turbulence.

As Volkman told me, half of his time at Michael Reese was spent treating patients, while the other half was spent conducting research on the treatment of strokes. And as he told it, during this research he made a discovery about combining two existing drugs as a "remarkably effective" new treatment for hemorrhagic strokes, when a blood vessel ruptures in the brain. With great excitement, he said he wrote up his findings and sent them to the leading journal in the field, the *Journal of Neurosurgery*, which, in his telling, loved the article and accepted it immediately with few changes. It was, he told me, a "very significant paper . . . with major implications."

But there was a catch.

The head of Volkman's department had been away on vacation while he had worked on the paper. And since this administrator led the division that had conducted the research, his name would need to appear on the paper. But, as Volkman told me, when this higher-ranking doctor returned from vacation and learned about Volkman's research, he "couldn't understand it, didn't agree with it, didn't like it, didn't trust it," and refused to sign off on its publication.

There was apparently nothing Volkman could do to convince this supervisor otherwise, and he said that he was forced to withdraw the article. "I worked for two years on a project and got it approved by a major journal and wound up not being able to publish it," he said. It was, in his telling, a shattering blow that influenced his career trajectory. He would later write, "In utter disgust, I gave up any plans to spend my life in medical research."

But when I spoke with Dr. Ronald Albrecht, who was the head of anesthesiology at Michael Reese Hospital and the lab director who Volkman claimed had spiked his paper, his memory was significantly different from Volkman's.

The differences started with Volkman's overall portrayal of himself at this time. Volkman had described his post-medical research career as "brilliant" and said that his research for the article about strokes was "major," "significant," and "revolutionary." Albrecht remembered nothing of the sort.

He described Volkman to me as a "nebbish," which made him the second person who knew Volkman at that time to use that word, after my father. Of Volkman, he said, "If he didn't open his mouth, you wouldn't be able to distinguish him from the wallpaper."

When it came to Volkman's academic prowess, Albrecht told me that there are two main measures of a medical researcher's success: publishing articles and securing grant funding. He recalled that Volkman hadn't done much in either category. And he certainly didn't remember the young doctor producing anything on the "revolutionary" level that Paul described.

What Albrecht *did* recall was that Paul had been keen on making money at the time and that he had frequently worked additional shifts in local emergency rooms. Albrecht believed that this work outside of the lab was a contributing factor to Paul's lack of productivity. He recalled having a conversation in which they mutually decided that Paul ought to resign, and he was unaware of any incident involving a brilliant research article that he had torpedoed.

The next time Albrecht heard about Volkman was decades later, when he read about his criminal case.

Whatever the exact circumstances of Volkman's exit from Albrecht's department, it marked the end of his time in academic medicine. The career that he had trained for, in a prestigious, government-funded program, was over less than a decade after his graduation. On his CV, Paul's last affiliation with an academic institution was his residency at Loyola Medical School in 1979. His last research-related position ended with his exit from Michael Reese Hospital in 1981. His name appears as an author or contributor on just eight publications between 1975 and 1979, including letters and articles to the journals *Neuropharmacology*, *Neurology*, the *Journal of Pediatrics*, and *Annual Review of Pharmacology and Toxicology*.

For comparison, many of Volkman's MSTP classmates would go on to decorated and prolific careers in academia. His colleague J. Ross Milley would coauthor four book chapters and more than thirty articles in peer-reviewed journals over the course of his career. Milley spent a decade as chief of the division of neonatology in the pediatrics department of the University of Utah's school of medicine. My dad published or copublished more than forty-five peer-reviewed articles in journals such as the *New England Journal of Medicine* and the *Journal of Clinical Endocrinology and Metabolism* and, at one point, had a six-month visiting professorship at Harvard Medical School. The "Published Work" section of Richard Pauli's CV is twenty-two pages long and includes more than 150 peer-reviewed articles. Another Volkman classmate from the University of Chicago, Dr. Jeffrey Kant, went on to teach at the University of Pennsylvania and then the University of Pittsburgh. In 2012, the College of American Pathologists gave him a Lifetime Achievement Award.

THE PEDIATRICIAN

Following his exit from the world of research, Volkman opened a solo pediatrics practice in Chicago in 1981, the year he turned thirty-five. Interviews about this part of his career were the most positive that I had. It seemed that, despite the doubts of his colleagues, Volkman had a genuine talent for the specialty.

One of the people I interviewed was a woman named Ellen Leahy, who took both of her children to Volkman's pediatrics office. Leahy was a Chicago native who worked downtown as a secretary for an investment firm. She and her husband had bought a house not far from Midway Airport, and she first went to Volkman in 1984 following the birth of her first child. His office was in a street-level building behind a grocery store that was close to her daycare provider. "I was basically doctor-shopping and thought I'd give him a try," she said. She later brought her second child to his office as well.

Leahy's impressions of Volkman were strongly favorable. His office was clean and the waiting room was outfitted with toys and kid-sized tables and chairs. Between vaccination appointments and trips to the doctor for her kids' frequent ear infections, she saw Volkman dozens of times.

During those visits, he struck her as both a "good doctor and a lovely man," she said. He had a gentle manner with the kids, and she found him kind and reassuring in their interactions. She said that he was "one of the least arrogant doctors I had come across."

He also seemed to genuinely like children. She remembered in 1990, when he met her second daughter for the first time, he entered the exam room with a smile on his face and said, "Who is this little peanut?"

In 1992, Leahy's family moved to a Chicago suburb, at which point the distance to Volkman's office became an inconvenience and she transferred her kids to a new practice. But she said that she was never as comfortable with their new doctors as she had been with Dr. Volkman.

Jean Martinez, who worked for Volkman as a part-time office assistant from 1988 until the early 2000s, also spoke well of him. She had first heard of Dr. Volkman because she was looking for someone to pierce her infant daughter's ears. And when she found him, and noticed how busy his office was, she mentioned her previous medical-office experience and interest in a job. He hired her almost immediately.

Volkman struck Martinez as quiet, mild mannered, and calm. He loved classical music, had pictures in the office of his kids, and he would sometimes leave work early to drive to Winnetka to coach his son's soccer team. She remembered the doctor teaching her that it was helpful to smile in a pediatrics office because it put the patients and their families at ease. He treated his staff well and gave them bonuses at Christmas. She said that he struck her as a "good role model [of] what you would want to see in a pediatrician."

Martinez viewed Volkman as more book-smart than street-smart. Once, when they were discussing the Vietnam War, she was struck by how little he seemed to know about it. (The reason, she guessed, was that he had been totally engrossed in medical school.) "He didn't even realize there was a war, practically," she told me. Another time, when she mentioned that she was going back to school, he asked if she was going for her master's degree. She was amazed that he didn't realize she hadn't completed college.

But overall, she found this naïveté harmless. At a basic level, it seemed to her like he loved the job and that he was good at it. "My experience with him was . . . nothing but good," she said.

Volkman told me that he enjoyed practicing pediatrics. But he also described the financial side of the specialty as "the rock bottom of medicine." And so, at some point early in his career, he struck a compromise: Instead of giving up the practice, he cut back his hours and went to work in local emergency rooms to generate more income.

Moonlighting in emergency rooms was something that he had first done during his medical training. On his CV, he lists two local hospitals — St. James Hospital, in Chicago Heights, and Mercy Hospital, in Chicago — where he worked as an ER physician between 1975 and 1979. And his tenure at a third hospital — Holy Family, in the suburb of Des Plaines — began in 1979 and extended into the early 1980s. In 1981, he also appears to have begun work as an attending pediatrician at Chicago's Children's Memorial Hospital, although it's unclear whether he was based in the ER.

By 1987, according to court documents, Volkman had clocked more than seven thousand hours of emergency room experience at hospitals around Chicago and had received board certification in the specialty. "All told, as of December 2, 1987, Dr. Volkman had nine or ten years of emergency room experience and had spent 12 years taking care of pediatric patients," one document reads.

Those documents come from a malpractice case filed against Volkman after the death of a one-year-old pediatric patient. The child's name was Amanda Frey, and her parents had brought her to his office when she hadn't slept well during the previous night.

MALPRACTICE, PART I: THE CHILD IN THE WAITING ROOM

On the morning of December 2, 1987, George and Cynthia Frey took their daughter, Amanda, to their pediatrician's office. Amanda was a little more than a year old, and she had visited Dr. Volkman numerous times for routine checkups, immunization shots, and blood tests. In addition to her poor sleep the previous night, she had also been upset earlier in the morning. Her parents thought that perhaps she had a cold, and when they called Volkman's office, an employee told them to bring the child in.

At some point after the Freys' arrival, Amanda's condition deteriorated rapidly. She began wheezing and taking partial breaths. Her lips and fingertips turned blue. She developed a high fever. As her condition grew more dire, Volkman was summoned to the child's side, where he examined her, recognized the symptoms, and diagnosed her with epiglottitis, a swelling of the small flap of cartilage covering the windpipe.

Epiglottitis, though treatable, could develop into a life-threatening blockage of air to the lungs. And Volkman believed he needed to act fast. He told someone in the office to call 911 and to instruct the paramedics to bring equipment for an intubation, which he felt was necessary to save the girl's life. He also personally placed a call to Children's Memorial Hospital, the nearest hospital that he felt was equipped to handle a patient in Amanda's state, and requested a transport team that could move her once he had gotten her stabilized.

At 12:45 P.M., the City of Chicago received its first 911 call from Volkman's office. The first two paramedics arrived within minutes.

The events that followed would be the subject of considerable disagreement in the ensuing years. Witnesses would offer differing testimony both about what *should* have happened and also some basic facts about what did. But there would be no dispute about the day's main — and devastating — events.

Following the arrival of the paramedics, Amanda was intubated. And at around 1:25 P.M., the transport team from Children's Memorial Hospital — which included a physician, a respiratory specialist, and two nurses — arrived and took over care of the child.

In the transport team's initial assessment of Amanda, they described her as cyanotic, meaning that she was deprived of oxygen — though at that time she was still responding to pain and her pupils were reacting to light, which indicated that she was neurologically intact. Not long after the team's arrival, however, the child went into cardiac arrest. CPR was performed, during which her breathing tube became dislodged. When she was reintubated and stabilized by around 1:55 P.M., her pupils were dilated and no longer reactive to light. She had stopped moving spontaneously. She was eventually transferred to Children's Memorial Hospital, where she died two days later.

Within weeks of the incident, Amanda's parents filed a lawsuit seeking damages from the City of Chicago, which employed the paramedics who, the complaint alleged, had reported to the scene with faulty equipment that contributed to the day's outcome. Volkman was later added as a defendant.

On a basic level, the significance of this event is self-evident.

A couple brought their child to Volkman's office, with no apparent idea that her illness could be life threatening. And within days, their child was gone, claimed by a condition that was nonfatal in the overwhelming majority of cases. Their loss must have been shattering.

When I reached out to various members of the Frey family for this book, I received no response. And though this was journalistically disappointing, I find it, on a human level, completely understandable. They don't owe me, or anyone else, their words about this tragedy.

And yet, for the story I'm telling, it's important to look more closely at the details of Amanda's death. Because, in addition to its intrinsic importance, the event had major implications for Paul Volkman. The Frey case pushed Volkman into a new phase of his career, during which, over fifteen years, he was sued by at least three other patients or their families. The Frey case would result in a $2.5 million verdict against Volkman, after a two-week trial in December 1993. (The City of Chicago was not found liable.) And this judgment, plus a subsequent jury verdict and two settlements, would eventually render Volkman unable to obtain malpractice insurance, which in turn prompted him to take a job at a cash-only pain clinic in southern Ohio in 2003. There, according to prosecutors, he became a prolific and deadly dealer of prescription drugs. Viewed in the context of his entire career, the Frey case is the first event in a domino-like sequence that led to many more deaths and Volkman's prison sentence.

From my research into the entirety of Volkman's life, I also know that his response to allegations of negligence in the death of Amanda Frey offers a grim preview of his later refusal to admit any fault or responsibility in Ohio.

Paul Volkman attributed the death of Amanda Frey to bad luck and the incompetence of others.

As he told it, his misfortune began that morning when Amanda's mother (whom Volkman once said "wasn't too smart") thought to bring the child to the office, and his secretary encouraged her to do so.

And in his telling, the situation got worse from there.

He said that, due to his experience in both pediatrics and emergency medicine, he recognized Amanda's condition almost immediately and knew how urgent it was. In one telling of the story, he described Amanda as "dying of epiglottitis." Based on his assessment, he felt that there wasn't time for the baby to be safely transported to a hospital for treatment.

Volkman also felt that he had the skills to perform the highly difficult intubation of a child with a swollen epiglottis. He said that he had performed numerous intubations on children in his hospital work "without a miss."

And he told me that, in this situation, he was "as good, if not better, than anyone else at doing that kind of thing." He has said that, therefore, based on the facts as they appeared to him, "I knew that I was the only one who could save this baby."

But although he believed that the child needed to be intubated on-site, and that he ought to perform this procedure himself, Volkman said that he also knew that he didn't have the equipment to execute his plan. This was his reason for requesting specific equipment from the paramedics who had been dispatched to the scene.

This was where, in his telling, things went sideways. When emergency personnel reported to the scene, he has said that they "wasted precious time" by arguing with him that the baby should be transported instead of intubated on the premises. And when they did finally give in to his arguments, he said, they provided numerous pieces of faulty equipment. The suction device that was necessary to keep Amanda's breathing tube clear of fluid and secretions had a dead battery. The adhesive to keep her breathing tube secure wasn't the right kind of tape. And the oxygen tanks needed to assist Amanda's breathing were empty. As he told it, it was due to these failures, not his own, that the child died. In fact, he once described his actions in his office that day as "literally heroic."

From Volkman's perspective, the situation only got worse from there. After Amanda's death, he said that he spoke with a Frey family attorney who apologetically explained that, though the family had no desire to go after him legally, they were compelled to do so because, without Volkman in the courtroom, he would be blamed for everything that had happened. Volkman said his lack of any culpability was reflected during the trial when none of the witnesses spoke critically about his actions. As he once told me, "Nobody said a word about it."

And yet, he said, the case took a bad turn when, just as the jury was getting ready to deliberate, the judge informed jurors that, due to some legal technicality, the paramedics were shielded from responsibility. In Volkman's words, "The judge told the jury that the city could not be sued."

In his telling, this left the jury with a painful decision. He has described their thought process as, "Well, here's this cute little baby who is now dead and we can't quite understand what the doctor did, but he's the only one left in the lawsuit."

This, he said, was how he wound up with a $2.5 million judgment against him.

———

Upon hearing Volkman's tale, I was eager to see what I could learn and verify for myself. But researching this case turned out to be a challenge. When I began to dig, I learned that many key documents, including the trial transcript, were either lost to time or trapped behind layers of bureaucratic red tape.

I also found that, despite a gap of more than thirty years since the initial events, many parties involved in the case were unwilling to speak to me. The City of Chicago declined to give its blessing to lawyers who had worked on the case to speak with me, citing legal concerns and the case's overall sensitivity. Another person whom I queried — an eyewitness to many of the events at Volkman's office — initially expressed a strong desire to talk and described how they had been haunted by the day's events. But they subsequently changed their mind.

For a long time, I was left with only Volkman's version of events.

But then this changed.

First, I got my hands on 130 pages of single-spaced legal filings from the appeals portion of the case, which described both the day's events and the subsequent trial in detail, from the perspectives of each of the three parties: the Freys, Volkman, and the City of Chicago. Then, by reaching out to people who were named in those documents, I spoke with three people who were either direct eyewitnesses to the day's events or who had testified as experts in the trial.

After reading the court documents and conducting those interviews, my picture of what happened that day became much clearer. It also got significantly more damning toward Volkman.

Documents from the posttrial appeals stage of the Frey case do, indeed, include support for some of Volkman's assertions.

While reading them closely, I learned that, in addition to Volkman, one other witness — Amanda's father — had testified at trial that the suction device provided by paramedics failed and that the oxygen tanks brought to the scene were empty. Meanwhile, the testimony of a third trial witness affirmed Volkman's claim that the paramedics' disagreement with him about whether Amanda should be transported had delayed the child's care. This third witness further testified that the argument represented a breach of the paramedics' standard of care because of their standing orders to defer to a physician's opinion.

The appeal-related documents also mentioned an experienced and board-certified pediatrician who had testified at trial as a medical expert on Volkman's behalf. This doctor approved of Volkman's refusal to transport the child to a hospital before her airway was secured and approved of Volkman's decision to intubate the child on-site. He also approved of Volkman's resistance to having Amanda transported to the nearest general hospital, as the paramedics were encouraging, because the expert agreed with Volkman that a specialized children's hospital was better suited to handle a patient in Amanda's condition. This medical expert testified that he believed the failed suction device and insufficiently filled oxygen tanks had been the cause of the child's death and testified that Volkman had not deviated from the standard of care in his actions that day.

But my reporting about the case revealed numerous other instances where witnesses and experts dramatically contradicted Volkman's story.

For instance, a cornerstone of Volkman's story was that the day's outcome was due to two catastrophic equipment failures: the malfunction of the suction device provided by paramedics, and the oxygen tanks that were, in Volkman's words, "empty" upon their arrival. But the filings I reviewed indicate that, during the trial, at least six witnesses testified that there were no problems with the equipment of the kind that Volkman alleged. Those witnesses included two paramedics who first reported to the scene, a firefighter who arrived shortly thereafter, and three members of a team from Children's Memorial Hospital (two nurses and a physician) who also arrived at the scene.

The filings also indicated that *Volkman's own notes* from the day of the incident did not mention an equipment malfunction and that his first allegations about failed equipment came nine days after the incident, when he wrote a letter to the Illinois Department of Health. As the City of Chicago wrote in one of its filings, "Before writing that letter, Volkman had met the defense counsel who was with the Frey family at the hospital where Amanda had been transferred, and knew that the family was contemplating a medical malpractice action." From what I can tell, the only other trial witness to testify that the equipment malfunctioned was Amanda's father.

The trial records also included ample evidence that contradicted Volkman's portrayal of himself as a blameless party who became tangled in the lawsuit due to a formality. In one instance, Volkman wrote to me that "the family sued the city and the CFD [Chicago Fire Department].

Then added me to the suit, because the lawyer apologetically said it was necessary for me to be in court, or the city would simply blame me." Years later, he added "the sleazy lawyer added me to the lawsuit, probably aware that the suit against Chicago would go nowhere because of a law indemnifying the medics."

But both the court records and my interviews indicate that, in fact, Volkman was not just a hapless party who was improperly lassoed into a legal dispute; his actions were central to the legal dispute. And while, certainly, there were trial witnesses who discussed the paramedics and their equipment, there were also many who focused primarily on Volkman's conduct.

These same records also decisively debunk Volkman's claim that "nobody said a word" about his actions during the trial. This is simply false. In fact, *many* words were said in criticism of Volkman's actions.

Perhaps Volkman's most controversial decision on that day was not to allow the child to be transported to be intubated at a hospital instead of on-site at his office. This was not just the recommendation of the two paramedics who first reported to the scene, who asked Volkman repeatedly to agree to let the child be transported; it was also the opinion of the nurse who answered Volkman's call from Children's Memorial Hospital. According to a summary of their conversation included in the court records, "Volkman told her not to worry about it — he had had two years of experience in anesthesia — and he hung up the telephone." Volkman's opposition to allowing the child to be transported also differed from the phone operator at a *second* local hospital that paramedics called after Volkman refused their suggestions, who also believed the child ought to be transported before being intubated. When the paramedics reported this second opinion to him, he once again refused.

It's worth noting that all of these paramedics and nurses had less training than Volkman and were thus advised to defer to his higher rank and expertise. But during the trial, two expert medical witnesses also affirmed that the intubation Volkman attempted at his office ought to have been performed by trained experts in a controlled hospital setting. Dr. Lynn White, who testified on behalf of the city, disagreed with Volkman's assessment that there wasn't time to safely transport the child, a crucial decision that set the stage for the disastrous events that followed. She also disagreed with Volkman's decision to intubate the child when she was still breathing on her own.

Separately, a medical expert for the Frey family was critical of Volkman's refusal to move the child to a hospital. And this second expert was also critical of Volkman's refusal to even move the child a short distance from his office to a nearby ambulance, where a steady supply of electricity was available that would have made Volkman's complaints about the suction device's failed battery moot. This expert testified that epiglottitis becomes fifty to a hundred times more dangerous when a patient's airway is not properly managed.

Reading posttrial filings from the case, I also learned about a failed procedure that Volkman had tried during his attempts to intubate the child.

In his accounts of the events that led to Amanda's death, Volkman had said that it took him two attempts to successfully intubate her, and, after his second attempt, "she immediate[ly] got pink instead of blue." But he didn't mention that, between the first and second intubation attempts, he had tried to perform a cricothyrotomy.

A cricothyrotomy is an emergency procedure during which a small incision is made in a small soft spot on a patient's neck between two pieces of cartilage to create an airway. It's somewhat similar to a tracheotomy, though simpler, which makes it preferable for emergency situations. To pull it off, however, the person performing it must be acutely familiar with the patient's anatomy to know the exact target for the incision.

During his testimony at trial, Volkman admitted that he had never performed this procedure before that day in his office and also that when he attempted it, he inserted the needle in the wrong place. The procedure failed. And one medical expert testified that Volkman's botched attempt at a cricothyrotomy likely made the situation worse, because it agitated the inflamed area and made it more likely that the child's airway would close further.

Volkman would routinely describe his actions at different times in his career — actions that were often harshly criticized by others — as not just appropriate, but exceptional. And he described his actions on the day Amanda Frey died as "heroic." Even before I set out fact-checking the details of her death, I found it odd and tasteless that he would use such a word, given the day's outcome.

Among those who disagreed with his characterization was the Illinois Department of Professional Regulation, which in 1990 filed a complaint against him seeking to have his medical license "suspended, revoked, or otherwise disciplined." The complaint stated that Amanda Frey was not in respiratory distress when paramedics arrived, that intubations for children are "very difficult," and that the decision to perform an intubation in his office without the proper equipment was "extremely dangerous and reckless." Elsewhere, the document said Volkman's actions that day were "unprofessional," grossly negligent, and careless toward Amanda's well-being, noting that they "resulted in the death of a patient."*

But an even more powerful rebuke to Volkman's "heroic" characterization came from the three people I interviewed about the case. One was Dr. Lynn White, the expert witness who had reviewed records from the case and testified on behalf of the city. The other two were emergency workers who reported to Volkman's office that day and later testified at the trial. Both preferred to remain anonymous due to the sensitivity of the case and the fact that they were still employed in the same, or similar, positions. One, who said that it was okay for me to describe her as an emergency transport nurse, I'll call ETN. The other, who was among the emergency personnel who reported to Volkman's office after the 911 call, I'll call EP.

Dr. White told me that she was alarmed when she first reviewed the files detailing the day's events. And she was unequivocal in her view that Volkman's actions that day were outside the standard of care. To her, the proper course of action in such a situation was obvious: Call an ambulance, don't move the baby and risk agitation and further closure of the airway, and transport the child on the mother's lap to a hospital where a trained anesthesiologist can manage the patient's airway and where surgeons are standing by if a tracheotomy is needed. White rejected Volkman's notion that there wasn't time to transport the child. And she described his decision to try to intubate the child in his office in various disparaging ways, including "completely ill-advised," "reckless," "unprofessional," and "straight-up malpractice." This was clearly a "scoop-and-run situation," she said.

White also found Volkman's claim that he was equally skilled at intubation as anyone at the hospital preposterous. Anesthesiologists are the elite airway experts of any given hospital, she said, and she found it "impossible" that Volkman would have been better.

---

* Volkman told me that he spent $45,000 in legal fees fighting the charges. After a disciplinary hearing — the records of which were, unfortunately, not available to me — he somehow succeeded at beating the charges. In June 1991, the agency withdrew its complaint and notified him that he remained in good standing.

Overall, she described the child's death as unnecessary and prevent-able. In her view, it was clear that the paramedics and the city were not at fault, but being the deep-pocketed party, they — not Volkman — had been added to the case for frivolous reasons. The paramedics, she said, "just responded to a situation that was already out of control."

The emergency responder whom I'm calling EP told me that, when he first arrived on the scene at Volkman's office, he would have never imag-ined the situation resulting in the death of the child. But he said that he watched with alarm as the doctor's incompetence made the situation worse. EP agreed with White that the obvious thing for Volkman to have done was to jump into an ambulance with the child and go to a hospital. He told me, "I don't know another doctor that would have done what he did."

He said that, although he urgently disagreed with Volkman's decision to try to intubate Amanda on-site, he was unable to stop the doctor because Volkman outranked him. He did admit that when the situation deterio-rated, he had thoughts of snatching the child and placing her in the ambu-lance himself. "It was just tragic to . . . watch a baby die, right in front of you," he told me.

Like White, EP was also convinced that Amanda's death was prevent-able. And he, too, felt that the city had been added as defendants in the lawsuit due to their potential as big payers, not because of actual fault.

EP was still shaken by the event when I spoke with him decades later. "I can close my eyes right now and see the same little child, as I did thirty-five years ago," he said. He believed that Volkman didn't just deserve to be sued for what happened that day; he felt the doctor should have been criminally prosecuted.

In my reporting, I also spoke with ETN, the nurse who fielded Volkman's initial call requesting a transport team from the children's hospital and who, later, was a member of the group dispatched to his office. She told me that the call was unusual because generally the hospital got requests from other hospitals, not individual doctors' offices. And she knew as soon as she got the call that this was a serious situation. This nurse knew that a child's airway was a small target to begin with and that the airway of a child with epiglottitis could become dramatically swollen, which made intubation even harder. Performing such a procedure in an office struck her as a very bad idea.

Her concerns were magnified by Volkman's arrogance and dismissive-ness during their phone call. When she implored him to transport the child to a hospital, he was defiant. And for reasons that she didn't understand, he didn't seem particularly scared by epiglottitis. The combination of the situation's high stakes and Volkman's arrogance disturbed her; she remembered looking at the clerk next to her when the call ended and saying, "God, I hope I don't lose my license over this." After speaking with her medical director, they decided that it was best for a team from the hospital to go retrieve the child.

ETN told me that the fact that the child went into cardiac arrest after the transport team's arrival made her believe that Volkman's second intubation hadn't actually succeeded, as he claimed. If it had — that is, if Volkman had successfully bypassed the blockage and opened Amanda's airway — she saw no reason why the child's heart would have stopped. Whatever the exact cause of the cardiac arrest, her team sprang into action: performing CPR, attaching IVs, and administering drugs. As a number of different people worked to try to stabilize the child inside the crowded exam room, she said that she noticed Amanda's father was standing next to her and she thought, "Oh my God, no one should have to watch this." The team was able to secure an airway and revive the child. But by this point it was too late: Amanda had suffered catastrophic injuries from the loss of oxygen.

This transport nurse, like the other two people I personally interviewed, was harshly critical of Volkman's conduct that day. She had seen successful transports of children in similar situations to the hospital, and she, like Lynn White, believed that in this case there was time to do so safely. If Volkman had agreed to this instead of choosing "be the savior and intubate this child," she felt the outcome would have been dramatically different.

"I feel that he is directly responsible for that child's death," she told me.

Beyond my familiarity with the facts of the day and the ensuing legal battle, I have only hints of how these events affected the Frey family.

The emergency responder whom I interviewed described Amanda Frey's parents as a "young, happy couple" who initially expected that they would bring their daughter home that day. As the events unfolded, he remembered them being stunned.

"It's a shame because they trusted this doctor," he said. "That's what we all do."

In addition to this account, one of the Freys' posttrial legal filings includes a brief, but poignant, glimpse of the family after Amanda's death.

"The evidence in this case showed that when Amanda was alive, [her brother] George Jr. spent considerable time playing with her," it reads.

The document continues:

> Amanda liked playing with her big brother. George Jr. was very happy to have a little sister and was very protective of her. George Jr. was always telling Amanda that he loved her and she was always kissing him.
>
> At the time of this incident, George Frey Jr. was almost five years old. He remembers being at the hospital the night his sister was taken there and seeing his mom and dad crying. One of the doctors let him go in to see Amanda.
>
> George Jr. still talks a lot about his sister. He is mad about what happened to her. When his friends come over he tells them that Amanda is in the picture that is over their mantle.
>
> George Jr. misses his sister. He goes with the rest of the family to visit Amanda's grave. However, he is reaching a point where it is difficult for him to go because it hurts him.
>
> Charlie Frey was born a couple of months after Amanda died. But, his mother talks to him about Amanda and Charlie tells her that he feels bad for Amanda. He also shows his friends the picture over the mantel and tells them that it is of his sister.
>
> Charlie once told his parents that he wanted to leave his radio at the grave so that Amanda could have some music. Charlie tells his mother that he wishes his sister was there.

LOCUM TENENS

The term *locum tenens* originates in medieval Latin, meaning "one holding a place." But by the late twentieth century the phrase had acquired a much more specific connotation, especially in the world of American medicine. If you heard someone refer to locum tenens after, say, the 1980s, they were likely referring to a doctor or other healthcare worker who was working somewhere on a temporary basis. *Locum tenens* was a fancy way of saying "rent-a-doc."

The concept got its start in the 1970s, with a program at the University of Utah called the Health Systems Research Institute. HSRI aimed to offer continuing medical education for rural doctors, and so it launched a system of providing temporary fill-in physicians for the doctors undergoing training. Two doctors involved in HSRI saw the broader potential for this service, and in short order each founded a company that brought it to a wider market. Comprehensive Health Systems was founded in 1979, and KRON Medical followed, in 1980.

As it turned out, the practice of sending doctors on temporary assignments offered rewards for nearly everyone involved. The communities that received the out-of-town doctors liked it. If a doctor fell ill, retired, went on vacation, or took a maternity leave, locum tenens doctors helped to meet the region's need. In 1994, a spokesman for the Kansas Medical Society explained to a newspaper reporter, "You've got physicians in underserved areas working, on average, 70 to 80 hours a week . . . Locum tenens doctors are the only opportunity for them to get some much-needed rest."

The doctors who went on the assignments benefited as well. If a young doctor was just starting their career, locum tenens work allowed them to try out different locations. It also offered a way for doctors to ease into retirement. One newspaper article from 1994 profiled a sixty-three-year-old doctor for whom locum tenens medicine meant driving around the country in an RV and practicing medicine along the way. "I stamp out fires wherever doctors are burning out," he said.

And for the professional matchmakers who connected doctors with temporary assignments, there was an enormous business opportunity. By 1990, CompHealth employed more than one thousand physicians who provided tens of thousands of temporary coverage days per year across the country. By this time KRON Medical had annual revenues of $25 million. By the early 2000s, annual industry-wide revenues topped $2 billion. In 2002, a spokesperson for a Texas-based locum tenens staffing company told the *New York Times* that more than twenty-five thousand doctors — close to 5 percent of all physicians in practice in the country — were employed on short-term assignments. The same *Times* article reported that the percentage of doctors who had previously worked temporary jobs had tripled since the late 1980s.

Paul Volkman was one of those doctors.

For years, Volkman had supplemented his pediatrics income with shifts in Chicago-area emergency rooms on nights and weekends. And in the 1990s he remained interested in making additional money.

The question of who, exactly, was behind this drive to earn more money yields different answers. Paul told me once that "I had a wife who liked nice clothes and nice furniture and thought she had a right to a nice life-style, after all, [being] married to a doctor."

But Paul's daughter, Jane, told me that she sees her dad as an equal part-ner in the endeavor. "He wanted a rich man's living," she said. At another point, she said that she believed providing money was a way for her dad to get her mother's approval in a relationship that didn't have many other sources of emotional intimacy. Meanwhile, Paul's son Adam offered a third explanation. In Adam's telling, his parents had an "inability to . . . coexist harmoniously." He recalled frequent arguments between his parents "about nothing in particular" that lasted for hours and often included threats of divorce. Their marriage was a "war zone," he said. And he felt that this was as much a reason for his father's locum tenens work as any other.

Whatever the exact motivations, Volkman found, somewhat counter-intuitively, that he was able to make more money by traveling outside the big city where he lived. In his explanation, Chicago, with its dense population and cluster of medical schools, had a robust supply of doctors, which pushed down the rates for emergency room work in local hospi-tals. But if he was willing to venture into smaller towns outside the city, or even a few hours away, he could find more available shifts, at a signifi-cantly higher rate.

In 1990, when the locum tenens industry was booming, he said that he took his first temporary job at an emergency room in Marion, Indiana, a town of around thirty thousand located 170 miles southeast of Chicago. And in the ensuing years, he became a regular on the locum tenens circuit, taking temporary jobs for days or weeks or months at a time to support his life back home.

I never got an exact number of the different places where Volkman worked as a locum tenens emergency room physician. And I'm not sure Volkman even knew himself. He once told me that, over the years, he had worked at "probably fifty" different hospitals. At another point, during sworn testimony for a lawsuit, he confirmed more than twenty specific locations where he had worked. Some of the jobs were in larger cities like Cleveland, Dayton, and Milwaukee. But the bulk of the work took place in small towns like Michigan City, Indiana (population 32,033); Belleville, Illinois (population 41,751); and Pomeroy, Ohio (population 1,556).

In that same sworn testimony from 2002, he described how the locum tenens process worked. He was not personally responsible for finding the temporary gigs; one of the various staffing companies with which he worked would do that. They would keep copies of Volkman's paperwork on file, including his med school diploma, his medical licenses, and info about his board certifications. And when a hospital somewhere had an opening — say, because a doctor was going on vacation for two or three weeks — that hospital would contact the staffing company, which would send over Volkman's paperwork. If a hospital approved of his credentials, Volkman got the gig.

During one of our interviews, Volkman explained the logistics of these temporary jobs. He told me that he would schedule two or three ER shifts in a row, and he would drive to the place from Chicago, report for work, and afterward go to a motel or extended-stay hotel and sleep. He would repeat this cycle of working and sleeping until it was time to return home. Some of these jobs lasted months (during which, I gather, he would return home for weekends). Others spanned just a few weeks.

Volkman once told me that the territory he covered was determined by his ability to fly or drive home with relative ease. Using Google Maps and twenty-eight hospital locations that I gathered from various records, I have mapped that territory. What emerges is a region that stretches across the Upper Midwest, extending as far north as Appleton, Wisconsin (a hundred miles north of Madison); as far south as Paducah, Kentucky; as far east as Cleveland; and as far west as Quincy, Illinois (about 115 miles east of Des Moines).

Another way to picture his locum tenens career is by tracking the years that he obtained medical licenses in various states. From publicly available databases, I know that he was first licensed in Illinois, in 1975, shortly after completing medical school. Then came Indiana in 1989, and later, in rapid succession, Iowa (1996), Ohio (1996), Wisconsin (1997), and Kentucky (1999).

Volkman described his work in these far-flung small towns as a mix of the mundane and the exciting. He explained to me that, due to federal legislation that prevented hospitals from turning away patients based on their inability to pay, emergency rooms had become one of society's safety nets. Thus, the majority of patients he saw in these emergency rooms were walk-ins who didn't have serious injuries or illnesses or who were, in Volkman's words, "just there because it's cold outside."

But he also said that, around once a month — or in what he calculated to be around one in every five hundred patient encounters — there would be a patient for whom he needed to make split-second life-or-death decisions. He told me about a time when he was working near Indianapolis and EMTs brought in a thirteen-year-old girl who had attempted to hang herself. He said that he successfully intubated the girl without aggravating any neck injuries and then put her into a barbiturate-induced coma, which he said protected her brain from a lack of oxygen. He told me she was flown to a children's hospital in Indianapolis, where she later survived with no permanent damage. "She would have been dead from brain damage, and I basically saved her," he said.

He also described another instance when an elderly woman had attempted suicide by swallowing all her antidepressant pills, which Volkman knew had the potential to cause an unusual and potentially fatal irregular heartbeat. (Volkman said that, given his background in pharmacology, he was particularly adept at treating overdoses.) In this case, he knew that the antidote to this woman's condition was the seizure medication Dilantin. So he administered some of the drug, and the woman's heartbeat returned to normal and her blood pressure stabilized. "So that was fucking incredible, basically," he told me.

As Volkman told it, working in emergency rooms was generally thankless, characterized by long drives and unglamorous surroundings. But it could be intellectually stimulating based on the sheer variety of patients and their conditions. Working in isolated hospitals meant that he encountered plenty of traumas (stabbings, gunshot wounds, car accidents) and acute illnesses (heart attacks, seizures, strokes). He also saw unusual cases, like syphilis, untreated broken bones, or abscesses caused by tuberculosis. Such work was inherently unpredictable, and it demanded access to a wide breadth of medical knowledge on a moment's notice. He told me that he enjoyed this aspect of the job.

Even though these far-flung hospitals provided him with considerable income, during our conversations Volkman often spoke of their surroundings with contempt. He called Marion, Illinois, a "dreadful little place." He said that it would be "pretty hard to find a worse place" than Gary, Indiana. He called the town of Portsmouth, Ohio — where he worked for a stint in the 1990s before later returning as a pain doctor — a "shitty area" and a "godforsaken place."

And he was similarly dismissive when describing the level of medicine that he encountered during his locum tenens work. At one point, he described "the laziness, sloppiness, and callousness of local small-town docs" with whom he worked. In another instance, he described one specific small-town hospital as having "incredibly bad" physicians who practiced an "awful brand of medicine."

Due to the nature of emergency room work, his interactions with patients tended to be brief and impersonal. And in the instances when he had pulled off what he described as miraculous feats, there were few people, beyond perhaps a nurse or two, who could even recognize what had occurred. But this didn't matter much because, as Volkman told me, he did it for the patients' sake, and for his own satisfaction.

"Plus," he said, "it turned out to be the only way I could make a living."

Volkman would later tell me that life on the locum tenens circuit was never particularly dependable, and it involved searching for a new job as soon as he finished the last one. "I generally managed to find enough jobs to keep going," he told me. "But it was always kind of a scrambling thing."

But as haphazard as this part of his career may have been, it paid well. And the Volkman family lived well as a result. In 1989, at around the same time as Volkman's first locum tenens assignment, the family moved from an apartment in Chicago to a rental house in the posh suburb of Winnetka, fifteen miles north of downtown. Winnetka was a small town of just over ten thousand, and yet it was home to one of the densest concentrations of wealth in the country. Around the time when the family moved, a *Forbes* list of the four hundred wealthiest Americans included four Winnetka residents.

Volkman later described the move as a roundabout cost-saving measure, because it meant that he could now send his kids to local public schools and save the money he and Nancy had been spending on tuition. (He framed his previous decision to send his kids to private school in Chicago as a necessity rather than a choice, because the public schools were "horrific.")

But those savings came with a palpable uptick in social pressure. Volkman described his family's lifestyle in those years as "very average middle class or somewhat less," which, by almost any standard — statistical, sociological, common sense — is a pronounced understatement. And yet it is a revealing admission about how those years *felt* to a man who was still living job-to-job, schlepping from one forgotten midwestern town to another.

In Winnetka, the Volkmans were "surrounded by extraordinarily wealthy people, who went to France and Italy for Christmas ski vacations, or Hawaii or the Caribbean," he told me.

He added, "We were definitely the poor people from the wrong side of the tracks."

MALPRACTICE, PARTS II–III: EMERGENCY ROOMS

In my attempts to independently fact-check Volkman's account of his locum tenens years, I emailed several hospitals seeking details about his time working there. And in some cases, during my trips to the Midwest, I personally visited hospitals to see what I could learn. These efforts mostly came up empty. In one instance, a communications staffer at a hospital responded to my query by saying that he wished he could help, but personnel records of the hospital where Volkman worked had not been transferred when the institution was sold to a larger hospital system. And since then, the hospital had been sold again, "making the likelihood of finding those records even more challenging," he wrote.

But there were a few notable exceptions. And as with other points of Volkman's career, these accounts were dramatically different from the stories he told.

One of those glimpses into Volkman's work as a locum tenens doctor happened unexpectedly, while I was interviewing a children's hospital nurse who was part of the transport team that reported to Volkman's pediatrics office for the Amanda Frey incident. That day's events, and Volkman's role in them, had haunted her. And when she encountered Volkman for a second time years later, it stayed in her mind.

The nurse told me that, at some point in the 1990s, she had received a call from an emergency room in northern Indiana about a young girl with asthma symptoms. This wasn't a particularly unusual occurrence, she explained; asthma cases were one of the most frequent reasons for general hospitals to request a transport to a hospital specializing in pediatric care. And this particular case didn't seem to be life threatening. The nurse gathered that the patient simply required a level of expertise that the general hospital didn't feel equipped to provide. During this call, the doctor on the phone mentioned his name: Paul Volkman. The nurse remembered thinking: "Oh, my God. This is that guy again."

As this nurse told me, she and her team headed to the hospital, and when they arrived the situation, as expected, didn't seem particularly dire. The girl was receiving a breathing treatment while her mother and grandmother sat by her side. She said that her team had begun switching over the girl's equipment in preparation for the transport when Volkman arrived at the bedside. And it soon became clear that he believed that the situation was much more severe than the transporting team did. In fact, he said that the girl needed a dose of intracardiac epinephrine.

At this point in her story, the nurse paused to say that she had never in her career been in a situation that required an intracardiac epinephrine injection, which is, in essence, a shot of adrenaline to the heart. Not only was such a maneuver not a treatment for asthma, it was a treatment used in only the most extreme situations. The only time she had ever even heard of an intracardiac epinephrine dose being used involved full-on cardiac arrest. "We don't inject drugs right into the heart," she told me. "I mean, nobody does that!"

And this child was certainly "not even close" to needing such treatment, she said. Volkman's suggestion was so extreme and over the top that it alarmed her. And the bedside nurse who witnessed the conversation seemed equally startled.

The transport nurse told me that, in response to Volkman's suggestion, she wanted to discuss the situation with her supervisors back at the children's hospital. When she made that call, she spoke with the same medical director she had worked with during the Frey incident and explained the situation. Her director advised her that she needed to get that child out of that hospital. With that encouragement, the transport nurse crafted a plan.

She decided that she was going to act as if she were complying with Volkman's orders, and so she asked the hospital nurse to go retrieve the requested shot of epinephrine. At some point Volkman, who was apparently satisfied that the situation was proceeding according to his directions, walked away. The hospital nurse nervously asked the transport nurse if they were really going to go through with Volkman's orders. The transport nurse explained that they were not; the hospital nurse was going to take her time getting the epinephrine, while the transport team was going to move quickly. After the hospital nurse left the bedside, the transport team hurried to grab the girl's chart and "ran out of the ER."

In the nurse's telling, it wasn't just a story about a doctor with a wildly overaggressive plan for treatment that alarmed the other professionals who witnessed it. It was also an anecdote about how, during the incident, she had seen Volkman assure the girl's loved ones that he would save their child. The same doctor who posed a direct threat to this child's well-being could also instill confidence that he had the knowledge and expertise to handle the situation.

She had never forgotten it.

Two other glimpses into Volkman's locum tenens years come from malpractice lawsuits, both of which were settled by Volkman's insurers before they went to trial. But each case produced enough documentation, or pointed me toward enough people other than Volkman, that they offered an alternative perspective on his work in emergency rooms.

The events that led to the first lawsuit took place on the morning of June 28, 1991, when Volkman was working at St. Therese Hospital, in Waukegan, Illinois, a city of seventy thousand located between Chicago and the Wisconsin border. That morning, a fifty-five-year-old woman named Mary Cooper, who had recently been diagnosed with non-Hodgkin's large cell lymphoma, arrived at the hospital with significant pain in her right shoulder, arm, and hand. Volkman saw Cooper in the emergency room, and she was discharged three hours later, at 11:15 A.M.

After her discharge, the pain in her arm worsened, and she went to her oncologist's office. At this point, according to legal documents, Cooper's hand was "blue [and] nearly pulseless"; her doctor examined it and recommended that she immediately go to a hospital. Within an hour, at a second hospital (not the one where Volkman had seen her), she underwent emergency surgery to remove a blockage in an artery in her wrist, a procedure known as an embolectomy.

Cooper remained at the second hospital, and a few days later, her hand's condition began to worsen once again. On July 5, one week after her first trip to the emergency room, she underwent a second emergency embolectomy, which led to slight improvement in the hand. But doctors ultimately deemed that an emergency amputation was necessary, and on July 8, her arm was amputated just below her elbow.

About a year later, Cooper filed a lawsuit against Volkman and the physicians' group that had employed him at the time. The complaint alleged that he had been negligent in his failures to adequately examine her, to order appropriate diagnostic tests, to consult with a vascular surgeon about her condition, and to diagnose the embolism in her arm. The complaint further stated that, due to this negligence, she had "suffered severe, permanent and irreversible damage both of a pecuniary and personal nature." Later, in amended complaints, the surgeon who performed the two emergency embolectomies that preceded Cooper's amputation (and who, allegedly, discontinued Cooper's regimen of anticoagulant medications at a critical time), was added to the list of the lawsuit's defendants.

In the years following the suit's filing, Volkman's insurance company filed for bankruptcy, and his coverage was transferred to an entity called the Illinois Guaranty Fund, which settled the case for $300,000 in February 1995.

I have spoken with Volkman repeatedly about this case. And in those conversations, he described the lawsuit as — like the Frey case before it — a meritless action brought by an unscrupulous attorney.

In those conversations, he told me that he dismissed Cooper from the hospital after examining her and receiving the go-ahead from her doctor to send her home. He also said that, after Cooper's surgery later on the same day that he saw her in the ER, her hand was fine for months before the problems that necessitated the amputation.

He further claimed that the lawsuit — which was brought by, in his words, "a sleazy Waukegan lawyer" — took place after his insurance company went bankrupt and was motivated by the lawyer's belief that Volkman's new insurer would put up less of a fight. He said that the settlement was reached "as soon as the lawsuit was filed" — which, he implied, was an indication of the fund's eagerness to settle and its failure to put up a proper defense on his behalf.

Overall, the case was "an easy day's work for 350K" for the attorney who filed the suit, he once wrote.

As with all of Volkman's malpractice cases, I did my best to independently piece together a picture of what happened. This meant speaking with the clerk's office of the county where the lawsuit took place and learning that, miraculously, decades after the events in question, there were still more than a thousand pages of documents related to the case on file. And those pages, though they turned out to be grainy and hard to read, contained some of the answers I was looking for.

The documents did confirm some of the facts of the story as Volkman had relayed them. One also indicated that, at some point in the lawsuit's progress, there was an expert, or multiple experts, who reviewed the facts of the case and "opined that there was no deviation from the standard of care by Dr. Volkman and any delay in the diagnosis had no effect on the ultimate amputation."

And yet, once again, many aspects of Volkman's account of the case were not supported by the facts. In Volkman's telling, one of the reasons he dismissed Cooper from the emergency room was because he spoke on the phone with her doctor, who told him to, in his words, "send her home." But the documents I received from the county clerk's office include no mention of Volkman receiving a go-ahead from her doctor to send her home. In fact, the language of one document suggests that he specifically "failed to call in a vascular surgeon for consultation, and also failed to inform Mary Cooper's treating physician of his findings or his differential diagnosis of compromised circulation to Mary Cooper's right hand," which suggests that no such call took place.

In Volkman's telling, after Cooper's initial surgery, her hand was "okay" for a period of months before it deteriorated to the point where an amputation was necessary. But the legal documents indicate that just ten days passed between Volkman's release of Cooper from the ER and her amputation, and just seven days passed between their encounter and her second, pre-amputation surgery.

Volkman also claimed that Cooper's lawsuit was filed *after* his initial insurance company went bankrupt and his coverage had been transferred to the Illinois Guaranty Fund. The timing of these events is critical because, in his narrative, Cooper's lawyer figured that his second insurer was likely to settle the case without much of a fight. Thus, it was this presumed easy payday, rather than Volkman's own negligent actions, that was the suit's true motivation. To bolster this aspect of the narrative, Volkman claimed that this second insurer handed over a settlement check to Cooper's attorney "as soon as the lawsuit was filed."

But neither of these things appears to be true. Documents indicate that Volkman's first insurer went bankrupt two years *after* Cooper's complaint was filed, which means that the plaintiff's lawyers would have had no prior knowledge of Guaranty Fund's involvement. The documents also indicate that a settlement wasn't reached in the case until February 6, 1995, more than two and a half years after Cooper filed her initial complaint on June 11, 1992.

As a final note: By the time I looked up the "sleazy Waukegan lawyer" who had brought the suit against Volkman, that lawyer (who declined to comment for this book) had won $1.3 billion in verdicts and settlements for his clients and had served as both chairman of the Law School Advisory Council for the University of Notre Dame Law School and the president of the Illinois Trial Lawyers Association.

Mary Cooper herself had long since passed away by the time I researched her lawsuit against Volkman. But I was able to connect with her daughter Dale, who told me a bit about her mother and the case.

Dale said that her mother grew up in a "big southern family" in Mississippi and later found her way to the small town of Zion, Illinois, located just south of the Wisconsin border. Mary worked for decades in two local factories: first at a television manufacturer in Zion, and later at a manufacturer of electrical machinery components in nearby Waukegan. She was, in Dale's telling, a smart, kind, fun-loving, hardworking woman with a "sweet smile" who was meticulous about her appearance, especially her hair and nails.

Dale didn't know enough about the events that preceded the amputation of her mother's lower arm to offer an account of Volkman's exact role. She had been in college in Arizona at the time and had arrived home in Illinois only after those initial events had occurred. But she did feel comfortable making a few general statements about the lawsuit.

First, she wanted me to know how awful the experience had been for her mother. She used the words "horrible" and "nightmare" to describe it, and she recalled how "shut down and just scared" her mother seemed before the amputation took place. Dale also remembered that because the affected hand was her mother's dominant one, Mary was forced to feebly write an "X" in lieu of a signature on presurgery paperwork. The scene struck Dale as dehumanizing.

Dale had the sense that her mother's amputation was preventable. She felt that whatever had happened in the lead-up to her mother being sent home from the emergency room on the day she saw Volkman, the process seemed flawed. She recalled hearing that her mother was clearly in pain from the moment she had come home from the ER, which, in Dale's eyes, seemed to indicate a lack of proper care and attention from whoever had treated her at the hospital. She did not believe that the lawsuit was frivolous, as Volkman claimed.

Whatever the exact events that had preceded the amputation, Dale told me that the aftermath was devastating. Her mother was forced into an early retirement by the surgery and had to learn to live with one arm. Mary struggled afterward with phantom limb pain. And due to the financial hardship of the situation, she had to sell her home and move in with Dale's sister in Missouri. All of this was on top of an existing cancer diagnosis. Dale said that during the last decade of her life, her mother was isolated and depressed. "She lost everything she had worked for," she said. The event "completely changed" her mother's life.

After hearing all of this, her already-modest $300,000 settlement seemed even smaller to me.

A second lawsuit from Volkman's locum tenens years originated in the early-morning hours of April 14, 1995, in an emergency room in Decatur, Illinois.

Volkman had signed a locum tenens contract in late 1994 to work in Decatur for a rate of $130 for every hour of active work in the emergency room and $100 for every hour he spent on call. Other documents from the case indicate that he was working around five shifts per month at the hospital at the time of the incident.

At around 1:20 A.M. during one of those shifts, a twenty-six-year-old man named Todd Kirchhoff arrived at the emergency room. Earlier that evening, Kirchhoff had been involved in some kind of altercation in the parking lot of a local bar. And during that encounter, he was hit in the face, knocked down, and his head struck the ground. At the emergency room, Volkman diagnosed him with intoxication and trauma to the head and face and eventually sent him home.

In the hours following Kirchhoff's discharge from the ER, however, his condition worsened, and he eventually went to another hospital, where he was diagnosed with a subdural hematoma — bleeding in the brain — which required emergency surgery. In the time that had elapsed between the injury and its treatment, Kirchhoff sustained damage to his mental capabilities. After the hematoma and subsequent surgery, Kirchhoff's father, Roger, was named his legal guardian. Five months later, Roger filed a lawsuit against Volkman on his son's behalf.

The lawsuit alleged that Volkman had failed to perform a proper neurological exam, failed to order and/or perform a computerized tomography (CT) scan, failed to diagnose and treat Kirchhoff's subdural and intracerebral hematomas, and discharged Kirchhoff without properly monitoring him. As a result of this negligence, the complaint alleged, Kirchhoff suffered permanent injuries, pain, and suffering and would need "great sums of money" to pay for his medical care, while being deprived of future earnings due to his disabilities.

The case worked its way through the court system for years. Depositions were taken. Motions and responses were submitted. A trial date was set. Then, in September 1999, as a trial approached, a settlement was reached for $950,000.

Once again, Volkman's malpractice insurer paid the bill.

Volkman's take on this case was, again, aggressively defensive. During an in-person interview, he described the lawsuit as "bogus" and a "pile of shit." Years later, in an email, he said that Kirchhoff was a "a mildly retarded hot head 24 year old" who had previously scored seventy-eight on an IQ test in high school. He said that Kirchhoff had come into the ER with a nosebleed, refused to cooperate with the X-rays that Volkman ordered for him, and later left the hospital against medical advice, but "the nurse forgot to have him sign an AMA [against medical advice] form."

He claimed that the surgeon who later operated on Kirchhoff testified that the hematoma had had "no effect . . . at all" on the young man. And he also said that he was sued by an "impoverished lawyer" and that the company settled for "$900,000 of Other People's Money."

I reached out numerous times to Todd Kirchhoff and his father, Roger, as well as other family members, but received no response. I did, however, speak with the lawyer who represented the Kirchhoffs, and he told a strikingly different story from Volkman's.

When Volkman spoke of this case, he portrayed this attorney as hapless, broke, and sleazy. And yet when I looked up Steve Jambois, I saw that he worked in a sleek, glass-lined building squarely in Chicago's downtown loop, for a firm — at which he was a partner — that apparently led Illinois in successful personal-injury cases. By the time I spoke with him, in 2021, Jambois had worked for thirty-five years, in more than twenty counties in Illinois, and secured $200 million in verdicts and settlements. "Impoverished" he was not. When discussing Volkman's description of his financial status, he said, drily, "We're all good there."

Jambois described Volkman's account of the Kirchhoff case as "completely inaccurate." He said that Kirchhoff did not previously have a notably low IQ and had not been enrolled in any special-education programs. He also disputed Volkman's categorization of Kirchhoff as a drunk and belligerent patient who refused treatment. As Jambois told it, Kirchhoff's condition had deteriorated *during the hours* he spent at the hospital. And he explained that, in the case's records, the hospital's intake nurse made no mention of strong signs of intoxication or trauma upon Todd's arrival, and yet, hours later, those symptoms were pronounced enough that he was unable to sign his own name. This was the opposite of what should have happened if he were merely drunk, Jambois said, and he said that should have been "easily diagnosed" by anyone treating him.

When it came to Volkman's assertion that the hematoma had had "no effect on him at all," Jambois said that Kirchhoff was, in fact, severely affected by the injury. Before the incident, he had a job; afterward, he couldn't maintain his own finances, and his father had to serve as his legal guardian. "Was he heading to get his Harvard PhD?" Jambois said. "No. But he was certainly a normal, functioning person before, and then was not afterward."

At the time of our interview in 2021, Jambois noted that Illinois state laws had changed since the Kirchhoff case to make hospitals more liable for malpractice or negligence by doctors they employ. Had this case occurred more recently, he said he wouldn't have settled for just $950,000. He would have sued the hospital as well, and he estimated that the institution would have likely contributed another $2 million.

During our conversation, Jambois told me that he didn't find Volkman's revisionist account of the case unusual. After years in this line of work, he was used to doctors' tendency to believe that they had been screwed over in such cases. "They don't want to brush their teeth in the morning knowing that they've killed . . . or seriously harmed someone," he told me.

But even if he didn't find Volkman's denials notable, he did mention two things about the case that stuck out. The first was a phone call he had received from Volkman shortly after the lawsuit was filed. At that time, Volkman's son Adam was, by coincidence, friends with Jambois's much younger half brother. And Volkman was calling Jambois to remind him of this fact and to strongly imply that, due to this personal connection, Jambois ought to drop the case.

Jambois had no intention of doing this. And he recalled explaining to Volkman that a doctor in Volkman's position wasn't even supposed to be speaking with the attorney of the person suing him; that was his own attorney's job. Jambois told me that it was the only time in his decades as a litigator he had received such a call from a defendant. "It wasn't a long conversation, but it was a very unusual one," he said.

The second thing that stuck with Jambois was Volkman's peculiar career arc. Here was a guy with what Jambois described as a "fantastic résumé" who lived in one of Chicago's most affluent suburbs and yet was working as a locum tenens ER physician in a small city three hours away from home.

"It just didn't make any sense [that] somebody who was as polished as he was on paper would be practicing medicine in Decatur, Illinois," he said. "It struck me as incredibly odd."

MALPRACTICE, PART IV: BANKRUPT

On February 27, 1998, at 3:43 P.M., Paul Volkman filed for federal bankruptcy protection. The records he filed that day, signed under penalty of perjury, offer a window into his life at the time.

According to his filing documents, Volkman lived in a house in Winnetka, Illinois, that he rented for $2,950 per month. His income for the two previous years had been $215,506 (in 1996) and $236,618 (in 1997). He listed his employer as "Weatherby Healthcare," a locum tenens staffing company. Among his assets, which amounted to $118,868, were two retirement funds totaling $113,768; a $1,500 security deposit on his rental home; and a five-year-old set of golf clubs worth $200. Meanwhile, his liabilities added up to $2,633,524 from judgments or potential judgments in multiple malpractice lawsuits, including the Frey case and the Kirchhoff case. On a page for describing personal items that would be exempt from his creditors, he listed household furniture worth approximately $2,000 and a wristwatch worth $300.

In our later conversations, Volkman did not describe this bankruptcy filing as an emergency measure he took due to the consequences of his own actions. Instead, as he explained it, it was a practical, sensible way to protect himself from malpractice judgments that he believed to be manifestly unfair.

As he told it, his appeals of the Frey verdict failed. And though his insurer paid $100,000 to the family, there was still an open possibility — according to what Volkman claimed to have been told by a lawyer — that one of Amanda Frey's siblings could decide to sue Volkman after they turned eighteen. And so, as a preventive measure, he filed bankruptcy to, in his words, "vacate the judgment."

During one of our in-person conversations in 2009, Volkman scoffed at the implication of a news report about his indictment that referred to him as a "once-bankrupt Chicago pediatrician." As he saw it, he had been sued unfairly and then used bankruptcy to deflect the unjust verdict.

Problem solved.

But was that really how the system worked?

Volkman's bankruptcy was one of many points in this project when I reached out to an expert for a crash course in a topic about which I had little prior knowledge. In this case, I got in touch with Bruce Markell, a professor of bankruptcy law at Northwestern University's law school who had spent years as a federal bankruptcy judge in Nevada, authored or coauthored numerous articles and books on the subject, and taught at a number of different law schools, including Harvard.

During our interview, Markell explained the idea underlying bankruptcy laws: that people sometimes find themselves in financial troubles that aren't necessarily their fault, and, in such a case, they deserve a second chance. He also said that, although Chapter 11 is more widely known due to news coverage of companies that file for bankruptcy protection, the vast majority of US bankruptcy cases involve individual people. He told me that most of those personal bankruptcy cases yield zero dollars to creditors, either because the person filing has no assets to be distributed or because what they do possess — such as a car, home, furniture, appliances, and clothing — is exempt from seizure or repossession.

Markell told me that the United States is one of the more liberal countries in the world when it comes to assessing and granting bankruptcy-related discharges like the one Volkman ultimately received. He explained that — crucially, in this instance — negligence, malpractice claims, and other claims related to unintentional harm, are usually among the debts that can be legally discharged in a bankruptcy proceeding. "It's a complicated system," he told me. "But in essence, if someone who harmed you filed bankruptcy . . . you're screwed."

When I asked Markell to help me decipher the specific documents from Volkman's case, he said it seemed that Volkman, through his bankruptcy filing, had successfully gotten past or pending judgments against him discharged or enjoined them from proceeding any further. In essence, he confirmed Volkman's description of what the bankruptcy had accomplished.

But Markell did add an important point that Volkman left out.

Markell told me that in 2005 Congress passed a set of laws that made the bankruptcy system stricter, particularly for those who earned more per year than the median income of their state. Under the new rules, higher-earning bankruptcy filers were placed on a multiyear plan to pay monthly installments to creditors from *future* earnings instead of having their debts wiped entirely. This would have included someone like Paul Volkman, whose filing mentioned his six-figure income from the previous two years.

In fact, Markell said that Volkman's case offered an example of why these reforms were passed. He said that the doctor had encountered a system that, in essence, told filers to "give us your present assets, and we'll take care of your present debts. The future is yours."

If Volkman had filed that same bankruptcy claim a decade later, he would have gotten a different result.

As I was closely reading Volkman's bankruptcy paperwork, an entry caught my eye in a section titled "Creditors Holding Unsecured Nonpriority Claims." On the page, which tracked various parties to whom Volkman owed, or could potentially owe, money, was an entry I didn't recognize. The amount was $30,000, and it was labeled "Possible Judgment in Lawsuit." The creditors were listed as Margaret O'Leary, Joanne DeMasi, and Nicole Demasi, a "Minor."

It would take a fair amount of digging, but I eventually heard the story behind these few lines of text. Margaret O'Leary was a personal injury and malpractice attorney in Chicago. And Joanne De Masi (the spelling of her name on the filing was incorrect) was the mother of Nicole De Masi, who was one of Volkman's former pediatric patients. At the time of Volkman's bankruptcy filing, the De Masis were attempting to sue Volkman, with O'Leary as their lawyer.

Over the years I knew him, when Paul Volkman told the story of his career, he acknowledged that he had been sued for malpractice a number of times. But he insisted that all those lawsuits were without merit, and, in our conversations and correspondence, he offered his accounts of those cases.

Still, he never volunteered an account — however misleading and factually unsound — of the De Masi case. And if I hadn't seen it in his bankruptcy filing, it's likely I would have never learned about it. It was, in a sense, a hidden case, perhaps because it didn't result in a settlement or verdict.

But as I would learn, there was a lot of pain and anger behind that story. And there was a woman who felt that Volkman had altered her life for the worse and had never been held to account.

The story began in the mid-1980s in Chicago, when Joanne De Masi was looking for a new pediatrician for her two kids. She had heard good reviews of Volkman, and his office was close to where the De Masis lived. So she decided to give him a try.

Her initial impressions of him were positive. Volkman wore khakis and sweater vests and struck her as being "a little on the geeky side." But that was hardly a problem. He was clearly intelligent, and she found his office to be clean, modern, and appealing.

The De Masis' first few years as Volkman patients went smoothly. Joanne said that her kids were generally healthy. They went to the doctor for regular shots and annual physicals. And based on those early experiences, she said she would have never thought he was a bad doctor.

The problem started around when Joanne's daughter Nicole was twelve years old, and Joanne noticed that Nicole's school uniform wasn't fitting properly. It seemed lopsided. And when Joanne looked more closely, she saw that Nicole's hips didn't seem to properly align. So she took her daughter to see Volkman, who referred them to a surgeon specializing in scoliosis. When the De Masis went to see the specialist, his prognosis was alarming.

The surgeon took X-rays that showed that Nicole's spine had a pronounced S-shaped curve, and he informed them that she was an urgent candidate for surgery. During those conversations, Joanne learned that if the problem had been caught earlier, it could have been treated with just a back brace. But now, the doctor told them that if Nicole didn't have surgery, the curvature in her spine would progress and begin to compress her right lung. If the condition continued untreated, by her early twenties, Nicole would have a hard time walking up stairs.

This conversation marked the moment when Joanne began to wonder about Dr. Volkman's competence. During all of Nicole's routine checkups, he had never mentioned scoliosis. Now her condition was apparently obvious and quite urgent. How had he missed this so badly?

The scoliosis diagnosis was the beginning of a medical nightmare.

A few months after her initial consultation with the specialist, Nicole underwent surgery to have two 16-inch metal rods implanted in her spine. During the ten-hour surgery, one of the machines meant to monitor the connection between her brain and spine malfunctioned, which meant that the surgical team had to reverse her sedative drugs, mid-procedure, wake her up, and have her wiggle her fingers and toes to indicate that she was okay, before they put her back to sleep. This double dose of anesthesia weakened her lungs, which led to her being placed on a ventilator for two days in the ICU after the surgery. Joanne told me that she was "furious" to see her child suffer on a ventilator.

The surgery was followed by a painful recuperation during which Nicole, who had recently turned thirteen years old, couldn't bend over or carry anything more than a few pounds, including her schoolbooks. She was essentially homebound.

Eventually, Nicole healed from the surgery. But then, after a few years, she noticed a lump on her back near the point of the surgical incision. The lump, she learned, was due to an extremely rare allergic reaction to the metal of the implanted rods, which meant she had to go back for another surgery in her late teens to have the hardware removed. Some of the wiring couldn't be removed because it was wrapped in scar tissue and too close to her spinal cord. So the surgeons took out what they could. It was around the time of this second surgery that Nicole's parents decided that her former pediatrician ought to pay for his missed scoliosis diagnosis.

They eventually found Margaret O'Leary, who was an experienced Chicago-area attorney for plaintiffs in malpractice cases. But as it turned out, the lawsuit that they hoped to file could get no traction. Joanne recalled O'Leary telling them that Volkman had no insurance and no money to pay, which meant that he wasn't worth suing. "And that was the end of that case," she said.

I spoke to O'Leary, who confirmed De Masi's account and gave me a bit more detail. She explained that the lawsuit never made it past the preliminary stages because Volkman's bankruptcy filing prohibited it from proceeding. There were no depositions. There was no settlement. And there was no trial.

The De Masis never saw a dime.

When I asked him about the case, Volkman told me that he hadn't seen Nicole in the three years before the scoliosis was spotted and that scoliosis "hardly ever manifests before puberty." He said that the reason the lawsuit didn't proceed wasn't due to his bankruptcy but because a surgeon whose testimony would be necessary for the plaintiff's case had told Joanne that she would have to pay him $10,000 to compensate him "for lost OR [operating room] time, to give a deposition." He characterized the case, overall, as a "total disgrace by an unscrupulous money grubber."

But once again, Volkman's account of this case diverges from others' in virtually every way. Both Nicole De Masi and Joanne De Masi insisted that Volkman had, in fact, seen Nicole during the years preceding the discovery of her diagnosis. And Joanne had no memory of a doctor refusing to testify due to money he would supposedly lose by taking time away from the operating room. When it comes to Volkman's claim that scoliosis "hardly ever manifests before puberty," a specialist from Johns Hopkins told me, "I would correct Dr. Volkman and say that Scoliosis USUALLY manifests itself before puberty."

The notion that the lawsuit was a "money-grubbing" "disgrace" was also at odds with the descriptions I heard from Nicole De Masi, her mother, and their lawyer. Margaret O'Leary felt that the case absolutely had merit, and she recalled just how unwilling to admit error Volkman had been in her interactions with him. She said that Volkman struck her as someone who was book-smart but "careless" when dealing with patients and "not necessarily rigorous with doing those things that he needed to do."

Joanne De Masi was still troubled by the lawsuit when I interviewed her decades later. She said that she wondered what would have happened if she hadn't spotted something amiss with Nicole's uniform. She also thought: How many of Volkman's other patients had issues that the doctor didn't spot?

Although the lawsuit never resulted in a payout, she recalled describing to O'Leary what, in her mind, justice would have looked like. She wanted Volkman to be forced to pay Nicole $5 per week for the rest of his life, "so he never, ever forgets her, and what he's done."

When I spoke with Nicole, she, too, believed that her surgeries and complications would have been prevented if Volkman had promptly caught her scoliosis. And she described a harrowing string of consequences that stemmed from that one mistake.

Twice, her life had been thrown off course by major surgeries: first to implant the metal rods, and then to remove them. During recovery for the second surgery, she needed antibiotics to be administered intravenously three times a day, and as a result, she couldn't work or go to school. She had to put her college studies on pause. While her friends were out having fun, going to college, and living normal lives, she told me, "My life stood still . . . for the second time."

When we spoke in the fall of 2022, Nicole had just had a third surgery on her back, and she was still in constant pain. This sometimes affected her mood and her parenting ability. She couldn't ride a bike. She couldn't walk very far without getting tired. She said that she was not a normal, healthy mom. She recalled that, when she first learned about the scoliosis, she hadn't realized how life-changing the news would be. Now, decades later, she knew that it was going to, in her words, "cost me till the day I die."

Nicole seemed particularly angry about how vulnerable she had been at the time of the missed diagnosis. "Pediatricians are supposed to look out for kids," she said. "That's why we went to the doctor: to make sure we were okay."

She was also stung by the fact that Volkman had never apologized, or even followed up, after initially referring her to a surgeon.

"There was no remorse," she said.

THE EXPERT WITNESS

Filing for bankruptcy protection does not seem to have significantly altered Paul Volkman's lifestyle. In fact, in the year after the successful discharge of his case, he and his wife moved back to Chicago to a conspicuously upscale address: 3240 North Lake Shore Drive.

The building was a twenty-story brick Renaissance Revival structure, operated by a high-end real estate company and staffed by a small army of doormen, maintenance workers, and valet attendants. The apartment to which the Volkmans moved, 9D, was "enormous," Volkman's daughter Jane told me. It had three bedrooms, a living room, and a dining room, all of which were soon furnished with the help of an interior decorator. The apartment's signature feature was its series of large windows overlooking Lake Michigan, with Belmont Harbor — a protected inlet where dozens of sailboats docked — in the foreground. Rent was around $4,000 per month.

When I spoke with Volkman about his financial decisions, he frequently placed the blame on his late wife, Nancy. And when he wasn't deflecting responsibility for his lifestyle, he tried another tactic: downplaying it. In one conversation, he described the family's standard of living, which included many years of private school for his two kids, as "very average middle class or somewhat less." At another point, he said, "We didn't live in any kind of extravagant way." When summarizing his career, he once told me, "I needed to make a decent amount of money as a doctor so I could support my family."

By the time the Volkmans moved to Lake Shore Drive, Paul had an additional income stream to help pay for their expensive tastes: expert testimony in malpractice lawsuits.

Experts play an integral role in the world of malpractice litigation. When patients allege that negligence or malpractice has occurred, their lawyers will need to secure experts to testify about what happened and explain how, exactly, the accused doctor's actions fell outside the realm of proper practice. In response, the defendants will call their own experts to opine about why the doctor's conduct was proper and within the standard of care. These experts are paid for their review of the documents in question, and for their subsequent depositions or testimony.

At the time that Volkman first began dabbling in this kind of work in the mid-1980s, the expert-witness marketplace was surging. One *New York Times* article from 1983 reported: "If the legal process reaches virtually every cranny of our culture, so, too, does the expert witness. There are authorities on children's toys, flaming desserts, depilatories, grain dust explosions and more." In another article from the *Times* in 1987 — headline: "Expert Witnesses: Booming Business for the Specialists" — the paper quoted a Yale Law School professor who called it "an escalation on the level of military preparedness."

It's easy to see why Paul would have been drawn to this work and why the industry, in turn, would be drawn to him. He was constantly looking to bolster his income, and reviewing medical records was a quick and relatively easy way to do that. At least two people I interviewed remembered him speaking favorably about his expert-witness work. His son Adam told me that he remembered how his dad was "always really jazzed about" the cases he got paid to comment on. And an office assistant in Volkman's pediatrics practice told me that she remembered him laughing after getting off the phone for a lawsuit-related conversation and saying something like, "Well, I just made $1,000 on that ten-minute phone call."

And there's little doubt that, on paper at least, Volkman made an appealing expert. Not only did he have two degrees from a prestigious institution, but he also had firsthand experience in multiple medical specialties. During one of his expert-witness depositions, when he was asked about the kinds of cases he worked on, he said, "I review cases with regard to pediatrics, emergency medicine, family practice, and pharmacology and toxicology."

Records from these cases are a bit tough to access. But I did find indications that Volkman once served as an expert witness in a case concerning an infant who suffered from cognitive issues, muscle problems, and a seizure disorder, all of which, the plaintiffs claimed, were due to an improperly performed spinal-tap procedure at an Ohio hospital. In another case, he worked as an expert on behalf of Dorene Ready — the wife of Major League Baseball player Randy Ready — who suffered a heart attack and a catastrophic brain injury after being improperly prescribed diet pills. After she sued the doctor who prescribed the medication, the case resulted in a $24 million verdict, the highest in Wisconsin history at the time.

Volkman has offered varying accounts of how much expert-witness work he did during his medical career. In an email to me in 2014, he said that, starting in the mid-1980s, he began "doing a few cases a year, making about 10k [annually]." But earlier statements that he made under oath indicate that the number was significantly higher. During one sworn deposition in 2001, he estimated that he offered expert testimony in "approximately eight to twelve cases a year." And in sworn courtroom testimony the following year, he said that he had testified in depositions "two to three hundred times." In the deposition from 2001, he said that he had testified in court "about fifteen" times, including cases in Ohio, Wisconsin, Illinois, Oklahoma, and Maryland.

Volkman never gave me a sum of what he made as an expert beyond his "10k" annual estimate. But using numbers that he cited under oath, it is possible to get a ballpark figure. Under questioning in one sworn deposition in 2001, he reported that his fee for his initial review of that case was $1,000; generally, if he agreed to take a case, he charged $3,000 for a deposition, regardless of its length, and $4,000 per day, plus costs, for any kind of trial testimony.

At this rate, factoring in an initial review and deposition, if he offered testimony in "eight to twelve cases a year" (as he said elsewhere) then this would have earned between $32,000 and $48,000 per year. And if you were to take his $3,000-per-deposition rate and apply it to his total estimate of "two to three hundred" instances of testimony, the sum is well into the hundreds of thousands of dollars.

This information is noteworthy on its own. But it's also helpful to remember when hearing Volkman's attacks on the medical malpractice system. The same system that he viciously criticized for targeting him was one that he was all too happy to partake in when it was aimed at someone else.

Volkman's frequent expert-witness testimony, and the sums that he made from it, are also important to remember when considering his later criticism of various experts who testified against him in his criminal case. These doctors were, as he once put it in a letter to me, "whores."

MALPRACTICE, PART V: ANGIE AND THE G-TUBE

Marion, Illinois, is a small town located 320 miles south of Chicago, where the state's borders narrow into a wobbly-lined U shape. The city has a prison, a Pepsi bottling factory, and a ninety-three-foot brick clock tower.

In 2001, Marion's population was around sixteen thousand. That year, in the early-morning hours of October 29, Paul Volkman was working an overnight shift at Marion Memorial Hospital when an eighty-four-year-old woman was brought to the emergency room from a local nursing home.

Angie Williamson was born and raised in Arkansas. After she married her husband, Jack, in 1944, the couple later moved to southern Illinois, where Jack practiced law and Angie taught in local elementary schools. They had one child, a son named James, who practiced law alongside his father and eventually became a judge.

Angie was a petite woman who stood about four feet, eleven inches tall. She enjoyed painting and was a member of numerous women's organizations, including the Women's Methodist Society and the Daughters of the American Revolution. Her granddaughter told me that it was a testament to her energy and curiosity that, after her retirement from decades of teaching, she returned to school to complete her previously paused college studies. She graduated from Southern Illinois University in 1974, in her late fifties, with a bachelor's degree in elementary education. After her husband's death in 1986, she remained independent, driving herself to the mall or to doctor's appointments. Her son described her as a "vibrant woman" who was active in her church and multiple book clubs.

In the late 1990s, as she entered her ninth decade, Angie started having health problems. She had spells of dizziness and began falling down. After a visit to a hospital and a series of tests, she was diagnosed with neuropathy (damage to her nervous system). For a time, despite her issues with balance, she maintained her mental capacity and was able to watch TV, talk on the phone, and make herself breakfast and lunch.

At some point, her son, Jim, the judge, began spending the night at her house to keep an eye on her. Her health issues got worse. After she suffered three falls in a single day in January 2000, she moved to a local nursing home. Two months later, she had a stroke.

By October 2001, the stroke had left her completely paralyzed on her right side, and she had only partial use of her left side. Her speech was limited, and she received close care from the staff at the nursing home. Her son visited her there every day after work.

But as hard as things had become for Angie, folks who knew her stressed that her life still had its small joys. She could smile and nod. She could say words like "Good" or make sounds to indicate her approval or disapproval. Although her food had to be pureed before she consumed it, she was, according to the nursing home's staff, one of the facility's best eaters. She could also be helped from her bed and into a wheelchair, which allowed her to go to the TV room to spend time with other nursing home residents, or be wheeled outside to feel the breeze on her face, which she seemed to enjoy. Her son would later testify that when he arrived for a visit at the nursing home, she would recognize him, and her eyes would brighten and she'd smile. "I had a feeling she was looking forward to me coming," he said.

Angie's first visit to the emergency room on the night of October 29, 2001, occurred at around 1:25 A.M. The reason was that her gastrostomy tube, which had been installed via a port in her abdomen to administer medication, had come out. The staffers at the nursing home were not qualified to replace the tube on-site, so she was brought to the hospital, where a doctor would do it.

Replacing dislodged gastrostomy tubes is a common task for an emergency room doctor. An attorney for Volkman would later say that, in his two decades of experience, he had replaced similar tubes "hundreds" of times. And in this instance, according to Volkman, he successfully replaced Angie's G-tube and sent her back home.

The precise way he confirmed the tube's placement would later become a matter of interest. Volkman testified that he used a technique that involves pushing air through the tube after it is placed inside the patient's abdomen. Using this method, if the tube is placed properly, the air makes a telltale gurgling sound that the person who has replaced it can hear via stethoscope. If the tube is in the wrong spot, there won't be a gurgling sound.

There are other methods that can be used to confirm a G-tube's proper placement. A doctor can request an X-ray for visual confirmation or, alternatively, can inject fluid into the tube and then draw it back to confirm that the returning fluid appears to have come from the stomach. But Volkman would later say that he didn't feel his replacement required any test beyond the air-gurgling technique.

After Angie returned to the nursing home, somehow, within a few hours, the tube once again became dislodged and she returned to the emergency room at around 5:50 A.M. Once again, she was seen by Volkman, and his notes from this second encounter indicated that Angie was "oriented x 3" — medical shorthand for a patient who knows who they are, where they are, and the approximate time. People familiar with Angie's condition say that this would have been impossible because she was not able to communicate in such a way. This seemingly impossible interaction recorded in the doctor's notes, in addition to those notes' general lack of detail, were two subjects that Angie's lawyer would later mention.

Volkman would deny that he was tired when he saw Angie for a second time, or that he was frustrated to see her return for a similar problem. He would also deny that the second placement of her G-tube was anything other than successful. In his telling, he once again properly reinserted the tube, confirmed its placement, and sent her home.

The next twelve hours passed without incident, and notes made by nursing home staff during that time indicate that the tube was functioning properly. But at around midnight on the day of Angie's early-morning ER visit, attendants noticed blood around the G-tube's entry point in her abdomen. After she began vomiting blood, she was taken back to a hospital, where she was seen by a general surgeon named Clay DeMattei.

After examining Angie, DeMattei suspected that her feeding tube was not in its proper place. X-rays confirmed his assessment. DeMattei was an experienced surgeon who had previously seen a number of cases where misplaced G-tubes required reparative surgery. And he recognized Angie's condition as serious. She had arrived at the hospital exhibiting signs of sepsis (a dangerous condition brought on by the body's response to an infection), and he believed that she needed surgery to save her life. He spoke with her son, Jim, to inform him about the situation and advise him that there was a chance his mother wouldn't survive the surgery. But DeMattei would later say that his "hands were tied"; the situation called for urgent measures.

As the surgery began, DeMattei was able to get a better view of Angie's internal injuries. He saw a mess of damaged tissue and observed that the wall of her stomach was clotted and swollen. He later explained that the damage was so extensive that he had to take half of her stomach out and "put her back together" before replacing it. He would also report that he had never seen, or even read about, a situation quite like this one, where the tube had been placed between the inner lining of the stomach (called the mucosa) and the thin layer of muscle beyond it (called the muscularis).

DeMattei would later say that, among all the G-tube-related injuries he had previously seen and operated on, he had never seen one that had been the result of the tube being pulled *out*. Every G-tube-related injury he had operated on had been the result of an error in pushing the tube *in* by the person installing or replacing it. This case struck him as no different. Most of the injuries that he saw during Angie's surgery were located between the layers of the stomach, and as he later testified, "there is no other way for that tube to have gotten in that position."

DeMattei had not seen the moment that Angie's injuries had occurred. But he firmly believed that Angie Williamson's extensive — and, ultimately, life-threatening — injuries had been caused at the emergency room, by the doctor who had twice replaced her tube in the early morning of October 29.

After the surgery, Angie remained on a ventilator for three days, and she stayed in the hospital for a week. She was eventually discharged but returned with nausea, fever, and vomiting. After being diagnosed with pneumonia and, later, pancreatitis, she returned to the hospital twice more in the coming weeks. Then, in late December, she underwent a second surgery to remove her gallbladder. People close to her felt that this string of incidents all traced back to that initial misplaced G-tube at the emergency room.

After those arduous weeks of medical care, Angie's previous quality of life had evaporated. She could no longer be fed orally; all food now went through her feeding tube. And this new permanent feeding situation meant that she needed to be hooked at all times into an electric machine that required a nearby outlet. As a result, she could no longer be wheeled around the nursing home with relative ease. She was essentially bedridden.

Nurses at the facility later testified that her smiles and small comments ceased. "She just appeared sadder to me," one said. Another added, "She [didn't] verbalize at all anymore."

Her son, Jim, also reported that after the stomach surgery and ensuing issues, his mother seemed far less emotionally expressive. He would talk to her and ask how she felt, but she mostly just stared at him in response. She seemed despondent; sometimes, he noticed tears in her eyes. Eventually he reached out to a local personal-injury attorney named John Womick who had experience with medical malpractice cases.

In response to the judge's query, Womick did some preliminary research, including requesting Angie's medical files and speaking with DeMattei, whom Womick said was "outraged" by what he believed were Volkman's actions. Womick agreed to take the case.

Womick later explained to me that representing an elderly client like Angie was a bit rare in personal-injury and malpractice work. Unlike, for instance, a young man or woman with a career's worth of lost income ahead of them, there was less of an argument to make to a jury about lost income and quality of life as the result of the malpractice. But the judge was a friend of his. And once he dug into the particulars of the case, he said that he viewed the situation as such a "god-awful, smacks-you-in-the-face, clear-cut case of negligence" that he decided to proceed. He said he had no idea that the doctor had previously faced malpractice cases. To him, Volkman was simply "what I perceived to be, not a very conscientious ER doctor."

The lawsuit against Paul Volkman was filed in December 2001, around two months after Angie's early-morning visit to the emergency room. The complaint stated that, in his capacity as an emergency room physician, Volkman had a legal obligation to "apply the knowledge and use the skill and care of a reasonably well-qualified emergency room physician," and that, numerous times that morning, he had failed in that duty. First, the complaint stated that he had improperly inserted a tube that was "too short for its intended purpose," an error that, within hours, prompted Williamson to return for a second replacement. Then, during that second replacement, he had improperly placed the tube between two layers of her stomach, rather than in the stomach itself. This error had caused a large tear in her stomach tissue, which led to subsequent health issues. According to the complaint, Volkman had failed to properly confirm that the tube was in its proper place and had failed to consult with a radiologist about the placement of the tube.

The complaint alleged that as a direct result of these acts of omissions and negligence, Williamson had suffered an injury and had been forced to undergo surgery; had incurred, and would continue to incur, medical expenses; and had experienced pain, suffering, and a decreased quality of life. She was now, via her son, who was acting as her legal surrogate, seeking a monetary judgment.

The *Williamson v. Volkman* trial began in Marion on December 11, 2002, almost exactly nine years after the start of Volkman's first jury trial for malpractice in Chicago. Once the jury was selected and sworn in, John Womick began by showing a video clip of Angie Williamson, who was not present in the courtroom but who was, he said, "the real plaintiff in this lawsuit." He described her health issues before the G-tube incident and its fallout, and the small sources of happiness in her life at that time. This was a case about the "catastrophic" toll of her treatment in the emergency room, he said.

Replacing a G-tube of the kind that Angie had was "not a difficult procedure," Womick said. But Paul Volkman had botched this procedure in such a way that, within days, Angie's life was in peril. Angie, at her age and condition, was not the kind of person whom you would want to undergo major abdominal surgery, he said. But she had no choice. And this surgery had led to a "cascade of events" that permanently changed her life, including pneumonia, pancreatitis, and, eventually, a second surgery to remove her gallbladder. None of this would have happened without the initial misplacement of her feeding tube in the emergency room, he said.

Womick explained to the jury that negligence occurs when a doctor doesn't meet the standard of care in his or her treatment of a patient. He argued that Volkman had been negligent both in his placement of Angie's tube and his failure to take proper steps to be sure that the tube was in the right place. He said that after witnesses had been called and evidence was shown, he was going to ask jurors to demand that the doctor pay damages representing what this woman had lost. He knew that money wasn't sufficient. "But there is no other substitute in our system for an individual who would like to recoup what she lost," he said.

In the defense's opening statement, Volkman's lawyer mentioned his client's degrees from the University of Chicago, his board certifications in pediatrics and emergency medicine, and his twenty-five years of emergency room experience. Paul Volkman had probably replaced hundreds of gastronomy tubes, he said.

He went on to describe the testimony that the defense's witnesses would offer, which suggested that the injuries seen by Dr. DeMattei during surgery could not possibly have been the result of an erroneous placement of a tube and also that records indicated there was no blood seen around Angie's G-tube port until more than twelve hours after she had returned to the nursing home. This, he said, was proof that the insertion had been proper, and whatever happened to cause Angie's internal injuries had taken place *after* she left the emergency room. The experts who had reviewed the case believed that Volkman's care was appropriate, he said. And this was why they would be asking for a verdict in the doctor's favor.

The question at the heart of the trial was about how Angie's injuries had occurred. Had Volkman, the experienced emergency room physician, acted within the standard of care to carefully reinsert her tube and confirm its proper placement? And thus were Angie's injuries self-inflicted after she returned to the nursing home and yanked the tube out herself?* This was the defense's suggestion.

Or had Angie's injuries been the result of a careless doctor who was sloppy in his notetaking, who had improperly reinserted her feeding tube, and who had declined to take extra steps to make sure the tube was properly placed before sending her home? This was the story the plaintiffs presented.

During the plaintiff's case, DeMattei testified that his thoughts about the origin of Angie's injuries hadn't changed since the day he first treated her. Improper placement of the tube was the most common cause of such an injury, he said. And all the cases that he had seen in his fifteen years of surgery had, like this one, occurred within a relatively short time after the placement or replacement of the tube. Based on what he saw during the surgery he performed, he believed "there is no other way for that tube to have gotten in that position."

---

* When I spoke with Angie's granddaughter Sarah, she told me that her grandmother had, in fact, pulled out the tube prior to the events discussed at trial, a fact that seems to bolster the defense's side of the case.

Another plaintiff's witness, Jim Williamson, explained that his mother was "completely paralyzed on her right side," which included her right arm. And he said that her use of the hand on her left side — the side of the tube's placement — was "very, very limited." She couldn't raise that arm or grip with it, he said, which implied it was physically impossible for her to have pulled out the tube herself, let alone with the force to cause the injuries she suffered.

In response, Volkman's lawyer called the doctor himself to testify. Prompted by questioning from his attorney, Volkman proceeded to walk the courtroom through the process of how he replaced the tube and confirmed its placement.

"You believe that's a fail-safe method?" Womick said during cross-examination.

"Nothing is fail-safe," Volkman responded. "But I believe that that is very reliable."

The defense also called two expert witnesses. One was a professor of emergency medicine from the University of Michigan who testified that Volkman had replaced the tube in "the usual and customary way" that met the specialty's standard of care. This witness was deeply skeptical that the replacement of the tube could have caused the injuries in question. Given the softness of the tube, the nature of injuries, and the gentle pressure involved in its replacement, he said it would be "medically impossible" for the injuries to have occurred due to the replacement. And he added that, in three decades in medicine, he had never seen, heard about, or read about such an event.

The other expert witness was a board-certified gastroenterologist and professor at the Washington University School of Medicine in St. Louis who testified that, based on the information he had reviewed, he believed the feeding tube had been manipulated at some time after Volkman had sent Williamson home. This, he said, was the reason for the blood that appeared around the G-tube's port in Angie's abdomen, and it was also the reason for her internal injuries. During his testimony, he pointed to the extent of the injuries that had been identified inside Williamson's stomach. To him, this disproved the notion that Volkman's improper replacement was to blame. "If the tube never made it to the inside of the stomach how could the damage occur on the inside of the stomach?" he asked.

But the trial was about more than just the placement of a gastrostomy tube. In presenting Angie's case, Womick adopted a strategy of arguing that his local, unpaid medical witness was more credible than the defense's highly paid witnesses from out of town. When it came time to cross-examine the first of the defense's experts, the Washington University gastroenterologist, Womick made a point of bringing up the hourly rates that the doctor had disclosed during direct examination: $350 per hour for reviewing documents, and $500 per hour for testimony in court or a deposition.

"Let's talk about money," he said. When he tallied up the work that the doctor had done for the case, he said that he was up to about $12,000.

The witness responded that he hadn't been keeping a running total.

A short while later, the lawyer asked, "And if you didn't have an opinion that Dr. Volkman met the standard, then that would drop down to about 500 bucks, wouldn't it?" The implication was clear: The expert witness had a financial interest in the pro-Volkman testimony he was presenting to the jury.

This issue also came up in the cross-examination of the defense's other expert witness, who had disclosed during direct examination that he had previously reviewed documents in around fifteen hundred cases and testified more than 150 times. At one point, Womick asked the doctor to estimate how much he would be making for his work on this case. The answer, the doctor said, was somewhere between $5,000 and $7,000.

This line of attack extended to Volkman himself. During his cross-examination of Volkman, Womick asked Volkman to confirm that he, too, had worked as an expert witness in "over 200 or 300 cases."

"Correct," Volkman said. "Over about, well, 18 years."

The foil to all this highly paid expert-witness activity was the plaintiff's star witness: Dr. DeMattei. In direct examination and opening and closing arguments, DeMattei was portrayed as a bright guy who had returned to work in his hometown, despite having the skills and smarts to go elsewhere. This doctor, who had saved this old woman's life with his surgical know-how, had never before worked as a paid expert witness, nor was he paid for testifying in this case, which marked his first time as a witness in any malpractice case. At one point, he described himself as a "small-town doctor."

When it came time for closing statements, Womick told the jury that the standard of care in Marion was "not what a paid hired gun from Ann Arbor says it is." And he proceeded to place the case on DeMattei's shoulders.

"Dr. DeMattei did not come here with an agenda," he said. "[He] did not come here with a paycheck. Did not come here about an interest, except one thing: to tell the truth."

At another point, he added, "Tell me why Dr. DeMattei would lie. I mean, why [would] a general surgeon at Marion Memorial Hospital . . . voluntarily make up all of this story against an ER doctor at that hospital?"

Another one of Womick's lines of attack was to not so subtly prompt suspicions about Volkman's career as a roving emergency room doctor. This became clear during Womick's cross-examination, when he asked Volkman where he had worked prior to his stint in Marion.

Volkman responded by naming three locations: Cleveland; Milwaukee; and Michigan City, Indiana. But Womick drew him out further, prompting the doctor to explain that before those jobs, he had worked in temporary positions for several years, through numerous locum tenens staffing companies. "I would work [at] 10 or 15 hospitals, two or three shifts at each one," Volkman said.

From here, Womick, who had clearly prepared for such a moment, asked Volkman to confirm that he had worked at individual hospitals, ringing off names in rapid-fire fashion: Ball Memorial Hospital in Muncie, Indiana; Belleville Memorial Hospital in Belleville, Illinois; St. Katherine's in East Chicago; St. Joseph's in Fort Wayne, Indiana; South Lake in Merrillville, Indiana; Decatur Memorial in Decatur, Illinois; West Suburban, outside of Chicago.

At some point, the lawyer stopped naming hospitals and just listed towns: Appleton, Wisconsin; Dayton, Ohio; Defiance, Ohio; Millersburg, Ohio; Pomeroy, Ohio; Quincy, Illinois.

Volkman confirmed all of them.

After naming twenty hospitals and towns where the doctor had worked, Womick said, "That's not all, is it?"

"Nope," Volkman said. "That's just a partial list."

"Didn't stay any place very long, did you, Doctor?" Womick said.

"That's the nature of temporary assignments," Volkman said.

"Well, is it?" Womick responded. "I have been at this awhile. Don't a lot of doctors stay with the same group for years and years?"

"You can be with the same group and be at many different hospitals," Volkman said.

"Not fifty," Womick replied.

Volkman's attorney had apparently anticipated such a strategy, and in his opening statement, he described his client's traveling lifestyle as "not an unusual situation at all." In his closing statement, he returned to the subject to say that this was the first trial he had been involved in where a man had been condemned for traveling long distances, and going from place to place, "to work to put food in his own family's stomachs."

Womick, in his own closing, said that he had never condemned Volkman for making a living. He was simply stating questions that jurors were surely already asking in their heads.

"Why Marion?" he said. "Why six hours from Chicago? Why Waukegan and Provident and Sinai and on and on and on and on and on and on?"

In his closing arguments, Volkman's attorney acknowledged that he and his client were facing an uphill battle. He said that he knew how hard it would be for jurors to watch the videos of Angie and hear from her son and then decide that the plaintiff hadn't met the burden of proof. "That takes guts," he said.

Yet that is exactly what he was asking them to do. He argued that the record showed that the injury had not occurred in the way DeMattei assumed it had — that, in fact, the injury occurred after Volkman dismissed Williamson from the hospital for the second time. He argued that Paul's treatment of Angie was within the standard of care and that he bore no responsibility for her emergency surgery and the health issues that followed.

Womick, meanwhile, ended by reminding jurors of the gravity of the case. He said that, because of the failed insertion of her feeding tube on the morning of October 29, Angie Williamson had almost died and had needed lifesaving surgery. He called it an "extraordinarily important case" and said that he considered it an honor to represent the judge and his mother.

In his closing arguments, Womick also portrayed Volkman as exasperated and resentful over the fact that this elderly woman had come to the emergency room twice during the same overnight shift. "That's why we are really here, because that was his attitude then," he said. He argued that Volkman's care was a reflection of his attitude.

He reminded the jury that Angie's right side was totally paralyzed and that she was unable to use her left hand, which made it impossible that she could have pulled out the tube herself. Paul Volkman, on the other hand, had worked inside her stomach twice that night. At one point he suggested that even a veterinarian could have replaced these G-tubes properly.

"The question," he said, "is in Marion, Illinois . . . does life have value? Dr. Volkman did not give her the quality of care that he could have."

He finished with a final jab at Volkman, who, according to Womick, would have rather spent his overnight shift sleeping on the night he treated Angie Williamson.

"Maybe if you have got to drive to Chicago, that's how it is," he said.

The jury was dismissed for deliberations shortly after closing arguments. After around three hours, they returned a unanimous verdict in favor of Angie Williamson. The damages of $354,016 that they assessed were the sum of three parts:

- $121,016 for past and future medical care;
- $100,000 for pain experienced in the future; and
- $133,000 for loss of normal life experienced and likely to be experienced in the future.

Those funds would not come out of Volkman's pocket; they would be paid by his malpractice insurer. Yet the consequences of that verdict would be life altering — for Volkman and, later, for dozens of people in an Ohio town four hundred miles to the east.

UNINSURABLE

The Marion lawsuit marked a turning point for Volkman. Afterward, he found himself unable to obtain malpractice insurance, which had drastic implications for his medical career.

The exact details of when and how he was informed of this development are still murky to me. And because this notification wasn't included in court records from his civil or criminal cases, I'm left to rely mostly on his account of how it happened.

Volkman has described this event in a few different ways.

In one conversation, he described waking up on the morning after the Williamson verdict to the news that he was no longer insured to work in emergency rooms and "couldn't get any" insurance if he tried. He said that he never received a formal letter informing him of his banishment; he just found himself unable to obtain insurance.

Later, he elaborated. "The insurance industry kept track of these case settlements," he wrote in 2014. "If the total amount was over a certain (unrevealed) amount throughout a doctor's career, his ability to secure malpractice insurance was abruptly terminated without any possible recourse, as was his ability to work as an emergency medicine physician."

At another point, however, he offered a slightly different account. In a 2019 essay about his life and career, he wrote that after the Williamson case, "several insurance company settlements against me made malpractice insurance prohibitively expensive for continued work in emergency medicine." This wording suggests he was *priced out* of the market, not blacklisted, as he had previously implied.

The exact timing of this event also remains unclear.

Based on his CV, Volkman's uninsurability doesn't seem to have taken effect immediately after the filing of the Williamson lawsuit, in December 2001. Nor does it seem to have been triggered by the verdict, in December 2002. Instead, according to his CV, his last emergency room job (in Gary, Indiana) ended in August 2002, four months before the Williamson trial began. Why he would stop working in emergency rooms *between* the filing of the lawsuit and the arrival of the verdict is a mystery to me, since it suggests that neither event prompted his expulsion from the market.

Regardless of whether Volkman was locked out or priced out of the market for malpractice insurance, he did not think that he was in any way responsible for the four malpractice cases that led to that moment.

He believed, instead, that he was a casualty of a system oversupplied with lawyers who were, as he said, "sitting in their expensive offices wearing three-piece suits having absolutely nothing to do . . . and having bills to pay." He was not a bad doctor; he was a victim of what he called "hungry lawyer syndrome." As he once put it, the malpractice lawsuits against him were "all cases without any remotely cognizable negligence . . . filed by ethically-challenged, financially struggling barristers in hopes of an easy payout of Other People's Money."

The fact that he was further penalized by the insurance marketplace was, to him, yet another injustice.

How plausible is Volkman's tale of repeated victimization in the world of litigation and malpractice insurance?

Before I share what I heard from experts, it's important to remember the harm at the heart of these cases. In one case, a child died from a serious but treatable illness. In another case, a woman lost her arm below the elbow, which forced her into an early retirement, among other hardships. In a third, a young man's cognitive functions dropped so severely that his father was appointed his legal guardian. In a fourth, an elderly woman had to undergo emergency lifesaving surgery, which led to subsequent complications that, all told, dramatically reduced her quality of life.

In his complaints about the unfairness of his treatment in the malpractice courts, Volkman rarely, if ever, acknowledged the devastating events that prompted these lawsuits. But these were not mere inconveniences. They were profound, life-altering injuries and traumas.

And when I looked more closely at Volkman's account of his supposed victimization in the malpractice courts, I found other instances where the story was skewed, was misrepresented, or didn't align with the opinion of experts. For instance, Volkman had written that "emergency medicine is well known as an area of medicine highly exposed to malpractice litigation." But people who study the relative litigation risks of different medical specialties place emergency medicine closer to the middle of the pack. According to a 2019 article in the journal *International Review of Law and Economics*, ER medicine carries far lower risk of a paid malpractice claim than various surgical specialties (including general, orthopedic, plastic, cardiovascular, and neurosurgery) as well as other nonsurgical specialties, including obstetrics and gynecology, urology, and anesthesiology. One of the authors of that article — Georgetown University law professor David Hyman, who holds degrees in both law and medicine, teaches classes on medical malpractice law and has written a book about malpractice litigation — described it to me as a "moderate risk" specialty.

I also learned that plaintiff's attorneys are, in fact, quite selective when screening potential malpractice cases. This is, in part, because juries tend to like and trust doctors and rule in their favor the majority of the time. It's also partly because many prospective malpractice claims, however valid and painful they are for the patient, may not have a potential payout that makes it worth the costs of proceeding. As Hyman explained, plaintiff's lawyers have to decline a large number of prospective cases "because either the damages aren't large enough, or the evidence of causation and negligence is weak."

As John Womick, the lawyer who sued Volkman in the Williamson case, told me, malpractice cases require hiring experts to review the materials and sometimes deliver depositions before a case can proceed. The attorneys for such cases work on a contingency basis, meaning that they only get paid if they win. To Womick, Volkman's notion of an "impoverished" or financially struggling malpractice lawyer was an oxymoron. "You have to have sufficient funds to finance the case," he said.*

And there were other aspects of Volkman's account that didn't withstand closer scrutiny. When he narrated his malpractice woes, Volkman portrayed his insurers as spineless, plaintiff-friendly companies that rushed to settle the cases against him regardless of those cases' underlying merit. But this, too, was at odds with what I heard from people who actually work in, or study, such cases. Hyman told me that insurance companies generally "don't pay money unless they feel like they have to."

I also spoke with Tom Baker, a professor at the University of Pennsylvania's law school, who has studied malpractice lawsuits in depth and wrote a 2005 book called *The Medical Malpractice Myth*, which debunked prevailing misconceptions about an out-of-control, doctor-unfriendly court system. Baker agreed with Hyman and told me that the idea that insurance companies would settle a case with no evidence of liability on the physician's part is "just wrong," he said. The industry, in general, is "absolutely not out to get doctors" he said; if anything, there's grounds to critique the industry on being *too aligned* with the interests of doctors. He added that cases where companies decide to settle generally indicate that the company didn't want to spend money defending what it believed to be a losing claim.

During these conversations with experts, I also got answers to questions about the events that led to Volkman becoming uninsurable.

When I told Baker that Volkman had been the subject of two settlements, two jury verdicts, and a fifth case that was deflected by his bankruptcy, he described it to me as a "very unusual" number of cases and said that it was "incredibly unlikely" that a doctor would be wrongly accused five times. Hyman had a similar response. "You don't get four paid malpractice claims through bad luck, even practicing in a high-risk specialty," he told me. "Especially when two of them are the result of jury verdicts."

---

* Womick's comments align with those of two veteran Boston-based malpractice attorneys who were interviewed in the publication *Medical Economics* in 2000, around the time of the Kirchhoff and Williamson cases. One of the lawyers explained that her firm reviewed dozens of cases for every case they accepted, while the other attorney estimated that it costs at least $20,000 to $30,000 to bring a case to trial. "Given the economics of malpractice law," he said, "any lawyer who takes frivolous cases is going to go bankrupt."

It was due to the unusually high number of verdicts and settlements against Volkman that neither Baker nor Hyman was surprised to hear that the doctor had wound up uninsurable. Baker brought up the analogy of the car insurance marketplace where, if a driver gets into a certain number of accidents, they might, quite understandably, find themselves locked out by most insurers. Volkman's exclusion from the malpractice insurance market didn't strike him as unfair or unjust. It sounded like the system operating as designed.

Hyman added that, given the usual slowness of state medical boards to crack down on problematic doctors, a lockout from the insurance industry was one of the few existing mechanisms for dealing with problematic doctors, short of a criminal investigation.

He, too, didn't think that Volkman was the victim of any kind of malevolent insurance-industry conspiracy.

"It's just that his insurer said, 'Enough already,'" he said.

MILWAUKEE

By the early 2000s, Dr. Paul Nausieda was a nationally renowned specialist in the treatment of Parkinson's disease and sleep disorders. He had published dozens of articles in scholarly journals; coauthored a booklet called *Parkinson's Disease: What You and Your Family Should Know*, distributed by the national Parkinson's Foundation; and served as chairman of sleep disorders medicine for the American Academy of Neurology. In the previous two decades, his regional research and treatment center in Milwaukee had flourished. Nausieda saw approximately 150 patients there each week and kept tabs on a number of others who were involved in research trials for new drugs. In 2002, St. Luke's Medical Center, where the center was located, described it as the "largest comprehensive Parkinson disease center in the world."

It was around this time that Nausieda received a phone call from one of his old University of Chicago classmates: Paul Volkman.

Back in medical school Nausieda had taken some of the same classes as Volkman. And after graduating, they spent some time in the same research lab at Michael Reese Hospital, in Chicago. One journal article from that time — "Lergotrile in the Treatment of Parkinsonism," from a 1978 issue of the journal *Neurology* — lists both of their names among five coauthors. Not long afterward, Nausieda moved to Milwaukee and had fallen out of touch with Volkman. At the time of his phone call, Nausieda hadn't spoken to his old colleague in years.

Volkman was calling to see if Nausieda knew of any jobs in the pharmaceutical industry for someone with a doctorate in pharmacology. Nausieda didn't have much to offer in that regard; he had worked with pharma companies during clinical trials but wasn't closely involved with their research-and-development departments, which is where he thought Volkman would find such a job.

But when Volkman explained that he was looking for a job, Nausieda had an idea. Given how busy his own practice was and the fact that Volkman's background was reasonably compatible with Nausieda's work at the clinic, perhaps he could come to Milwaukee to treat Parkinson's patients.

Volkman began the job in August 2002.

The Milwaukee position marked yet another professional pivot for Volkman. He had conducted research in pharmacology. He had practiced pediatrics and family medicine. He had worked in dozens of emergency rooms across the Upper Midwest. He had been an expert witness for malpractice cases of various kinds. And he was now, as his CV later noted: "Evaluat[ing], treat[ing] and continuing care of 1400 Parkinson/Alzheimer patients using sophisticated combinations of drugs . . . combined with pallidotomy and deep brain stimulation."

According to Nausieda, the new job was a good fit. The ninety-mile distance between Milwaukee and Chicago, and the fact that the job required Volkman to be away from home for a few days at time, didn't pose much of a hurdle. (Volkman was, after all, quite used to traveling from his years of locum tenens work.) And Nausieda and Volkman got along well. When I spoke with Nausieda in 2011, he recalled that he and his wife had hosted Volkman for dinner a few times, during which they talked about books, music, and their shared interest in the history of medicine.

When it came to the work itself, Volkman struck Nausieda as someone with a better grasp of medical theory than of hands-on medical practice. But this was a minor quibble. Volkman seemed happy to read up on his new area of focus. And Nausieda would later describe Volkman to me as a "typical, successful physician who gets along great with their patients" and who struck him as "perfectly appropriate" in the role. At one point Volkman even suggested a yoga program for Parkinson's patients, which became a permanent part of the center's offerings.

There was just one problem.

For Volkman to remain at the center on a long-term basis, he would need to be granted admitting privileges at the hospital so that he could share the burden of off-hours on-call work with Nausieda's team of physicians. This distribution of labor was a major reason for bringing him on in the first place, and without those privileges, his continued employment wouldn't make economic or practical sense. Nausieda told me that when Volkman first applied for those privileges there was a bit of delay, which wasn't too surprising to Nausieda, who knew that paperwork can sometimes move slowly through a hospital's bureaucracy. But when the delay continued for months, Nausieda inquired with the hospital administration.

The answer he received was that Volkman's application was being intentionally blocked by someone in the hospital's administration. And though he never learned exactly who was causing the holdup, he did hear that the person was unlikely to change their mind. When Nausieda pressed for more detail he learned that the veto traced back to when Volkman had previously worked as a locum tenens physician in the hospital's emergency department and, in Nausieda's words, "had a run-in which left this other person with a really bad taste in their mouth." That was the extent of the explanation.

When I spoke with him in 2011, Nausieda was still a bit puzzled about the incident. He said that if Volkman had made some kind of disastrous medical error, it would have likely shown up in the local courts or at least in the hospital's disciplinary committee. But he found no such paper trail. And he was at a loss for explaining what else may have prompted the blockade. "Whatever happened," he said, "somebody was royally pissed about something."

When I asked Volkman about this, he acknowledged that he was denied admitting privileges at the Milwaukee hospital, but he gave a different explanation. His rejection was not the result of a nasty impression he had left in the past; the problem, he said, was Nausieda's reputation within the institution. "Nausieda tended to provoke spiteful battles, and I was victimized," Volkman said.*

Whatever the exact cause of Volkman's denial, it was nonnegotiable: He

---

* It seems unlikely that an institution where Nausieda was as internally disliked as Volkman claimed, would, in its Winter 2002 newsletter, publish a lengthy feature article with his smiling face and the headline "Revolutionizing the Scope of Care for Parkinson Disease." But after our first interview, Nausieda declined to answer my additional questions, so I'm left with Nausieda's and Volkman's dueling narratives.

was never going to be cleared for staff privileges at St. Luke's in Milwaukee. And when this became clear, Nausieda had to tell Volkman that he couldn't afford to pay his salary.

When I spoke with Nausieda about this in 2011, the episode seemed to strike him as odd and a bit unfortunate. Nausieda acknowledged that, despite all of Volkman's training, he seemed like "a lost soul who never quite found where his niche was." But Volkman had struck him as a reasonable guy, and he would have kept him on his staff if the politics of the institution had allowed it.

The rejection in Milwaukee was catastrophic for Volkman. His employment options were significantly limited before the Milwaukee job, and when he lost the position in early 2003, it sent him into free fall. Without malpractice insurance, he was unable to get any kind of doctor job in the Chicago area, since, as he once explained, "even ghetto Medicaid storefront clinics required malpractice coverage."

He spent some time collecting unemployment compensation from the state. He even, as he once wrote in an autobiographical narrative, spent "brief stints chopping vegetables in restaurant kitchens." He would later say that this brief foray into nonmedical wage work "induced me to take any job I could get without insurance, as a doctor."

He was desperate.

Then, one day, while scanning the internet for potential jobs, an opportunity appeared. It was an ad for a pain clinic in southern Ohio in need of a physician. It was located in a town called Portsmouth, near the southernmost point of Ohio, just across the river from Kentucky.

He made the call.

— PART TWO—

CRIME SCENES

BOOMTOWN

The city of Portsmouth, Ohio, is located on the banks of the Ohio River, not far from the southernmost tip of the state. It is a region known among locals as the Tri-State Area, due to the proximity of Ohio, Kentucky, and West Virginia. For folks who live there, crossing from one state to another is a regular part of life.

Portsmouth is situated in the foothills of the Appalachian Mountains. These gently sloping green hills surround the town in a natural basin, and, across the river, in Kentucky, a ridgeline runs parallel to the river at a height of more than nine hundred feet. The hills are sometimes called the Little Smokies for the way that mist settles into their folds and creases.

Portsmouth's population has been less than thirty thousand for decades. And yet, because of the sparsely populated region that surrounds it, when you reach the city's limits, it feels as if you've arrived somewhere notable. The town is home to Shawnee State University, a multiplex cinema, a history museum, an imposing county courthouse, and a hospital with more than two hundred beds. When you drive down one of the town's main roads, Chillicothe Street, you pass enough multistory buildings that the term *downtown* doesn't just feel like a figure of speech.

For those who live elsewhere, the mention of Ohio might conjure mental images of flat cornfields and midwestern culture. But this part of the state is an exception. In the 1960s, the city of Portsmouth launched the tourist slogan "Where Southern Hospitality Begins." Step into one of the city's most beloved restaurants, the Scioto Ribber, and you'll find a menu of hickory-smoked ribs; sides of coleslaw, baked beans, french fries, and sweet potato; sweet tea; and homemade peanut butter cream pie for dessert. Speak to local residents and you'll notice more than a hint of a southern drawl. The name *Volkman*, when pronounced by locals, can turn into *Vokeman*. The term *pill mill* sometimes sounds like *peel meal*.

From Portsmouth, it'll take you about two hours to drive to Cincinnati or Columbus, but just under forty minutes to get to Ashland, Kentucky, hometown of famous country singers Naomi and Wynonna Judd as well as the Paramount Theatre, where Billy Ray Cyrus filmed the music video for his 1992 pop-country hit "Achy Breaky Heart."

Portsmouth was never one of Ohio's better-known places, but there are still a few reasons why you may have heard of it. Sports enthusiasts may know that the NFL's Detroit Lions franchise began as the Portsmouth Spartans in the early 1930s, or that Portsmouth is a few miles from the boyhood home of Branch Rickey, the Brooklyn Dodgers general manager who signed an African American second baseman named Jackie Robinson to the team in 1947, and thereby broke the sport's color barrier.

Pop-culture aficionados might know that Scioto County is where Leonard Franklin Slye — better known by his show name, Roy Rogers — spent some of his formative years. Before the fan clubs, the films, and the chain of fast-food restaurants, Slye lived in a six-room farmhouse in the nearby rural community called Duck Run. Today in downtown Portsmouth there is a plaza named in his honor with cement imprints of his hands and cowboy boots.

But for years, Portsmouth's strongest claim to fame was manufacturing.

In the late 1800s, the city became a hub of brick manufacturing, shipping thousands of bricks to booming cities around the country, including Boston, New York, Chicago, Philadelphia, Baltimore, and Washington, DC.

By the early 1900s, Portsmouth was home to six shoe factories that employed four thousand people who, cumulatively, produced fifteen thousand pairs per day. Around this time, when a reporter visited the headquarters of the city's Drew, Selby & Company, he was dazzled by the massive operation. "Hundreds of skilled operatives were seen working with nimble fingers, keeping time to the musical cadence of whirring machinery," he wrote. "Car loads of leather in the receiving room; cords upon cords of the finished products in the shipping room; thousands of orders in process of 'going through the mill' . . . whirr, buzz, energy, push, everywhere!" A promotional packet from the mid-1930s proclaimed: "Wherever You Go in the United States the Women Wear Shoes Made in Portsmouth."

And then there was steel. Thanks to its location near rich deposits of iron ore, Portsmouth was an early hub for metal manufacturing in the 1800s. Then, around the turn of twentieth century, a massive, two-hundred-acre steel-production plant was constructed along the Ohio River in the Portsmouth-abutting village of New Boston.

During the First World War, the plant churned out Howitzer shells and sheet metal for small boats called submarine chasers. In the 1930s, the factory's output included pig iron, galvanized sheets, metal roofing, steel barrels, rods, railroad spikes, barbed wire, and galvanized nails. During the Second World War, products included steel drums, bomb casings, and woven wire fencing. At the height of its World War II production, the steel plant had a bowling league, an employee band, and a monthly newsletter called *Portsmouth Plant News*. In 1949, a public report to shareholders noted that, during the previous year, the company employed more than four thousand people and took in net sales of nearly $60 million.

During these decades, the mill was a fixture of the local landscape, and its most distinct feature was a towering, hundred-foot blast furnace where iron ore was turned into pig iron, an ingredient of steel. Capable of reaching temperatures above thirty-five hundred degrees Fahrenheit, the oft-photographed structure was nicknamed Old Susie. During this era, one writer described "furnaces flaming by night and by day, the glow of molten metal illuminating for miles."

In these years of industrial success, Portsmouth had swagger and pride. Steamboats and locomotives arrived and departed throughout the day. The city had a bustling downtown, featuring a brick opera house, a beaux-arts-style Security Savings Bank & Trust Company building, and a nine-story Masonic Lodge completed in the late 1920s. At one point during these heady years, the local board of trade published a promotional packet trumpeting the city's prosperity. Portsmouth was "not a 'boom city,'" a page assured readers. "The growth has been steady."

Over the years, I've heard many explanations for the city's steep decline.

Technological change certainly played a part. In the early and mid-1800s, Portsmouth benefited from its location at the end of a canal that connected the Ohio River to Akron and farther on to Cleveland and Lake Erie. But with the advent of steam locomotives in the mid-1800s, this once-advantageous location became irrelevant. Railroads also helped spell the end of the steamboats that once chugged up and down the Ohio River. By the 1930s, demand for paving bricks dropped with the advent of cheaper and quick-to-produce materials, like asphalt and cement.

Other factors I've heard blamed for Portsmouth's decline include labor organizing and unrest that spooked potential employers, a catastrophic flood in 1937 that caused millions of dollars in damage and prompted one shoe manufacturer to move elsewhere, and the less-than-convenient distance between the city and Eisenhower Interstate System built in the mid-twentieth century.*

---

* The closest Eisenhower interstates are in Grayson, Kentucky (I-64, forty miles south), and Columbus, Ohio (I-71 and I-70, ninety miles north).

And, of course, Portsmouth's many manufacturers were heavily affected by the same outsourcing trends that hollowed out Rust Belt industrial cities from Michigan to western New York.* In 1979, one *Cincinnati Enquirer* reporter visited Portsmouth and offered a blunt assessment of what he found. "Portsmouth was once a boom town — steel, shoes, prosperity," he wrote. "Foreign imports killed things."

In late January 1980, things got worse. Two headlines blared from the cover of the *Portsmouth Daily-Times*, announcing the closure of the steel mill: "Mill Loss Would Cut 1,224 Jobs" and "Officials Trying to Estimate Tax Loss." The articles relayed a message from the plant's owners that the decision was not a labor issue; it was simple economics. The rise in iron imports plus a decline in iron usage had left the plant unable to sustain sufficient profits to keep it operating, they said.

At the time of the closing, the mill was still Scioto County's largest employer. And when the shutdown occurred, local governments lost almost $2 million in taxes. The emotional impact was no less devastating. The mill had been a place of employment for thousands with its own vibrant social ecosystem, including dinners, dances, parades, and picnics. After the closure, the sprawling complex of abandoned buildings remained on the eastern outskirts of Portsmouth, a cold and quiet reminder of the city's former glory.

In September 1989, *Life* magazine published a story about Portsmouth called "Children of Poverty." The article focused on the tenants of a two-story building located just blocks from town hall. The brown house — across the street from a motel and a used-car dealership and "bounded on three sides by vacant lots" — was in severe disrepair. The roof sagged. The paint was peeling. The walls, windows, and screens had holes. Life in this decrepit home was dire and bleak, and this was the point of the story. "From the children at 215 [Washington Street], we can get an idea of what it is like to grow up poor in America in 1989," the article read.

The following pages described how nearly every aspect of life in the home was a struggle. The kids fared poorly in school and experienced health effects due to malnutrition and elevated lead levels. They also missed out on many experiences that most American kids took for granted. "They have never been to a movie or taken a vacation," the article said. "They have never been on a plane, a train or a Greyhound bus. They never eat

---

* According to numerous maps of the Rust Belt, Portsmouth is located just inside the southern border of the region.

out—even at fast food places." One family of six eked out an existence on a monthly public-assistance income of just over $600. A family in another apartment had moved seven times in five years: from Ohio to Kentucky to Ohio to three different towns in Florida and then back to Portsmouth.

Black-and-white photographs accompanying the text showed ten-year-old Carrie Ellen Copas, a melancholic girl with wavy blond hair and big eyes. In one shot, she stood outside the house, picking at the peeling paint of the exterior and staring, unsmiling, into the camera. Other photos show the home's inhabitants clustered together for family portraits that gave a sense of the home's cramped confines.

Portsmouth was described in the piece as "both heartland and no-man's-land." The article reported that the unemployment rate was over 10 percent and around a third of the city's children lived below the poverty line. At one point, one of the kids told the reporter: "I don't want to live here. I want to live someplace where it's pretty."

The article was not well received in Portsmouth. A columnist for one local paper wrote a response arguing that the region "did not deserve nor need another negative story about a community that has been getting kicked plenty over the recent years." He said he was glad not to be associated with *Life*, which he called "a publication that deals in sensationalism to make their product saleable."

But even if locals were aggrieved by the town's portrayal, it was hard to argue with article's underlying conclusions. In the late 1980s, Portsmouth, like other communities in Appalachia, was a desperately poor place. And it had been for some time.

"THE OXYCONTIN CAPITAL OF THE WORLD"

David Procter was a native of Canada who received a medical degree from the University of British Columbia in 1976. After an internship in Nova Scotia, he arrived in eastern Kentucky in 1977. At first, he worked for another doctor. But within a couple of years, he set out on his own.

Procter established his medical practice in the tiny town of South Shore, Kentucky, directly across the Ohio River from Portsmouth. Someone once described South Shore to me as "just a little spot on the side of the road" with "nothing there but a few restaurants, a grocery store . . . and a ball field." In 1980, its population was 1,525.

Procter was technically a family practitioner, but over time he became known as a doctor with a loose hand for writing narcotic prescriptions. His practice was tremendously successful.

Procter was a colorful character. He wore fur coats. He bought a Mercedes, a Porsche, and a vintage red Corvette. In the mid-1980s he built a massive $750,000 mansion and decorated it with antiques, handwoven rugs, and what one newspaper later described as a "set of 7-foot-tall bronze storks valued at $1,800." In Greenup County, Kentucky, this was not how you blended in with the crowd.

In 1987, Procter caught the attention of regulators at the Kentucky Bureau of Medical Licensure (KBML), which disciplined him for a list of offenses, including a failure to maintain adequate patient records and administering narcotic medications to patients whom "he knew to be addicted to such drugs and who he had reason to know were not using such drugs in an appropriate manner." The board suspended his license for two months, fined him $5,000, and gave him five years of probation.

Procter was apparently undaunted. And in the coming years, both his personal and professional lives became more flamboyant.

At work, Procter's patient base swelled to more than four thousand people. A staffer who worked for him in the mid-1990s recalled how, once his parking lot became full, cars would spill over to nearby alleys and roads. "He'd see so many people in a day's time . . . you'd get back from lunch, there'd be ten people waiting for you," she said. After he moved to a shopping plaza in South Shore, nearby business owners described seeing patients sitting in cars and snorting crushed pills or waiting around with coolers and eating sandwiches, as if they were tailgating for a concert or football game.

The unusual activity spilled over into Procter's personal life as well. In 1993, he was indicted for pointing a pistol at a teenager who he believed had stolen a T-shirt from one of his sons. He was acquitted but later agreed to a $3,000 settlement with the threatened boy's father.

In late 1998, Procter was involved in a car accident in which he sustained a head injury. Due to ensuing issues with memory and concentration, he voluntarily stopped practicing medicine the following month. But even if the accident hadn't happened, he would have soon been forced to stop seeing patients.

In 1999, the KBML issued an emergency suspension of Procter's medical license. To justify its decision, the board released a fifty-page report from a physician who had reviewed dozens of records from Procter's patients.

At the top of that report were allegations of sexual misconduct relating to three patients. Patient A was a young woman whom he had first treated in the late 1980s, when, after hearing her report of stress, he wrote her a prescription for Xanax without seeing or evaluating her. She continued to receive this prescription for a year. Then, after a six-year gap, she returned and asked for Lorcet for headaches.* At this time, Procter began asking her to date him and, at one point, told her that she needed to come to his office after hours to have a mole removed. According to KBML documents, when she returned, he gave her an injection, removed the mole, turned off the lights, groped her, and "pulled his pants down and had her perform oral sex on him."

Patient B was a woman who first began seeing Procter as a patient after a car accident. She reported that Procter began kissing her during office visits, which, in later visits, escalated to sex, all while he continued to write her prescriptions for controlled substances. These visits involving sex and prescriptions happened approximately twenty times until, according to the report, the woman suffered a drug overdose in Procter's office and one of his nurses drove her home. She entered a rehabilitation program shortly thereafter.

A third patient alleged that, while she was a patient of Procter, he exposed himself to her. She declined his advances, but later returned for treatment for neck pain, at which point he gave her an injection that sedated her, and then, according to the report, "removed her underwear and had oral sex with her, while her child was in the examination room."

These disturbing allegations were, quite literally, just the beginning of the KBML report. The KBML's independent reviewer had also looked at the charts of numerous other Procter patients, and their assessment reads like a catalog of sloppy, dangerous, and unethical medical practices. Among the issues cited in Procter's charts were poor or nonexistent note taking; a lack of formal diagnosis for patients; a recurring lack of physical exams; a lack of consultation with other doctors; a lack of non-narcotic pain treatments, such as physical therapy or prescribing nonsteroidal anti-inflammatory medications; a pattern of heavy prescribing of opioids and sedatives, often with little apparent justification and for long periods of time; a failure to

---

* A painkiller that includes the opioid hydrocodone.

treat psychological conditions such as anxiety or depression; and a failure to refer patients to other doctors. In more than one instance, the consultant described what he believed to be "iatrogenic disability," meaning an illness or injury caused by the doctor's care.

In conclusion, the KBML consultant reported that, even setting aside the allegations of quid pro quo sexual impropriety — allegations that themselves "would be enough to constitute failure to comply with minimal standard of medical practice and constitute a threat to his patients and the public" — Procter still posed a "danger of the health, welfare and safety of the physician's patients and the general public." The consultant said the doctor's overall practice "clearly does not meet even the minimal criteria for the practice of medicine within the Commonwealth of Kentucky."

But while Procter was deemed unfit for the *practice* of medicine — first by a doctor who assessed his head injuries; then by the Kentucky Board of Medical Licensure, which assessed records from years of his practice — he did not step away from the *business* of medicine. Over the next few years, Procter hired doctors to work in South Shore under his guidance, management, and detailed instructions. In doing so, he transitioned from operating his own pill mill to becoming a kind of pill mill entrepreneur. In the 2015 book *Dreamland: The True Tale of America's Opiate Epidemic*, the author and former *Los Angeles Times* reporter Sam Quinones describes Procter as the "Godfather of the Pill Mill, the man who had started the first business and showed others how it was done."

Quinones is hardly alone in this assessment. According to a number of other sources — the *Louisville Courier Journal* and *Lexington Herald-Leader*; various local nurses, doctors, and public health officials — the tale of David Procter is where the region's story as a hotbed of illegal prescription drug trafficking begins.

The first post-head-injury doctor whom Procter hired, Steven Snyder, arrived in eastern Kentucky in 1999 with a history of legal and regulatory trouble. In the mid-1980s in Indiana he had faced numerous felony counts relating to illegal distribution of prescription drugs and illegal gun possession. Those charges were later downgraded to a single misdemeanor and dismissed. But Snyder remained under scrutiny by the Indiana Medical Board, which in one document described "serious question [about] his medical and/or physical capacity to practice safely." In 1989, he voluntarily surrendered his Indiana license — a move that he would later admit was partly due to his desire to avoid the board's recommended psychological counseling and addiction treatment. After a stint living and working in Florida, he found his way to Kentucky, where, in 1999, he was hired by Procter on a $2,800 weekly salary.

Snyder's tenure as a Procter employee was tumultuous and short-lived. It ended after eight months with an argument in which Snyder reportedly threatened Procter with a handgun. Snyder subsequently started his own clinic nearby. And in later documents from both his criminal case and the Kentucky Board of Medical Licensure, he acknowledged that during this time both he and his wife were addicted to narcotics. He also admitted that he wrote narcotic prescriptions for members of his wife's family who didn't need the medications; that he sometimes wrote scripts for patients he never saw; and that he also wrote scripts for other patients with an agreement that they would split the pills with him. In a plea agreement, he attested that he had prescribed more than thirty thousand narcotic pills over eighteen months between 1999 and 2000.

Snyder was federally indicted on weapons and drug charges in early 2001. In response, he pleaded guilty and surrendered his Kentucky medical license. He was eventually sentenced to thirty-five months in prison — a sentence significantly shortened by his cooperation with authorities' investigation of Procter.

After Snyder, Procter hired another out-of-town doctor named Frederick Cohn, who began working for him in September 1999. Cohn had an impressive résumé: He had gone to med school at the University of Pennsylvania and completed his internship and residency at Stanford. But while practicing in New Mexico in the 1980s, he had faced sanctions and a license suspension from the state medical board for what he admitted was grossly negligent treatment involving an abortion he performed on a sixteen-year-old patient. (He had diagnosed the teenager as six to eight weeks pregnant when she was, in fact, twenty-eight weeks pregnant.) Cohn began working for Procter in South Shore but, like Snyder, lasted less than a year before launching his own clinic in a nearby town.

Following complaints from both a local police department and a local physician, the Kentucky Bureau of Medical Licensure opened an inquiry on Cohn. And during a February 2001 search of his office, KBML investigators found prescription pads preprinted with entries for an opioid painkiller, a sedative, and muscle relaxers, along with patient sign-in sheets indicating that patient visits at the clinic were scheduled at three-minute intervals. Evidence indicated that Cohn had routinely seen more than 120 patients per day, and, in one case, saw 146.

A consultant for the KBML who reviewed more than fifty seized charts from Cohn's clinic wrote that the doctor's charts showed no evidence of even basic medical due diligence. There were no histories taken, no physicals performed, and no medications prescribed other than controlled substances and "an occasional Viagra." The consultant said that Cohn's practice posed a threat to the Commonwealth of Kentucky and added, "I greatly fear for the safety of all concerned."

Cohn's clinic was raided and shut down by law enforcement later in 2001, and he was eventually charged with illegal distribution of pills and Medicaid fraud. He pleaded guilty and was sentenced to three and a half years in prison and ordered to pay more than $160,000 in restitution. Before he was sentenced, Cohn told the judge that he was ashamed of his actions. He said that, while working in Kentucky clinics, he had seen more money than ever before in his life, he got "greedy," and his work became sloppy as a result.

"I rushed my patients through," he said. "My charts were incomplete, and I am guilty."

Rodolfo Santos was one of the last doctors hired by Procter after his injury-induced retirement. Santos arrived in May 2001 and started at a salary of $2,500 per week, which quickly rose to $4,000.

According to two employees who spoke with authorities, the doctor saw between forty and fifty patients per day, and the clinic was open from 8:00 A.M. to 6:00 P.M. State authorities later estimated that Santos wrote prescriptions for nearly three million controlled-substance pills during thirteen months of practicing. Eventually, Santos came under scrutiny from the KBML — prompted, in part, by a tip from a coroner across the river in Scioto County who reported that one of Santos's patients had been found dead with an empty bottle of sedatives prescribed by the doctor in their hand and that this death fit a "familiar pattern" for the office.

The KBML's file on Santos contains a remarkable summary of an interview in which Santos apparently told the investigator that "all of his patients were liars and drug addicts. 100% of his patients are addicts and he is educating them."

While speaking with regulators, Santos confirmed that his patients traveled a hundred miles to see him, but he maintained that he didn't know if patients were sharing or selling his prescriptions, because, as he said, "I am not the police." He told the investigator that he sometimes told patients to cut back on their dosages or dismissed them if they reached a certain ceiling dose. The investigator noted, "He stated that he is rehabilitating the patients and the Board should give him a medal." At one point during the interview, Santos left the office and came back three hours later, agitated and smelling of alcohol.

A separate inquiry by the Drug Enforcement Administration questioned whether Santos had misrepresented the cause of death on the death certificate of a fifty-nine-year-old patient to whom he had prescribed opioid painkillers by attributing it to "cardio-respiratory arrest" instead of an overdose, which the agency suspected.

Santos was indicted in June 2002. Forgoing a plea, he chose to proceed to trial, which included surprise, last-minute testimony of Procter, who had recently pleaded guilty in his own criminal case. Procter's testimony at Santos's trial was a remarkably candid account of how he ran his clinics after his accident. From the stand, he recalled explaining to Santos that, though he was no longer practicing, he owned and ran the clinic, made choices about personnel, and "controlled the practice and all administrative duties." He also recalled explaining to Santos that the doctor's job was simple: to write prescriptions.

Procter further described how he had explained to Santos that it didn't matter that most of the patients he saw at the clinic didn't need medical treatment or that many were chemically dependent on the drugs. Procter also admitted that he gave out cash bonuses based on the number of patients Santos saw and the prescriptions he wrote. "I told him he needed to see more patients and write more prescriptions so we could make more money," Procter testified.

Santos, in his own testimony, portrayed himself as someone who had tried to help a crooked clinic straighten out. As he told it, he had arrived at a clinic that was in a state of pronounced "disarray," including haphazard record keeping and patients fighting in the waiting room. He said he had dismissed hundreds of patients for selling their prescriptions or going to multiple doctors for prescriptions and had attempted to wean others off narcotics.

The jury didn't buy it.

The doctor was convicted and later sentenced to sixteen years in prison. At his sentencing hearing, the father of a thirty-five-year-old man who died of an overdose after receiving one of Santos's prescriptions said his son's death had been caused by the doctor's greed. He called Santos a "phony," a "quack," a "criminal" and a disgrace to the medical profession. He added, "This action has degraded our entire society and brought harm to us all."

In 2002, Procter was indicted, along with two female employees, on drug-dealing charges.

He eventually pleaded guilty to a number of those charges. And in his plea agreement, he admitted to prescribing excessive amounts of controlled substances to two female patients to maintain a sexual relationship with them. He also acknowledged that his offices were essentially a criminal operation that kept minimal medical records, performed little to no meaningful examination, and routinely prescribed controlled substances outside the bounds of legitimate medical practice.

And yet this was still not the end of his tale.

In August 2003, days before his sentencing, Procter and a female friend were arrested at the Canadian border in Detroit with luggage, more than $40,000 in cash, a fake ID, and plane tickets to the Cayman Islands, via Toronto. Charges stemming from the attempt to flee were laid out in a new, additional indictment the following month. Procter pleaded guilty to those charges, too.

In the end, Procter was sentenced to more than sixteen years in federal prison. At his sentencing, the judge described him as a man who "preyed on vulnerable people who are already hooked on drugs." The judge wondered aloud whether Procter had more money stashed in the Cayman Islands. But even if he did, he said, "there will be a lot of mold on it before you get to it." *Portsmouth Daily Times* coverage of the sentencing included a photo of the doctor being led from the courthouse with his head bowed and his wrists handcuffed.

By the early 2000s, David Procter was an infamous figure in the region: a gun-toting, flashy-car-driving, mansion-dwelling, pills-for-sex-trading, medical criminal who had tried, and failed, to make a last-minute dash for the border. But even as the saga of Procter and his proxy doctors was playing out across the river, Portsmouth had its own notorious physician.

Dr. John F. Lilly had graduated from Princeton University before starting his career in orthopedics. He had worked as a surgeon at a hospital in Salt Lake City, Utah, but after a series of internal investigations and at least one settlement in a malpractice lawsuit, he moved to Ohio, where he was issued a medical license in 1993. Lilly spent at least a few years on the staff of the Southern Ohio Medical Center, though he resigned in 1998.

Shortly thereafter, he opened a pain-management clinic in downtown Portsmouth, on the city's central thoroughfare, Chillicothe Street. According to investigators, payments at the clinic were made in cash, and Lilly wrote thousands of prescriptions for opioid painkillers and tranquilizers. The office became known for the crowds that assembled there in the morning before the doctor arrived.

Lilly's prescribing first raised concerns among local pharmacists, and law enforcement scrutiny followed soon after. Portsmouth police noticed an alarming uptick in the number of apparent overdose deaths after the opening of his clinic. And during Lilly's tenure, burglaries in the area increased 20 percent from one year to the next. "For a period of about three months, police records show, homes or pharmacies were being broken into and robbed of prescription drugs almost daily," one news article noted.

In March 2000, after an investigation involving local, state, and federal law enforcement, Lilly was charged with more than forty criminal counts, including drug trafficking, engaging in a pattern of corrupt activity, and carrying a concealed weapon. Later, authorities added an additional charge of involuntary manslaughter for the overdose death of a twenty-two-year-old patient.

Lilly was arrested while trying to purchase an automatic weapon from an undercover agent. After, when authorities searched his home and office, they found $497,000 in cash, some of it packed into shoeboxes beneath a set of stairs. The search of his office found beer cans in the waiting room and a nonfunctioning X-ray machine. His mug shot showed him with messy hair and a bushy goatee.

In his defense, Lilly said that his patients suffered from a range of painful ailments, including shoulder dislocations, knee problems, back pain, arthritis, and bone fractures. He said that his prescriptions were in fact "very common, acceptable prescriptions" for "right-out-of-the-book, normal dosages" and that his patients benefited from this care. He claimed he saw no signs that his patients were abusing the medication he prescribed, and he said that if patients sold their pills then that was their crime, not his.

Despite these claims of innocence, on the day that his trial was scheduled to begin in Portsmouth, he pleaded guilty to one of the charges against him. As part of the plea deal, Lilly paid a fine of $20,000 and agreed to permanently forfeit his Ohio medical license. And as the *Columbus Dispatch* noted, he was also ordered to forfeit "more than $500,000 in cash and possessions, including a forklift truck and a Bobcat loader that were purchased with money obtained from his illicit prescription business."

He was sentenced to three years in prison.

News coverage from this time was beginning to answer a question that would be asked for decades to come: Why was this part of the country such a hot spot for corrupt doctors?

One article by the Associated Press noted that many of the eastern Kentucky doctors who ran afoul of the law had been "recruited to work in the medically underserved region." Another article from the time pointed out that "South Shore's location, across the river from Ohio and just down-river from West Virginia, made it an ideal place for addicts seeking to visit doctors and pharmacies in different states to avoid detection."

Whatever the exact reason, in the years leading up to Paul Volkman's arrival in southern Ohio in 2003, Portsmouth and nearby Kentucky towns had acquired a reputation as a place where pills flowed freely and doctors were often hauled away in handcuffs. In 2000, most of the Kentucky counties with the state's highest per capita hydrocodone use were clustered in the eastern part of the state. And among those counties, Greenup — located just across the river from Portsmouth — ranked second.

One news article from this time captures the mood of Portsmouth almost two full years before Volkman arrived. On June 20, 2001, the top story on front page of the *Portsmouth Daily Times* covered the role of the local prescription drug problem in the city's mayoral race. The story began, "Portsmouth may be known as the 'OxyContin Capital of the World,' but mayoral candidate Franklin T. Gerlach said that will change if he becomes mayor . . ."

TRI-STATE HEALTHCARE

Denise Huffman — the pain clinic owner who hired Volkman to come to Ohio, employed him for more than two years and was eventually indicted alongside him — was born on April 23, 1953, in Portsmouth, Ohio. She was the second of four children. Her father, Herbert, was a Korean War veteran and electrician who died suddenly in 1976 at age forty-four of an apparent heart attack.

Denise grew up in Lewis County, Kentucky, a poor, rural county on the southern bank of the Ohio River, west of Portsmouth. She completed middle school, but dropped out of high school before the end of her freshman year. When asked about this decision during a 2006 deposition,* she said, "My parents were going through a divorce and it was a bad time . . . That's the best answer I can give you." Later, she would complete her GED. But she did not go to college.

At age seventeen, she married John Huffman and, a few months later, gave birth to a son, Paul. Four and a half years later, at the age of twenty-one, she gave birth to her second child, Alice.

The details of Denise's professional life before 2001 are a bit unclear. She was mostly unreceptive to my interview requests over the course of this project — although during sworn testimony as part of legal proceedings, she has described a series of odd jobs. She has said that she worked briefly as an aide at "two or three nursing homes." She also worked for some time in local factories, including the Williams Shoe Factory in Portsmouth; the Mitchellace shoelace factory (also in Portsmouth); and a metal parts manufacturer in Maysville, Kentucky. She has also mentioned stints working in at least two fast-food restaurants: the burger chain Rally's and Domino's Pizza.

Perhaps one reason for this scattershot employment history was that, as she explained in a deposition, shortly after getting married in 1970, she and her husband "traveled around to many states for many years" for his job as a union electrician. But beyond such broad descriptions, the details of John's career — how long he worked, where they traveled to, how long these stints lasted — are hazy.

At some point, John retired from his work as an electrician due to issues with his hips, his back, and arthritis, and he began collecting disability benefits. And Denise has described several of her own health problems. For years, she dealt with a heart condition, as well as an anxiety disorder. She has described undergoing multiple surgeries, for unspecified reasons. She was also in a car wreck in the late 1970s or early 1980s, which apparently led to some lingering pain problems. In 2005, she wrote in an online

---

* Denise's lack of cooperation during this deposition, and her inability to answer basic questions, was so pronounced that, at one point, the attorney questioning her paused to ask, "Is there some medical problem with you that would affect your memory or your ability today to relate events to us?"

chat forum, "I rarely ever have a day that I don't live with a slight head-
ache at my best and as I sit here and type my upper mid-back between my
shoulders burn[s] like fire."

Denise later cited her experiences as both a chronic pain patient and
the spouse of one when explaining why, at the age of forty-eight — with
no college degree, no medical training, and no experience owning a business — she decided to open a pain clinic. During her 2006 deposition she
said, "I've always been interested in the health field," and added that she
was a chronic pain patient herself. Later, during trial testimony, she said
that she had always wanted to be a nurse and explained that watching her
husband try to navigate the medical world as a worker's comp patient with
a number of ailments made an impression on her. She was struck, she said,
by the way he "suffered and dealt with a lot of things with paperworks
[sic] and different doctors and things." She has also said, under oath, that,
in 2001, in South Shore, Kentucky, she felt that a pain clinic "was a good
business that's needed for the area."

The story of a forty-eight-year-old high school dropout with no medical
training who was inspired by personal experiences to start a pain clinic
in a region rife with prescription drug abuse is dubious. And yet it is the
more flattering of the accounts of why Denise Huffman founded Tri-State
Healthcare in October 2001. Another explanation, which comes not from
Denise but from various other people and court documents, is that Denise
was yet another protégée of David Procter who, having learned the pill mill
trade from the "godfather" himself, decided to try her hand at the business.

For many reasons — a lack of access to key documents, Denise's unreliability, the refusal of other key players to speak with me — I was never able
to nail down the exact nature of Denise's connection to Procter. But given
the importance of the question, it's worth explaining what I know.

I know that Denise founded her pain clinic in the same tiny Kentucky
town of South Shore, where Procter had worked for decades, and did so a
little more than a year after Procter had agreed with the Kentucky Board
of Medical Licensure to forfeit his medical license.

I know that, at the time of the clinic's launch in October 2001, Procter
had already cycled through numerous proxy doctors at his clinic, and
John Lilly, another notorious pain physician, had recently pleaded guilty
to pill-related crimes across the river in Portsmouth. It's hard to imagine
that Denise would have been unaware of these events.

I know that, by Denise's own admission, she was a longtime patient of Procter. But she would later claim, under oath, that, on a personal level, she "probably . . . never had over five conversations with him." I also know that she has admitted, during that same sworn deposition, that she was friends with Procter's then girlfriend, Kathy Dials, who, after Procter forfeited his license, ran a clinic, staffed by locum tenens physicians, located in the same building as Procter's former office. Procter and Dials had a son together, and he was apparently a regular visitor at this clinic. Dials would later plead guilty to charges of wire fraud as part of Procter's criminal case. Regarding her friendship with Dials, Denise said that they "went many places together" and sometimes had meals together.

During her 2006 deposition, Denise explained that, at some point, in 1999 or 2000, following the death of her brother, she went to this Dials-owned clinic as a patient and struck up a conversation with Dials, who upon hearing about Denise's grief, encouraged her to get out of the house and spend some time at the clinic. It was in this capacity — apparently as a friend spending time at the clinic — that Denise said she stepped in to "give a few people receipts" at the clinic. She said that she did this as a favor to a friend, not as an employee. And she said this had nothing to do with her decision to start a pain clinic of her own in the same small town within two years.

But the Denise-Procter connections don't end there.

In 2004, the *Lexington Herald-Leader* published an article stating that Denise's daughter, Alice, who was among the first employees at Denise's new pain clinic, had previously worked for Procter. And there are also indications that Denise herself worked for Procter. In a motion filed by Volkman's defense team during the lead-up to his criminal trial, his attorneys sought to bar any mention of Procter during the upcoming trial. The document stated that "Dr. Proctor [*sic*] and . . . Denise Huffman shared an employer-employee relationship at a pain clinic long before Ms. Huffman's association with Dr. Volkman" and later described her as having a "close association" with him.

Denise also seems to have played a role in the criminal investigation and prosecution of Procter. One article from the *Lexington Herald-Leader*, published while the Procter case was unfolding, mentions the fact that Denise was scheduled to testify at Procter's trial (which never happened; he eventually pleaded guilty). And later, in 2003, Volkman would write in an email to a friend that "Denise has worn a wire into one of the drug mills and cooperated with local DEA and FBI agents to help convict Proctor [*sic*]."

In one strange, additional twist, at Denise's sentencing hearing in federal court in 2012, the judge mentioned a letter from Procter, who had written to the court, from prison, to share what he knew (or claimed to know) about Denise's criminal activity and to apparently encourage a stern sentence. This was perhaps an indication that he was still bitter about her role in his prosecution years earlier. At the very least, it showed his interest in her case that, while incarcerated for his own pain-clinic-related crimes, he sent a letter in opposition to leniency.

I wish I could more definitively describe Denise's connection to David Procter before she started a pain clinic in the same tiny town where he was infamous for pill mill activity. But she refused to answer most of my questions, Procter and Dials did not respond to my queries, and written records are inconclusive.

But I can say with confidence that Denise Huffman was a patient of David Procter. She was a friend of Procter's girlfriend at a time when the woman ran a pain clinic, where Procter was a visitor, and apparently spent time at the clinic. And there are enough connections between Denise and Procter that I understand why folks in the region view her as someone who followed closely in his footsteps.

Denise opened her clinic, Tri-State Healthcare, in the fall of 2001. From the beginning, it was a family business. One of the first employees was her twenty-six-year-old daughter, Alice, who helped to manage day-to-day business affairs of the clinic, including paying bills, purchasing office supplies, and helping patients with paperwork. Two of Denise's nieces, who each had training as medical assistants, helped with patient-intake activity. For its doctors, the clinic relied on locum tenens staffing companies, much like the ones that Volkman had used for years in his traveling emergency room work.

Denise has said that she initially tried accepting payment from patients who were covered by insurance or the Kentucky worker's compensation program, but she never got reimbursed. Alice has said that during those early days, the clinic couldn't afford to hire an additional staffer to track down payments from various sources. And so, in short order, Denise decided that her clinic would accept only cash.

During trial testimony, Alice shared her memories of the initial goals of the clinic. She explained that her mother wanted to open a clinic for longtime pain sufferers for whom various treatments and surgeries had failed to bring relief. Under oath, Alice said that, from the clinic's outset, "probably 90 percent" of its approach to treating pain was prescribing medication.

The first physician hired at Tri-State was a Colorado-based doctor named Richard Gritzmacher. Gritzmacher had a medical degree from the University of Wisconsin and a master's degree in public health from Yale. For nearly thirty years he had practiced family medicine in a small group practice in coastal Connecticut. After the death of his first wife in 1996, he had remarried, moved to Colorado, and started taking locum tenens work in Arizona, New Mexico, Colorado, and Washington, among other places. Over time, he acquired medical licenses in seven states.

Gritzmacher's tenure at Tri-State was short but eventful. The conditions he found after just five days of work were apparently alarming enough to prompt him to write a whistleblower letter to the Kentucky Board of Medical Licensure. In the letter, he said that he had been told before his arrival that Tri-State was an urgent-care facility that averaged around twenty patients per day. But within an hour on his first day, it was clear to him that the clinic was, in fact, "a store-front narcotic prescription outlet."

The doctor said that during the five days he stayed at the facility, he saw thirty to thirty-five patients per day, and only about "five or six" presented with an acute illness of the kind he had been told to expect. The rest were seeking refills for prescriptions of muscle relaxers, anti-anxiety medications, and narcotic pain relievers. He stated in his letter that, after realizing the true nature of the clinic, he canceled his second week of scheduled work. Still, even though he knew the operation was "not right," he felt compelled by his contract to complete at least one full week. He was writing to the KBML, he said, "in the hope that you may take action regarding this facility, so that other responsible physicians will not, like me, unknowingly become involved in its operation."

The letter was perhaps more effective at catching the KBML's attention than he intended. After receiving it, the agency opened an investigation into the clinic, and into Gritzmacher himself. And when representatives from the KBML approached the clinic with questions, Denise — in what would become a recurring strategy for her — claimed that it was the doctor, not the clinic, who was at fault. To assist with the KBML's review, she provided names and records for sixteen patients. The ensuing investigation found that "each and every chart" shared striking similarities. Each chart came from a patient's first visit. Each patient was prescribed the narcotic painkiller Lorcet and the sedative Xanax, and "most" were prescribed the muscle relaxer Soma as well. Most of the patients were under forty-five years of age, and many were in their twenties and thirties. All paid in cash, and none of the charts contained a proper patient history, examination, assessment, or treatment plan. The clinic, noted the KBML consultant who performed the review, "seems to attract a specific type of patient base that is given controlled substances with minimal resistance." The consultant concluded that Gritzmacher* was correct to call Tri-State a "Store Front Narcotic Outlet."

But the board's reviewer also faulted the doctor for his actions after arriving at the clinic. The board's consultant wrote that Gritzmacher had standards he ought to have upheld during his stint at the pain clinic, and he failed to do so by agreeing to write these prescriptions without taking proper histories, performing adequate exams, or providing a treatment plan. "I feel that Dr. Gritzmacher was a 'victim of circumstances' but that does not prevent him from meeting minimal standards of care," the KBML consultant wrote.

It would take years for the saga to come to a resolution. And eventually the he-said, she-said nature of the conflict spilled over into the press. In a *Lexington Herald-Leader* article about the KBML inquiry from 2004, Alice Huffman said that she was shocked by the doctor's allegations, described his letter as "totally bogus," and claimed that there was "nothing in that letter that was true, at all." She added, "We didn't knock him in the head and make him treat patients."

Denise, for her part, told the paper that she had hired Gritzmacher to treat patients, not violate rules, and said that Tri-State had always described itself as a pain-treatment clinic. She said that if the placement agency had misled Gritzmacher about her clinic, then that was "their problem, not ours."

Eventually, Gritzmacher reached an agreement with Kentucky Bureau of Medical Licensure stipulating that, for a period of five years, he could not legally practice medicine in Kentucky unless approved by a KBML panel. As part of that agreement, he submitted the opinion of a physician whom he would have called on his behalf if the matter had proceeded to a hearing. That witness stated that he believed Gritzmacher acted appropriately during his short stint at Tri-State and that the prescriptions he wrote — "for a defined, limited period of time, not to exceed 30 days, with no refill permitted" — met

---

* Gritzmacher had passed away by the time I researched this portion of the story. Otherwise I would have reached out to him for comment.

an "acceptable" standard of care. Gritzmacher's expert witness added, "He cannot be faulted for giving some of his patients the benefit of any doubt regarding their professed pain, especially considering that sudden withdrawal from their medications might have been dangerous and would have left these patients without effective means to treat their pain."

It was an inauspicious start to Denise's career running a pain clinic. The very first doctor she hired was alarmed enough by the clinic to alert the medical board, which (more than two years later) resulted in sanctions for him and unflattering press for the clinic.

But despite the damning findings of the KBML's report, Tri-State itself faced no criminal charges or administrative sanctions. The clinic remained in business — though the turbulence was far from over.

More than a year passed after the Gritzmacher incident. During that time, Denise apparently found doctors who were more amenable to the clinic's style of business. She would say that "seven or eight" doctors worked for her during this time. But then, in early 2003, the clinic once again made headlines.

The article — "Fake MRI Reports Get Drugs for Many: Patients Buy Documents to Support Pain Stories" — ran on the front page of a Sunday edition of the *Lexington Herald-Leader*. It was part of a series of stories about the "booming" illicit market for prescription drugs in eastern Kentucky.

This report focused on an illicit industry that had risen from the black market for pills: the production of fake MRI reports and other falsified medical records that were used to obtain illegitimate prescriptions. "Investigators say the emergence of such counterfeit documents shows the problem is becoming both more organized and more sophisticated," the article stated, explaining that records provided a cover for all parties involved in an illicit pain-clinic visit: the patient, the doctor who writes the script, and the owners of the clinic.

The article reported that some fake MRIs were being printed on letterhead paper from a hospital in Paintsville, Kentucky, while another source said that many of them were originating in Portsmouth, Ohio. The focus of the article, however, was the tiny river town of South Shore and, specifically, Denise Huffman's Tri-State Healthcare.

The paper reported that the operators of Tri-State had reported fifty-two alleged fake MRI reports to the Greenup County Sheriff. But as with the Gritzmacher incident, it was unclear just who, exactly, was blowing the whistle and who was actively involved in the shady activities. The article described one former patient who had been indicted after using a phony MRI report to receive prescriptions for a "variety of pain pills" from Tri-State and noted that the patient "appeared angry at clinic workers who, she said, accepted her $120 office fee before turning her over to police."

In the report, Denise and Alice once again presented themselves as honest actors who were trying to root out corruption in their midst. Alice told the paper that she dutifully notified the authorities about patients with falsified medical records. "We're a legal business," she said. "That's why we're still open."

According to the article, the clinic was under investigation. But a local prosecutor told the paper that he hadn't sought additional indictments on fake MRI charges "because the Tri-State clinic has had several temporary physicians, and he would have trouble contacting them to testify in court."

Once again, the clinic remained open.

Tri-State would have at least one more strange incident involving yet another temporary doctor before it moved across the river to Portsmouth.

During the early years of his career, Richard Ruhling had practiced medicine in at least four states, including California and New York, before he settled in Chattanooga, Tennessee, in the early 1980s. He stayed there for the next twenty years and made a living either partially or entirely from locum tenens work in area hospitals. In an interview, he told me that he especially liked working at small-town hospitals that were quiet enough that a doctor could spend most of a night shift sleeping.

Ruhling's pre-Tri-State career was notable for his public speaking and writing. For years, he delivered presentations about stress, quitting smoking, happiness, nutrition, and low-calorie diets. Often these presentations had strong Christian themes. In 1967, while he was an intern in Dayton, Ohio, he delivered a presentation called "Christ, the Way." In 1976, as part of a celebration of the seventieth anniversary of the Loma Linda Seventh-Day Adventist Church, he gave a talk titled "Practical Experiences in Medical Missionary Work." In 1981, while working in Upstate New York, he spoke on "stress and healthful living" at a local Seventh-Day Adventist church.

In addition to practicing medicine, he also acted as — there's really no other way to phrase this — a self-appointed apocalyptic prophet. In the mid-1980s, a Tennessee newspaper published an interview in which Ruhling said that a major earthquake would soon strike Southern California, a prediction he based on his "studies of the Bible, history and nature." He also told the paper that he was convinced that the end of the world would begin on the Jewish holiday of Yom Kippur.

That same year, Ruhling's name was mentioned in the *Miami Herald* as a purveyor of "apocalyptic pseudo-science." Ruhling had apparently sent the paper the same predictions of a major earthquake, along with a pre-written news story, which he hoped the newspaper would publish the following day, titled, "I Told You There Would Be an Earthquake."

It would be this same eagerness to share his religious views that got him into trouble at Tri-State. Ruhling came to Tri-State as a locum tenens physician, filling in when one of the clinic's longer-term docs was away. He started work in late February 2003, shortly after the fake-MRI report was published in the *Herald-Leader*. My understanding of what took place is drawn primarily from documents later published by the Kentucky Bureau of Medical Licensure.

Upon arriving at the clinic, Ruhling apparently told one or both Huffmans that he had some books and videotapes he was interested in selling to patients. The names of those books and videos weren't specified in KBML documents, although by this time he had published a book titled *The Bridegroom Comes!* that is described on Amazon as "explain[ing] how not to be left behind for biblical events that are imminent." In subsequent years he would publish books called *Exodus 2: A Christian Patriot's Answer to the Coming Civil War — Fight or Flight?*; *The Fall of Jerusalem 2023: How a 9-11 Event Will Bring Biblical End-Times*; and *Countdown to Armageddon: How Much Time Do We Have?*

Alice Huffman apparently agreed to allow Ruhling to sell his books to patients. But an issue arose when, during a lecture or discussion that Ruhling was leading with a handful of patients, Alice overheard him say, "Anyone interested in buying my books or tapes that wants an extra prescription please follow me to my office." She then apparently saw him accept money that appeared to be in exchange for books and written prescriptions. The following day, three patients came to the clinic and said that they were willing to buy Ruhling's books in exchange for extra prescriptions, at which point Alice attempted to fire Ruhling and told him not to return.

Ruhling apparently negotiated with Alice and promised that he wouldn't make anymore offers to patients if he could finish out the week. But the next day, Alice saw four patients who were carrying the books Ruhling was selling, and when she asked about them, they said they had been instructed not to tell her, but that Ruhling had sold them the books in exchange for prescriptions. Ruhling was then permanently fired, and the next month Alice filed a grievance with the KBML.

In a 2010 interview with a Tennessee newspaper, Ruhling denied that he had done anything wrong. He said that, during his time at Tri-State, he discovered that the patients were "mostly drug addicts" who had become addicted due to previous bad medical care and that, because he had experience helping people quit smoking, he had offered tips on withdrawal plus "a motivational book from a Christian perspective." He admitted that, as an incentive, he gave patients who bought his book an extra month of prescription refills. And he said that it was this proactively written refill prescription — which eliminated the need for a follow-up visit to Tri-State and thus deprived the clinic of a $100 visit fee — that had upset the Huffmans. During the interview, he added, "It has been more than 25 years since a malpractice suit was filed against me. I have never been the subject of medical discipline until this came up after my retirement."

In a 2021 phone interview with me, Ruhling took a similarly defiant approach, defending his books as affordably priced and "not doctrinal [or] denominational," despite their basis in the Bible. Throughout our conversation, Ruhling frequently veered off subject to deliver rants about prescription drugs, the supposed dishonesty of the Centers for Disease Control (CDC), the Bible, the benefits of a plant-based diet, and a "massive cover-up" within the federal government to hide the true dangers of the COVID-19 vaccine. Afterward, in response to my request to see his CV, he emailed me a document that read, in part, "I believe I can explain when the Big One is coming from biblical information that makes good sense, and I would be glad to share it by phone in 2–3 minutes for why it will be in 2023."

Alice's complaint to the state medical board prompted a KBML investigation that found that Ruhling's prescriptions-for-books scheme was, indeed, "unacceptable." Beyond that, the board found the doctor's overall activity at the clinic to be deeply suspicious. He had been hired, apparently, to "fill in as a prescription writer while the regular physician was away for a week," and he had dutifully filled that role, doing "nothing more than writ[ing] refills for . . . chronic medications," a reviewer for the KBML wrote.

In an echo of the KBML's investigation of the Gritzmacher allegations, the board's hired consultant wrote:

> The physician [Ruhling] alone does not constitute a danger to health, welfare, and safety of patients or public, but the clinic does.

There is no medical care, just narcotic prescriptions being written.
The physician is the vehicle that the clinic uses, and hides behind,
to generate revenue.

As a result of the KBML inquiry, Ruhling agreed to surrender his
Kentucky medical license. But yet again, Tri-State faced no sanctions from
the KBML or law enforcement.

It's not hard to understand why Denise Huffman would have been eager
to move her clinic out of Kentucky in the spring of 2003. In just a year
and a half since her clinic had opened, Tri-State Healthcare had received
unfavorable press coverage in one of the state's leading newspapers, and
the clinic's relationships with two of its hired doctors had imploded rather
spectacularly.

And all of this was taking place during, or shortly after, a flurry of indictments against doctors in the region, including Steven Snyder (January
2001), Frederick Cohn (August 2001), Rodolfo Santos (June 2002), and
David Procter (July 2002). From a purely self-preservationist standpoint,
Denise would have been keen to get a fresh start across the river in a different state, outside of the KBML's purview.

But this was not how Denise described the reason for her pain clinic's move to Portsmouth. Under oath, she has described the decision as a
matter of practicality and convenience. She said that one day she was driving through downtown Portsmouth when she was stopped at a red light
and noticed a vacant doctor's office on the side of the road. The building
looked like a good fit for her clinic, so she inquired about leasing it. When
she found the terms favorable, she signed the paperwork. And so, in April
2003, Tri State Healthcare moved to a location on Gay Street, in downtown
Portsmouth, a few blocks from the central post office.

But though she had secured a new office, Denise was also in need of a
new doctor, since one of her steadier locum tenens physicians planned to
take the summer off to tend to some home-improvement projects.

As it turned out, this problem was soon solved. Denise found a doctor
who was exceedingly qualified for the job of a pain-management physician. His name was Paul Volkman, and he had an MD and a PhD from the
University of Chicago.

FIRST IMPRESSIONS

Things went well in the beginning.

This is something that the three central players at Tri-State Healthcare seem to agree on.

Denise has said that Paul made an initially favorable impression on her in several ways. In addition to sharing his credentials, he told her that he had previously worked at Southern Ohio Medical Center and mentioned names of people he had worked with there that she recognized, so, as she once wrote, "it sounded legit to me."

Volkman was also apparently aware of Dr. Procter's reputation in the area and made it clear during his initial conversations that he was totally opposed to working at that kind of medical office. And she has said that at one point he wore a white coat with "the name of some place with Parkinson's Center" on it (presumably a leftover from his stint in Milwaukee) that added to the picture of legitimacy. Denise was apparently so comfortable with her newly hired doctor that she promptly became his patient herself. And in time, each member of her immediate family — her husband, her son, and her daughter — became a patient of Volkman as well.

Alice was also apparently impressed by the new doctor. She told me that when Paul started working at the clinic, he was friendly, asked a lot of questions, and seemed genuinely interested in the patients. He spent a "good bit" of time examining them and reviewing their records, she said, adding that he took thorough notes, recommended non-narcotic treatment methods like yoga and physical therapy, and seemed happy to treat patients' non-pain-related issues, such as high blood pressure. "He seemed competent and moderate in his prescribing," she told me. She liked him.

Volkman was also initially pleased with his new clinic. Before taking the job, he had made a trip to Portsmouth to survey the situation and he would later say that it "seemed legitimate and carefully and conscientiously operated." He told me that, during his initial conversations with Denise, she struck him as "reasonable."

According to Volkman, his due diligence included carefully questioning Denise about her involvement with David Procter. He claimed that she denied any ties to him or intentions to run a similar operation and assured him that her only goal was providing honest, reliable, and compassionate chronic pain care to people in the area who needed it. According to him, "she was aware of the illegal practices which had brought the DEA down on Procter, and she had never, and would never allow anything of the sort at her clinic." Later, in sworn testimony, he would admit that he "did not think" to ask Denise if she had the proper credentials to run a pain clinic.

Volkman apparently remained pleased with his new employer well after his arrival. In emails he sent in October 2003, six months after he began work at Tri-State, he spoke approvingly of the clinic, Denise, and his work in Portsmouth.

He wrote that southern Ohio was a deeply depressed place with little functioning industry and few employment prospects outside of the service sector. "Lots of car repair shops and fast food," he said. "Lots of drugs, prostitution, corruption, violence and despair." He mentioned three doctors, including Procter and Santos, who were recently convicted of illegal pill-related activity. He also said that it was "common knowledge" that there were still "several clinics" in the area that sold prescriptions for anyone with $250, despite no visit with a physician. One explanation for how such illegal activity continued was what he described as "levels upon levels of corrupt officials who [are] paid off to look the other way."

But in Volkman's telling, within this setting, he was carefully and cautiously pursuing the goal of relieving patients' pain. He described Denise as a "brilliant, tough matriarch who essentially runs a family business that keeps her dozen kids, nieces, etc., together." And he said that her reasons for starting the clinic were pure: She couldn't find a reliable physician to treat her own "severe neck pain" or the pain suffered by her husband ("a disabled electrician [with] terrible back and hip pain") and son ("terrible foot and leg problems after a botched orthopedic procedure followed by a severe wreck").

In these emails, Volkman said that his new clinic carefully screened prospective patients to confirm their honesty when reporting symptoms and remained vigilant after these initial steps via pill counts, urine tests, and active use of electronic prescription-monitoring databases "to detect multiple scripts and doctor hoppers." At one point, he mentioned that one of the ways he knew Denise was on the right side of this issue was that she had "worn a wire into one of the drug mills and cooperated with local DEA and FBI agents to help convict Proctor [sic]."

On the logistical front, Paul's new job required a lengthy and multi-legged commute between Chicago and Portsmouth that he completed twice a week. He would later explain to me what this four-hundred-mile journey entailed. After spending a weekend at home in Chicago, he would wake up around four o'clock on Monday morning for a flight from Midway Airport to Columbus. Once he landed in Ohio's capital, where he had left his car, he completed the two-hour drive to Portsmouth. He would spend the workweek in Portsmouth and then complete the same commute in reverse on Friday to return to Lake Shore Drive.

For another doctor, the length of such a weekly trek might have been a deal-breaker. But Volkman was apparently unfazed. Perhaps the desperation that preceded the new job provided a boost of motivation. And the salary — $5,000 per week, to start — certainly would have also helped. Anyway, by this time, he had more than a decade of experience traveling long distances for locum tenens jobs.

It's possible that the distance between home and work was even a perk of the new job. After all, it meant that nobody from his home life could casually swing by his clinic to see what was happening there.

And then there was his new specialty.

By 2003, Volkman had accrued an unusual array of professional experiences. He had worked briefly in medical research and coauthored articles in pharmacology journals. He had owned and run his own pediatrics practice for more than fifteen years, which he eventually expanded into a family medicine practice. He had spent more than twenty years working in emergency rooms. And he had, most recently, spent time working in a neurology practice that focused on Parkinson's disease. Now his new job in Ohio signified yet another pivot.

At Volkman's criminal trial, a professor and pain-management expert from Ohio State University would describe the complexity and risk that awaited a doctor in pain management. He explained that the ever-present risks of addiction, diversion, and overdose in the specialty made it a "very difficult thing to do." It was a field that required its practitioners to juggle numerous questions during the treatment of a given patient: Is this patient chemically dependent on the medication? Are they diverting their pills? Is the patient suffering from undiagnosed depression? Would surgery — or injections or nerve stimulators — be helpful?

But when I spoke to Paul about this transition, he recalled being undaunted. He said that, in preparation for the work at Tri-State, he read up on "all the literature" in the field, which included what he described as a "big fat book." He later attended a national meeting of the American Academy of Pain Medicine, which allowed him to be, in his words, "fully apprised of the current standards and practices, and regulatory and legal issues in the use of controlled substances in pain management." He also took a board-certification test, which he described as "pretty easy."

By all accounts, Volkman had never previously lacked confidence, and he certainly didn't falter now. In fact, given his background in pharmacology, he would later write that working in pain management was "the closest a doctor could get to practicing [my] unique specialty."

The facet of the new job that appears to have captured most of Volkman's attention was the *legal* landscape of pain management. He would later say that, in preparation for his new role, he read about the case of David Procter, as well as other cases around the country where doctors had been investigated and prosecuted for prescription drug dealing. He also went to significant lengths to study a recently passed Ohio law concerning the treatment of patients with intractable pain.

For more than a decade prior to Volkman's arrival in Ohio, state legislatures across the country had been discussing chronic pain patients and the doctors who treated them. The first state-level law that codified protections for both parties was the 1989 Texas Intractable Pain Treatment Act, which prohibited medical facilities from limiting or restricting narcotics on their premises, authorized physicians to prescribe controlled substances during the treatment of intractable pain, and prevented the state medical board for disciplining a doctor for prescribing narcotic pain medications in the course of legitimate treatment. It was designed, as one article in a Texas-based medical journal wrote, to "assure that no Texan requiring narcotics for pain relief, for whatever reason, was denied them because of a physician's real or perceived fear that the state regulatory agency would take disciplinary measures against the physician for prescribing narcotics to relieve pain."

Other states followed suit, including California, Oregon, and Florida. And by the mid-1990s, an article in the American Pain Society's newsletter praised these laws for giving "much-needed recognition to the necessity for better treatment of intractable pain and . . . help[ing] to correct past policy, which discouraged any use of opioids." By the year 2000, numerous states had passed laws designed to assure patient access to pain care. One was Ohio.

Ohio's intractable pain bill was first introduced in 1997 by a Republican state representative who told a reporter, "People should not have to suffer needlessly from pain." Like similar legislation from other states, the Ohio bill would protect doctors from sanction or discipline if their treatments adhered to guidelines published by the state medical board. Testimony in favor of the bill in the Ohio Senate argued that a large percentage of chronic pain patients didn't get the relief they needed. One state senator said, "We don't want physicians out there who are afraid to manage pain." The bill passed and went into effect the following year.

The law, as enacted, stated that doctors who prescribed narcotics for chronic pain would not face disciplinary action from the state medical board solely based on their medication regimens as long as they abided by certain conditions in their care. These included maintaining records about the patient's medical history; tracking the dates when medications were prescribed, dispensed, and administered; and keeping notes on the patient's response to that medication. According to the law, doctors were meant to feel safe — legally and professionally — if they diagnosed and treated patients "according to accepted and prevailing standards for medical care." Volkman would later say that he committed the Ohio Intractable Pain Act to memory and followed it "carefully" during his work at Tri-State. In years to come, he would refer to the law as if it were a coat of armor through which no federal law enforcement investigation ought to have been able to pierce.

And so, after completing his crash course in the medical principles of pain management, the region's history of criminal doctors, and the state law pertaining to prescribing narcotics, Volkman said he felt cautiously confident about his new specialty. As he later explained it: "I figured, 'OK . . . this is a very dicey area, but it's possible to tip-toe between the land mines. Make sure that you're careful and do what you're supposed to and it'll be alright.'"

Despite the comfort Volkman felt with the principles of pain management, Tri-State Healthcare ran into problems with local pharmacies almost as soon as Volkman arrived. Six pharmacists would later describe their concerns during the doctor's criminal trial.

Some pharmacists were alarmed by the quantities of medications Volkman prescribed and by the glaring similarities in prescriptions between patients. "Everybody got the same excessive quantities," one said. Another pharmacist noticed that Volkman's patients tended to arrive at the store in quick succession, what he described as "kind of a wave." Other pharmacists were struck by the tendency of these patients to pay in cash. This was not an area where people normally paid $500 or $600 in cash for a prescription, yet it happened with Volkman's patients.

One theme across numerous pharmacists' testimonies was a concern with the distance that Volkman's patients were driving to have prescriptions filled. A pharmacist at a Rite Aid in Grayson, Kentucky, found it strange to be presented with prescriptions from a doctor located forty minutes away. Another pharmacist in Kenova, West Virginia, thought that the long distance to the doctor's office was a sign that the customer had stolen a doctor's prescription pad.

Yet another red flag was how young Volkman's patients seemed, along with their apparent lack of the intense physical distress that their heavy-duty prescriptions suggested. One pharmacist later remarked that "in all honesty, they were in better health than I was."

The list of concerning factors continued. One pharmacist from a family-owned shop in West Portsmouth remembered patients calling and asking specifically if he filled scripts from Dr. Volkman, which he found unusual. Then, when the patients showed up, they were strikingly impolite. He recalled how, in one case, a patient entered the shop, cut the line, and threw the script on the counter and asked, "How much are these?" Another pharmacist remembered extreme behavior on the other side of the spectrum — aggressive friendliness — which also seemed odd. Some of Volkman's patients, whom he had never seen before, walked up to the counter and called him by his first name.

All of these strange incidents took place in a region with well-documented problems with drug diversion, addiction, overdoses, and criminal doctors.

Within weeks, numerous pharmacies refused to fill Volkman's scripts.

Volkman would remain unequivocally defensive about all aspects of his activities in southern Ohio. And this included the prescriptions that so alarmed the area's pharmacists.

Volkman maintains that regimens of medications he prescribed for Tri-State patients were individually tailored to each person. And having reviewed some of his patient records myself, I can attest that they show the occasional individualized prescription for non-narcotic drugs, such as the blood-circulation drug Trental; the heartburn drug Zantac; the airway-clearing asthma drug albuterol; the autoimmune disease drug Plaquenil; the antinausea and anti-allergy medication Phenergan; and, in one instance, the erectile dysfunction drug Viagra.

But despite these occasional exceptions, from his very first weeks working at Tri-State, Volkman's prescribing followed a clear pattern. For patient after patient, he prescribed three different types of medication: an opioid narcotic painkiller, an anti-anxiety sedative (benzodiazepine, sold under the trade names Xanax or Valium), and a muscle relaxer (carisoprodol, trade name Soma). In the case of the opioid painkillers, he was often prescribing two different drugs at once: oxycodone as well as another opioid for "breakthrough" pain. These four prescriptions — two opioids, plus a sedative and a muscle relaxer — would be described during his criminal case as a distinct and predictable "cocktail."

Volkman, for his part, stands by the legitimacy of each individual prescription, as well as the overall combination that so many patients received. He has said that the opioids were prescribed to treat the often-excruciating pain that patients reported. The sedatives were required because "virtually all of these patients needed medicine to help them sleep." And the muscle relaxers were because "almost [all] of my patients complained of severe muscle spasms usually radiating down one or both legs."

But as the testimony of pharmacists and other witnesses indicated, it wasn't just the *types* of medications that Volkman prescribed that prompted concern, it was also the amounts. Volkman himself has acknowledged that many of his patients were on regimens that involved taking twenty or twenty-five tablets per day. And records show that some patients' daily prescribed regimens called for even more pills than that. These records, which were admitted into evidence at trial and then later released to me, include handwritten dosage schedules written by Volkman that advise patients of how and when they ought to take the pills he prescribed.

The schedule for a Tri-State patient named Dwight Parsons, for example, was based on Parsons waking up at 7:00 or 8:00 A.M. and going to sleep between 9:00 and 10:00 P.M. In between, Volkman advised him to take medications at two-hour intervals — a total of seven different times — over the course of the day. Upon waking up at 7:00 or 8:00 A.M., Parsons was advised to take six pills: two Norcos (a painkiller that includes the opioid hydrocodone), one 30-milligram oxycodone, one Xanax, one Soma, and one Disalcid (a nonsteroidal anti-inflammatory pain medication). The rest of the regimen read as follows:

- At 10:00 A.M. he would take four more pills: two Norcos, one oxycodone 30, and one Soma.

- At noon, he would take four more pills: two Norcos, one oxycodone 30, and one Xanax.
- At 2:00 P.M., for his fourth dose of the day, he would take four more pills: two Norcos, one oxycodone 30, and one Soma.
- At 4:00 P.M., he would take five more pills: two Norcos, one oxycodone 30, one Soma, and one Xanax.
- At 6:00 P.M., he would take three pills: two Norcos and one oxycodone 30.
- And at 8:00 P.M., for his seventh and final dose of the day, he would take five pills: two Norcos, one oxycodone 30, one Soma, and one Xanax.

Parsons's total prescribed pill count for the day was thirty-one. And the daily totals for each medication were written by the doctor at the bottom of the schedule: fourteen Norco tablets, seven oxycodone, four Xanax, five Somas, and one Disalcid.

Parsons's regimen was not particularly unusual for Volkman's patients. Other patients who were discussed at the trial had daily regimens of twenty total pills, twenty-nine total pills, and, in one case, forty-two total pills. One document submitted at trial was a dosage schedule written for a patient who worked night shifts. In this schedule, Volkman advised the patient to take pills at eight intervals between 3:30 P.M. and 6:30 A.M. His daily dosage total was twenty-two pills: eight 30-milligram oxycodone tablets, eight Lortab (a pain reliever that contains the opioid hydrocodone) pills, three 2-milligram Xanax pills, and three Soma tablets.

Years later, the government would call three medical expert witnesses to testify at trial about Volkman's prescribing practices. And each of them expressed grave concerns with prescribing patterns that were evident from his first days on the job.

One expert, a toxicologist and emergency room physician, remarked that due to the muscle relaxer Soma's euphoric effects, the drug had a "highly abusive potential." He also expressed concern about Volkman's simultaneous prescribing of opioids and benzodiazepines, which, he said, increased patients' potential for overdose. He explained that very rarely do opioid-related overdoses trace back to just an opioid; more often, he said, "the combination of agents that we see, particularly when treating patients that have opiate related deaths, tend to be a combination of opiates and sedatives."

Another expert physician who testified for the government — the same pain-management specialist who had testified about the complexity and risk inherent in the specialty — said that he found the absence of time-release narcotics among Volkman's prescriptions to be an "extreme deviation from the established practice in the field of pain medicine." Prescribing controlled substances was a risky endeavor, he said. And based on the striking similarities across Volkman's prescriptions to different patients, among other factors, he felt that the combination and quantities of drugs being prescribed "was not consistent with the legitimate practice of the field of pain medicine."

A third expert, also a pain-management physician, was struck by the repetition of what he called Volkman's "basic cocktail" of two opioids, an anti-anxiety drug, and a muscle relaxer. He called Volkman's prescribing practices "chaos" and said that he didn't know of any legitimate doctor who practiced or prescribed in such a fashion. After reviewing some of Volkman's prescribing records and the corresponding patient health records, he said he saw no medical rationale for the prescriptions being written or the frequent escalations in dosages from visit to visit. It looked to him more like a simple business transaction: "Drugs for money."

In emails from the time, Volkman dismissed local pharmacists' concerns about his prescribing for various reasons. In one email, he attributed resistance to "deep and wide prejudice against chronic pain patients and the doctors who treat them" from people who believed such patients "should be able to bear the pain without complaining and without meds, otherwise they are weak or somehow immoral for needing narcotics."

If ignorance and bias didn't fully explain local pharmacists' concerns, he also suggested sabotage. In the same series of emails from 2003, he mused that perhaps "Proctor [sic] and his business associates" were helping to instigate the spread of "transparent lies" about his clinics among pharmacists. It was also possible, he wrote, that some pharmacists were "crooked" themselves and colluding against him. At other points, he blamed the Kentucky Pharmacy Board for "intimidat[ing] pharmacies from filling out scripts" and the Ohio Pharmacy Board for "harass[ing]" his patients and accusing them of dealing drugs.

At a basic level, Volkman clearly viewed pharmacists' refusal to fill his scripts as an outgrowth of *their* corruption or flaws, not his own. And he does not appear to have ever seriously considered stopping or altering his approach due to their concerns.

Later, in conversations with me, he remained defensive. He told me that his patients "almost all got those [drugs] because they almost all had symptoms requiring those." And he was adamant that no adverse effects could occur if his patients were honest about their symptoms and adhered to his regimens. "Real pain patients who take pain medicine under the careful supervision of their doctor <u>never</u> die as a result of their medicine taken according to directions," he once wrote.

And so he and Denise decided to launch their own pharmacy.

As surprising as it might seem, according to Ohio laws at the time, Tri-State was allowed to apply to establish an on-site medication dispensary. If approved, the clinic would need to keep close track of all controlled substances that moved through the dispensary and maintain detailed records in logbooks. And Volkman, under whose DEA registration the dispensary would operate, would be required to personally approve every tablet dispensed on the premises. But for Volkman and the Huffmans, these conditions were apparently preferable to moving the clinic some-where else (where pharmacists might be just as skittish about Volkman's scripts) or closing the clinic altogether.

And so, in mid-June 2003, after just two months of Volkman's employment at the pain clinic, he and the Huffmans filled out an Application for Registration as a Distributor of Dangerous Drugs form and sent it to the Ohio Board of Pharmacy. On the form, which was later submitted as evidence during Volkman's trial, Denise was listed as the owner of the clinic, Alice was described as "Office Manager," and "Paul H. Volkman MD" was listed as the pharmacy's main applicant. Volkman included his Social Security number and Ohio medical license number on the form.

In response to the application, the pharmacy board sent an agent to the clinic to inspect the premises and to carefully explain the conditions of the law to Alice and Paul. During that visit, the agent emphasized how stringent the rules were: If the license was granted, Volkman would be responsible for verifying every prescription filled on-site. The agent would later testify that, upon learning these conditions, most physicians decided it wasn't worth the hassle. But not Volkman. He signed the inspection report as the "Person In Charge," and that day — July 22, 2003 — Tri-State was issued a license to dispense medications directly to patients.

It was a major moment for Tri-State. Volkman and the Huffmans would no longer be hampered by the complaints of local (and not-so-local) pharmacists. Their clinic now allowed patients to see the doctor, receive a prescription, and fill that prescription all under one roof.

In an email from around this time, Volkman wrote to a friend, "We are striving to be totally self contained, by having our own pharmacy so it really doesn't matter what the local pharmacists think of me and whether they fill any of my scripts."

He added: "I think that is the only way for a pain clinic to operate."

THE DECADE OF PAIN CONTROL AND RESEARCH

It can be hard to remember just how enthusiastic the country was about pain treatment and opioids in the early 2000s. But such remembering is essential to understanding Paul Volkman's story. He arrived in pain management at a time of strong tailwinds for the cause of pain treatment and, specifically, the use of opioids. The momentum had been building for decades.

The origins of that movement trace back at least to the early 1970s, when pain was recategorized from being a symptom of other illnesses and injuries to a phenomenon worthy of study on its own. In 1973, an "International Symposium on Pain" was held at a conference center outside of Seattle, and, from that inaugural meeting, an organization called the International Association for the Study of Pain (IASP) was launched. The ensuing years brought the launch of the academic journal *Pain* in 1975 and the establishment of the American Pain Society in 1977.

The 1980s brought more changes to the medical world's approach to pain. In 1986, the World Health Organization published a report on cancer pain that called it "an important but neglected public health issue in developed and developing countries alike." The report said that more than three million people worldwide suffered from cancer pain every day, but many didn't receive adequate treatment. The reasons included a lack of systemic education about cancer pain management, a lack of concern from "most" national governments, and fears of addiction among both cancer patients and the general public if strong opioids were more widely prescribed. The report was an attempt to shift these trends. "It needs to be emphasized that relief is possible for the several million cancer patients who each day suffer unalleviated pain," it stated. The authors argued that painkillers, when administered correctly, were capable of controlling pain in more than 90 percent of patients. "Of particular importance are oral preparations of opioid drugs," they said.

The same year, two academic researchers published an influential report in the journal *Pain* about the opioid-based treatment of thirty-eight non-cancer patients with chronic pain. Their findings improved the reputation of medicines that generations of doctors had been taught to avoid due of fear of addiction. The researchers wrote, "We conclude that opioid maintenance therapy can be a safe, salutary and more humane alternative to the options of surgery or no treatment in those patients with intractable non-malignant pain and no history of drug abuse."

While some researchers gave doctors encouragement to prescribe opioids, another paper gave a clinical name to previous negative attitudes toward narcotic painkillers: opiophobia. The article stated that physicians in America undertreat pain because of an "an irrational and undocumented fear that appropriate use will lead patients to become addicts." A few years later, another term entered the medical lexicon: *Pseudoaddiction* described a phenomenon whereby a patient exhibited many of the recognized signs of addiction and yet was actually not addicted but simply undermedicated. One way to avoid pseudoaddiction was the timely administration of adequate pain medication, the authors wrote.

This push toward a more liberal approach to prescribing opioids accelerated considerably in the 1990s. While state legislatures around the country passed laws aimed at securing treatment access for pain patients, the American Pain Society embarked on a public relations campaign aimed at medical providers. For years, doctors and nurses had closely measured and monitored four key indicators in patients: body temperature, blood pressure, pulse, and respiration rate. In 1995, the APS suggested the addition of a "fifth vital sign" — a patient's pain level — that would be monitored with the same frequency as the others. The initiative quickly caught on. The nation's single largest health system, the Veterans Health Administration, added the "Fifth Vital Sign" in its communications to doctors. Other institutions and organizations followed suit. Dr. James Campbell, the American Pain Society president who came up with the "Fifth Vital Sign" idea, would later say that the campaign "transformed medicine."

An even bigger moment came in 1996, with the release of OxyContin.

Created by Purdue Pharma, a small Connecticut-based pharmaceutical company with a knack for marketing, OxyContin was intended as a single pill that patients could take for hours of pain relief, rather than swallowing a number of shorter-acting pills to achieve the same result. The time-release mechanism of the drug was located in its outer coating, which prompted the company to warn patients not to crush or chew the drug, lest they receive the full, whopping dose at once.

OxyContin was a new spin on an old substance. As the *New York Times* reported in 2001, "chemically, it is a close relative of every other opium derivative and synthetic: heroin, morphine, codeine, fentanyl, methadone." The drug did not perform particularly well, in terms of efficacy or safety, when compared with other similar opioid medications. What made OxyContin different was the *story* that the manufacturers told about the drug.

In advertisements, sales presentations, and face-to-face interactions with doctors, Purdue aimed to convince doctors that the drug was appropriate for arthritis, injuries, and other ailments that caused moderate pain. And they argued that, convenience-wise, the drug was far better for patients than shorter-acting opioids. At the same time, the company aggressively downplayed the risks of addiction that had previously prompted physicians to steer clear of opioids beyond narrow uses, such as postoperative pain or end-of-life care.

Purdue's marketing of OxyContin was an unprecedented blitz. The company held training conferences for doctors, nurses, and pharmacists at sunny resorts and paid for meals, travel, lodging, and other expenses. It hired scores of salespeople dedicated to convincing doctors to prescribe OxyContin and incentivized that sales force with lucrative bonus packages. It spent millions placing ads in medical journals and produced promotional videos to doctors, like one called *I Got My Life Back: Patients in Pain Tell Their Story*. In just a few years' time, through sheer capitalistic commitment and marketing muscle (and a glaring lack of caution about the downstream effects of such a misleading campaign), this one relatively small pharmaceutical company accelerated the shift in attitudes toward opioids within the medical profession. It did this through what *New York Times* journalist Barry Meier has called "the biggest and most aggressive marketing campaign for a powerful narcotic in modern pharmaceutical history." In the years following OxyContin's release, the number of prescriptions rose from around three hundred thousand in 1996 to more than seven million by 2002. Meanwhile, sales for OxyContin leapt to $1.5 billion in 2002.

The movement for aggressive pain treatment continued into the new millennium. In 2000, Congress passed a bill, which was later signed by President Bill Clinton, that included a short resolution that the decade beginning January 1, 2001, would be designated the Decade of Pain Control and Research.

An article in the journal *Pain Medicine* hailed that distinction as a "major accomplishment." And in March 2003, just a month before Volkman began working at Tri-State, a physician made this "Decade" the subject of his address at the annual gathering of the American Pain Society.

He told the crowd that the field of pain management had undergone a "revolution" in the previous twenty-five years. Pain was no longer just a by-product of disease, he said; it deserved diagnosis and treatment on its own. At one point, he said, "We should ask ourselves, 'What is going to happen if we do not seize this opportunity to make a difference in the remaining nine years of our decade?'"

AARON

The first of Volkman's pain patients to die was a man named Aaron Gillispie. He was thirty-three years old and worked as a maintenance man for the Portsmouth Housing Authority.

Or, at least, Aaron Gillispie's death is the first that investigators would later pin to Volkman.

In a story rife with competing narratives, few aspects are more disputed than the number of people who lost their lives due to Paul Volkman.

This number varies widely depending on the source. The indictment itself listed fourteen people who, authorities alleged, died because of medications that Volkman prescribed to them. Before the trial, prosecutors dropped two of those death-specific charges. As a result, during the trial, attorneys from both the prosecution and defense referred to allegations regarding twelve patient deaths.

But when the *Columbus Dispatch* covered the indictment, the article ran with a timeline of eighteen patients' deaths. And in two instances, I've seen estimates from DEA officials that are significantly higher. In 2012, a DEA official told the *Lexington Herald-Leader* that the agency had investigated thirty-four overdose deaths among Volkman's patients. According to another DEA agent I spoke to, the number of deaths investigated was actually thirty-nine.

Volkman, meanwhile, has remained consistent about the number of deaths he caused: zero. And during the trial, his lawyers called at least one expert witness — a seasoned forensic pathologist — who agreed with this assessment, at least based on the selected patient files that he had been asked to review.

My approach to this aspect of the story is partly dictated by practical factors. Although I fought fiercely for access to information about the Volkman trial (which included filing a Freedom of Information Act lawsuit against the DEA over its years-long refusal to release trial evidence), I never obtained detailed info about deceased patients who were *not* mentioned in the trial transcript or other court records. Thus, for most of the patients underlying DEA officials' remarks about thirty-four or thirty-nine deaths, I have no information. No names. No age. No place of residence or date of death. No details about visits to Volkman.

And even if I *did* have more information, it makes journalistic sense to focus on the people who were discussed in detail during his criminal case. For this, the number is thirteen: twelve patients named in specific counts of the indictment, and one additional patient who was mentioned in the indictment and discussed in trial testimony.

When discussing these thirteen people, it's important to note how much Paul Volkman acknowledges to be true. He acknowledges that these people were his patients, that he prescribed medication to them, and that they died during the time they were seeing him, often within days of their last visit to him.

For this facet of the case, the main areas of disagreement aren't so much about basic facts but about *cause* and *responsibility*. That is, *why* did these people die? And *who* was responsible?

Each of these questions yields other questions.

When discussing the reasons why Volkman's patients died, the testimony of various trial witnesses attempted to answer some of the following questions:

- Did these patients die because of an overdose of the medications Volkman prescribed to them?
- Did that determination of an overdose, when it was made by a coroner or forensic pathologist, properly factor in the physical tolerance to opioid pain medications that the patient might have developed from taking those medications for some time?

- Did they have other physical conditions, such as heart disease or cancer, that may have caused their death, instead of the medications?
- If no autopsy was performed, on what basis was the cause of death determined?

When the trial discussion turned to assigning responsibility for the patient deaths, other questions were asked:

- Did the deceased patients have documented histories of pain? And/or did they have a history of substance abuse?
- Were they being honest about their symptoms when they saw Volkman?
- Did Volkman have a legitimate doctor-patient relationship with this person? And were his prescriptions medically appropriate?
- Did the patient take their medications in the manner that he advised them to?
- Were they taking other substances — such as methadone, cocaine, or alcohol — that he didn't know about and that he never would have authorized?

Much of the testimony from the doctor's lengthy criminal trial in 2011 attempted to answer these complex questions.

When it comes to exploring these questions for myself, I have drawn on a large amount of material. Volkman was outspoken before and after his trial, so I have no shortage of *his* account of what happened. I will include excerpts from his remarks as I tell the stories of these patients. And as a factual counterweight to his claims, I have access to hundreds of trial exhibits and the testimony of eighty witnesses, totaling more than four thousand pages of transcript.

Beyond simply sifting through details of these folks' deaths, I have also gone to great lengths to learn as much as I could about their lives. This information comes from dozens of interviews with loved ones, as well as obituaries, photographs, Facebook posts, and other materials.

And this brings us back to Aaron Gillispie.

———

Aaron was born in Ashland, Kentucky, in 1969. He was a father to three daughters: Brittany (born in 1987), Kristen (1993), and Erin (1994). I saw more than one photo of him with arms wrapped lovingly around his blond-haired girls. In one, he's wearing blue jeans, a plaid shirt, a baseball cap, and work boots. In another, he's wearing a jersey for the San Francisco 49ers. One of those daughters, Brittany, told me that her dad "was always trying to make somebody else laugh."

Health records for Gillispie show that, at the time of an on-the-job injury in the mid-1990s, he was employed at a grocery chain warehouse in Florida. But he subsequently moved back to the area where he grew up. At the time of his first appointment with Volkman in April 2003, he was employed as a maintenance worker for the Portsmouth Housing Authority. Documents from his visits to the clinic state that he had recently missed work due to "severe pain in his lower back, neck, pain and numbness/ muscle weakness into both arms, and weakness in his legs at times."

Aaron's pain had prompted him to seek relief from numerous pain specialists over the years, including two pain clinics in Kentucky. Gillispie had been a patient at Tri-State, starting in October 2001, at its location across the river in Kentucky. And when the clinic moved to Ohio, he began making his visits there.

Volkman's notes from that first meeting described Gillispie as walking with a "visible altered/painful gait." And the doctor's initial summary of his symptoms — a multipage document that Volkman often dictated after his first appointments with a patient — indicated that pain was affecting nearly every aspect of Gillispie's life, including his sleep and ability to play with his children. Volkman's notes indicated that, though Gillispie denied any suicidal tendencies, the patient "has times of depressed mood and severe irritability with wife and children, [and] he says his pain keeps him from working or socializing."

Volkman's intake notes also mentioned the failure of previous, non-narcotic pain-relief attempts, including physical therapy and the use of over-the-counter drugs. As a result, under a section titled "Management Plan," Volkman included the note: "Use of chronic opioid therapy with objectives of improved sleep, reducing and controlling pain intensity, improving mobility, [and] improvement of concentration ability."

After his first visit to the doctor, Aaron was prescribed three different opioids: Tylox, OxyContin, and a Duragesic (fentanyl) patch. In a subsequent visit Volkman removed the patch, but then added a prescription for the sedative Xanax to his regimen.

Two days after that June visit to the clinic, Gillispie died at the age of thirty-three. An autopsy led a forensic pathologist to determine that he had died from the combined effects of the multiple medications in his system, including oxycodone, diazepam, and meprobamate.

Around two weeks after his death, the Scioto County coroner sent a formal letter to Volkman at Tri-State, requesting Gillispie's records. Citing state law, the letter read, in part, "You are hereby ordered to produce copies of any and all medical records on this patient by Friday, July 25, 2003. You may bring the records to the Coroner's office in the Courthouse, or you may mail them . . . Thank you for your assistance."

It would not be the last coroner's letter Volkman received.

DEA

In the early 1970s, while Paul Volkman was in medical school, three events occurred that would have a major effect on his life decades later.

The first was the passage of the Comprehensive Drug Abuse Prevention and Control Act of 1970, later known simply as the Controlled Substances Act. The law aimed to streamline an existing hodgepodge of federal laws pertaining to banned or dangerous substances. Under the CSA, substances would be neatly organized into categories, called schedules, based on their dangers and potential for therapeutic purposes. Some substances — like cocaine, marijuana, and LSD — that were deemed to have no legitimate medical use were classified as Schedule I and banned outright. Other substances, like opiate painkillers, which had recognized medical uses but also a risk of abuse, were classified as Schedule II through Schedule V, according to their risk level.

To prescribe a so-called controlled substance, a physician needed to be registered with the government. When they prescribed such a substance, they were required to include their registration number on the prescription so that the movement of the substance could be tracked. Patients, in turn, needed a valid prescription to possess such a controlled substance. Without one, possession of the substance would violate federal law.

Passage of the Controlled Substances Act was a milestone for federal drug-law enforcement. As the Drug Enforcement Administration later wrote in a self-published history of the agency, "this law, along with its implementing regulations, established a single system of control for both narcotic and psychotropic drugs for the first time in U.S. history."

A second key event came in June 1971, when, during a press conference about the nation's drug problem, President Richard Nixon used new language to describe how the federal government would address the issue under his leadership. "America's public enemy number one . . . is drug abuse," he said. "In order to fight and defeat this enemy, it is necessary to wage a new, all-out offensive." It was a noteworthy rhetorical shift, and it marked the start of one of the nation's defining domestic policies of the next half century: the War on Drugs.

A third event took place in 1973, when Nixon, through an executive order, created a new federal agency called the Drug Enforcement Administration (DEA). Before then, for almost sixty years, federal drug enforcement responsibilities had bounced between an ever-shifting array of government agencies. Now those activities would be consolidated under one roof and one name. Among the new agency's responsibilities, according to its founding documents, was the "full investigation and preparation for prosecution of suspects for violations under all Federal drug trafficking laws."

The story of what happened next differs depending on who's telling it.

If you ask employees of the DEA, or folks who are sympathetic to its mission, you'll hear about a heroic, hyper-capable agency that, for more than fifty years, has been bravely protecting the American people from coldhearted criminals, both foreign and domestic, who are eager to peddle dangerous substances. Those substances have changed over the years, from cocaine in the 1970s to crack in the 1980s and Ecstasy and methamphetamine in the 1990s and early 2000s.

Fans of the agency will tell you that, regardless of the foe, the DEA's efforts have been valiant and quantifiable. In 2003, the House of Representatives passed a resolution honoring the agency's thirtieth anniversary, which noted that between 1986 and 2002, DEA agents seized more than ten thousand kilograms of heroin, nine hundred thousand kilograms of cocaine, and 1.5 billion dosage units of methamphetamine. During that same time, the agency made more than 443,000 arrests of suspected drug traffickers.

"Since 1973," the resolution read, "the men and women of the DEA have served our Nation with courage, vision and determination, protecting all Americans from the scourge of drug trafficking, abuse, and related violence."

To the agency's critics, meanwhile, the DEA is a serially incompetent, corrupt, and largely unaccountable juggernaut that continues to belligerently pursue a failed drug war that has disproportionately affected marginalized groups and produced little proof of lasting success. It is an agency that has attempted to apply a Prohibitionist mind-set to an issue that demands nuance and compassion and has failed at virtually every step of the way. Opponents of the DEA aren't just outspoken critics of its policies; they often call for the agency's dissolution altogether.

Where you fall between these two viewpoints will depend on various factors, including your political leanings, your feelings about law enforcement, your views on drugs, and, if you're involved in healthcare, your personal experience with the agency. When researching the history of the DEA, I could have easily spun off and written an entirely different book focused just on the polarizing agency.

But it's also possible that — if you're like me before I began this project — you haven't spent much time thinking about the DEA at all. And this is perhaps the most salient fact about the agency: Despite its size (an annual budget that tops $3 billion, a workforce of nearly ten thousand, and offices across the country and around the world), it seems to mostly operate outside the national consciousness. As big and influential as it is, it remains overshadowed by its older, bigger, and more famous sibling agency, the FBI.

Whatever strong reactions the DEA inspires, on one point there can be little debate: By the turn of the millennium, the DEA's focus was changing.

Twice in 2001, DEA officials delivered congressional testimony about the growing problem of prescription drug abuse and diversion. And in June of that year, the agency took the unprecedented step of releasing an action plan responding to one specific drug: OxyContin.

In that document, the agency explained that OxyContin, which had been released five years prior, had a legitimate application for treating moderate to severe pain. But the drug's runaway success, including its exponential growth in prescriptions and annual sales, had led to alarming amounts of abuse. This was in part because the drug's signature time-release mechanism could be easily bypassed by crushing the pill, which unlocked a dose of opioids that surpassed any previously manufactured pill.

The plan stated that diversion of the drug was mainly concentrated in rural areas in the eastern part of the country, but the problem was expanding. And the drug had "been described by some local law enforcement officials as a national epidemic in the making," the agency stated. In some of the worst-hit areas, law enforcement resources were becoming depleted. "Continued increases in the diversion and abuse of OxyContin are considered likely unless firm and immediate action is taken," the report said. Thus, the agency announced it would be "using all available enforcement tools" to disrupt the illegal trafficking of the drug.

As promised, the next two years saw a sharp rise in enforcement activity related to the illegal distribution of prescription opioids. The DEA would later report that its OxyContin-focused cases increased fourfold from 2000 to 2001, and OxyContin-related arrests rose sevenfold in that same time.

The DEA had cracked down on the illicit use of prescription medications before, with Quaaludes in the 1970s and 1980s and anabolic steroids in the 1990s. But it had never engaged in a campaign as highly publicized as its efforts to rein in illegal use of OxyContin. And given how widely prescribed the drug had become among doctors, this was potentially dicey territory.

And so, in addition to the release of its action plan, the agency took another unprecedented step: the release of a statement, coauthored with twenty-one health organizations, called "Promoting Pain Relief and Preventing Abuse of Pain Medications: A Critical Balancing Act." With that statement, the agency linked arms with nurses, academic researchers, palliative care experts, medical ethics experts, and other medical specialists (oncologists, anesthesiologists, pain-management professionals) to publicly affirm two goals: treating pain and preventing abuse.

Among the points on which all parties said they agreed were:

- Undertreatment of pain is a serious problem in the United States . . . Effective pain management is an integral and important aspect of quality medical care, and pain should be treated aggressively.
- For many patients, opioid analgesics — when used as recommended by established pain management guidelines — are the most effective way to treat their pain, and often the only treatment option that provides significant relief.
- In spite of regulatory controls, drug abusers obtain these and other prescription medications by diverting them from legit-

imate channels in several ways, including fraud, theft, forged prescriptions, and via unscrupulous health professionals.

- Drug abuse is a serious problem . . . Focusing only on the abuse potential of a drug, however, could erroneously lead to the conclusion that these medications should be avoided when medically indicated.

To further assuage unease in the medical world, in early 2002, the DEA's then administrator Asa Hutchinson spoke at a gathering of the American Pain Society.

In his remarks, Hutchinson assured his audience that the DEA didn't select pharmacists or doctors to investigate at random; 90 percent of the time, he estimated, investigations began with tips from doctors, pharmacists, law enforcement, or family members of patients. He further noted that the vast majority of doctors would never see or interact with the DEA. In the previous year, he said, the agency initiated 861 investigations and took actions against 697 doctors from a pool of 900,000 DEA-registered physicians.

"I'm here to tell you that we trust your judgment," he said. "You know your patients. The DEA does not intend to play the role of doctor."

He added, "A physician acting in good faith and in accordance with established medical norms should be confident in their ability to prescribe appropriate pain medications."

Not everyone was convinced.

In a column for the *New York Times*, opinion columnist John Tierney wrote that he believed the DEA's strategy was less about addressing the new threat and more about pressure the DEA felt from Congress (to whom it had to annually plead its case for renewed funding) to produce tangible results in the War on Drugs.

"As quarry for D.E.A. agents, doctors offered several advantages over crack dealers," he wrote. "They were not armed. They were listed in the phone book. They kept office hours and records of their transactions. And unlike the typical crack dealer living with his mother, they had valuable assets that could be seized and shared by the federal, state and local agencies fighting the drug war."

It was in this context — an agency formed to enforce the nation's drug laws pivoting its focus to pharmaceutical drugs amid a rising trend of abuse and overdose, with murmurs of unease from some observers — that, in

June 2003, a DEA office in Columbus received a tip from a pharmacist in West Virginia about the amounts of controlled substances Paul Volkman was prescribing. In the ensuing months, DEA offices received numerous similar complaints from other pharmacies about the Portsmouth-based pain doctor.

After Tri-State opened its on-site dispensary, the nature of the complaints changed. Now it was Volkman's wholesale orders, not individual prescriptions, causing alarm. In August 2003, a medical supplier in Connecticut told the DEA that a Tri-State order for hydrocodone had exceeded the company's limits for ordering. The same month, another supplier notified a DEA office in Texas that Volkman had recently placed the largest order for hydrocodone the company had ever seen.

Those complaints from pharmacies and pharmaceutical suppliers were added to a growing file on Volkman. After the doctor's arrival in Portsmouth, the agency had also received calls from local law enforcement agencies, as well as notice that the Ohio Boards of Medicine and Pharmacy had also received tips about Volkman.

In September 2003, less than six months into Volkman's tenure at Tri-State, the DEA officially opened an investigation.

DANNY AND JEFF

Danny Coffee was a jokester.

His sister, Diana, told me that when they were kids, one of his gags involved pretending to run into a door, kicking it to produce a loud *thunk*, and then holding his head as if he were in pain. As an adult, he was known to ride a bicycle inside the house or mail his brother random photographs with no apparent focus or subject to them. His signature prank, which three separate people recalled during interviews, took place during family gatherings, when he would sneak off to a sibling's car, crank up the radio, and turn on the windshield wipers so that the next time the driver turned on their car, they received a multisensory jolt.

Danny was born and raised in Greenup, Kentucky, a small town on the banks of the Ohio River about twenty miles southeast of Portsmouth. His daughter Amanda compared the town to Mayberry, the idyllic, all-American fictional setting of *The Andy Griffith Show*.

Danny's father was a school bus driver who played bluegrass music in his free time. His mother worked at a grocery store and various nearby restaurants. The Coffees were, in the words of one family member, an "average blue-collar family."

Danny was the second youngest of six children. And while some of his siblings moved away, Danny stuck around Greenup, which earned him the nickname "boomerang baby." After working in a few wage-earning jobs over the years after high school, he was eventually hired as a custodian for the local public schools.

Danny was a trim guy who could eat heaping amounts of food and never gain a pound. He kept a neat appearance. He wore his blue jeans with a seam down the front, and he tucked in his T-shirt. He "never had a hair out of place," his daughter told me.

Danny had three kids: Amanda, Carley, and Adam. Carley told me that, after Danny and his wife split, on weekends he took Carley to the batting cages or to ride go-karts or to Pizza Hut for cheese sticks.

In my conversations with Danny's family members, I frequently heard about his sunny temperament. Carley said that she couldn't remember her dad ever being cruel or angry. His older daughter, Amanda, told me, "Everybody in the community absolutely adored him."

One day in the mid-1990s while Danny was driving, his car was T-boned at an intersection. Danny sustained a neck injury and required hospitalization. Once discharged, he spent months recovering and suffered from headaches and ringing in his ears. He would later have corrective surgery, but afterward, his pain remained. This was why he started going to local pain clinics.

Danny's first visit with Volkman took place in August 2003, about four months after Volkman's arrival. Records of subsequent visits were either lost or misplaced, so I don't know what Danny wrote on his patient-intake forms or what Volkman wrote in his notes from Danny's visits. What I *do* know is that Danny returned to Volkman regularly in the ensuing months, and he was prescribed lots of medication. His mother, Lena, would later recall telling him: "Danny, they gave you too many pills."

During the time of these monthly visits to the pain clinic, Danny's family members noticed a change in his behavior. Carley recalled weekends when her dad called to tell her he couldn't pick her up because he didn't feel well and other times when he fell asleep abruptly. In one case, he nodded off with a sandwich in his hand. Amanda also recalled finding him asleep and having to repeat "Dad! Dad! Dad!" to wake him up. It scared her.

Danny's brother, Lloyd, who lived out of state, remembered that during his visits home, his brother didn't seem as full of life as he used to be. He seemed tired. Whether it was more from the pain or the drugs or both, he couldn't tell, but he later told me that Danny's "apathy was palpable." When Lloyd spoke to Danny about the medication he was on, Danny said that he was taking the pills as the doctor advised. Lloyd didn't know if that was true.

Danny's sister, Diana, perhaps saw the worst of her brother's troubles. She told me that Danny cashed in his retirement savings and sold his car to continue to pay for his visits to Volkman. One evening, when she visited him at home, she found him "completely out of it" and put him in the backseat of her truck, activated the car's childproof locks, and took him to the hospital to get straightened out. Afterward, she went back to his home, scoured it for pills, and flushed them down the toilet.

She told me that, eventually, folks at Danny's job knew that he was addicted to drugs and saw him as a liability. They had to let him go.

In the fall of 2003, Danny was living in a trailer behind his parents' house in Greenup. And on the morning of Monday, November 17, 2003, he drove his son to school and returned home, where he made himself a sandwich for breakfast.

By coincidence, that same morning, his daughter Amanda had driven to her dad's house to tell him the news that she was pregnant with twins. When she got there, she sat in her car for a few minutes. She would later say that something — some unknown force — made her pause for a moment. She had a feeling something was wrong.

Eventually, Amanda got out of the car, walked to the door, and knocked. There was no answer. The door was unlocked, and she let herself in. At first glance, she didn't see Danny. She said that she called out, "Hey Dad, where you at?" and heard nothing.

Amanda figured that her father was next door at his parents' house, so she went over and asked her grandparents about him. They said they had seen him walk by a little while earlier, and Amanda figured that he might be in the shower. So she went back to the trailer and walked farther inside. Then she saw her dad on the couch. He wasn't moving, and his body was tilted over. His lips were swollen and blue.

Later that day, Danny's sister, Diana, was at work at the Greenup County School Board when she received a call from her father. He told her to come to the house, which was something she hadn't heard him say in years. When she arrived and got out of the car, she could hear her mother wailing.

By midafternoon, Greenup County Coroner Leslie Neil Wright arrived on the scene. When he got there, the television in Danny's trailer was still playing. He collected medications from the scene, including two bottles prescribed by Dr. Volkman. In his authorization for a postmortem examination, he wrote: "Found slumped over on the right side of the couch. Had fixed himself lunch and it was found next to him untouched. History of drug abuse and depression." An autopsy and toxicology analysis would determine that Danny's death was due to multiple drug intoxication from lethal amounts of hydrocodone and oxycodone.

Years later, when his mother was contacted by a reporter from the Associated Press, she said, "I'm sure the pills they gave him killed him . . . I think it was just plain murder."

One day after Danny Coffee's death, a patient named Jeffrey Reed had an appointment with Volkman at Tri-State.

Jeff was a carpenter who was born in 1965, in Troy, Ohio. He was one of seven children. His father was a US Army vet and truck driver.

In the summer of 1990, he married Cheryl Stiltner in Greenup County, Kentucky, and two years later their daughter, Amanda, was born. Photos from the time show Jeff looking tall, slim, and handsome, with sandy-blond hair and a mustache. In one photo, he holds his daughter in his arms and smiles at the camera. In another, he sits cross-legged on a patch of grass with his daughter in his lap and gazes down at her lovingly. His wife, Cheryl, would later describe him as a "very good person."

In March 1995, when Jeff was twenty-nine, he was working and fell from scaffolding onto a wooden porch, injuring his wrist. A week later, he underwent corrective surgery to install a screw and wiring into the injured arm.

Jeff couldn't work after the injury, and due to the pain, he began to go to local pain clinics for relief. During one visit to Tri-State in March 2002, a year before Volkman's arrival, he reported pain in his neck, wrists, and lower back, as well as insomnia. That day, he received prescriptions for Xanax and the narcotic painkiller Lorcet, which contains a combination of hydrocodone and acetaminophen.

Sometime after April 2003, when Jeff had his first appointments with Volkman, his wife noticed dramatic shifts in his moods. On days when he was scheduled to see the doctor, he'd seem energized and excited. But when his pills ran out a few weeks later, he would lie on the couch, lifeless and sick, and take trips to the bathroom due to diarrhea and vomiting.

Things got worse.

His wife, Cheryl, said that Jeff was so overmedicated that he nodded off at odd times. He would pass out while eating and she would have to take food out of his mouth so he wouldn't choke, or he would fall asleep with a lit cigarette in his hand that she would remove. She would later testify that, sometimes, "he would just be sitting there and just fall over."

Meanwhile, his efforts to get cash to see the doctor and buy pills became more extreme. He took items from his own home to sell for cash. He pawned VCRs, guitars, and his daughter's TV.

At one point, Cheryl counted the pills Jeff received after a trip to Tri-State; there were more than six hundred for a single month. She didn't think it was possible that a person could safely take that much medication, and she was further alarmed by the distances Jeff was driving to get those prescriptions filled. One pharmacy was in Paintsville, Kentucky, an hour-and-a-half drive away from where they lived, in Greenup. When she asked Jeff about this, he told her that Volkman said that this was the closest pharmacy that would fill his scripts.

Cheryl was so alarmed that she made a call to the clinic herself and asked to speak with the doctor. She was told that he wasn't available, but she left a message. "I just want to tell him that you cannot give one person that many pills," she remembered saying. The person at the clinic hung up on her.

Months passed with Jeff returning to Volkman for regular visits. After one appointment in August, he received scripts for 450 pills: 180 Lorcets, 180 oxycodone, and 90 Valium.

On November 20, 2003, two days after one of Jeff's visits to the clinic, Cheryl woke up around six thirty in the morning. When she walked to the bathroom, she found the door locked. She figured that Jeff had passed out or taken too many pills, which wasn't particularly unusual, so she decided to go make coffee. After a few minutes, she tried again and called his name. There was no response. She started to think that something bad might have happened.

Cheryl's cousin, who lived next door, helped her get into the locked bathroom. Inside, they found Jeff sitting on the floor, cross-legged, and leaning forward with his head over his lap. When they hoisted him up, they saw that his face was blue. There were three pill bottles on the vanity; all had been prescribed by Dr. Volkman.

On the day after her husband's death, Cheryl called Tri-State for a second time. Once again, she asked to speak with Dr. Volkman. And again, she was told he was unavailable. This time she said, "Well, I just wanted . . . to let you know that you helped kill my husband and you're responsible for his death."

The man on the other end told her not to threaten him. She responded that she wasn't threatening anyone. Then, she said, the man from the clinic hung up.

1219 FINDLAY STREET

In the fall of 2003, around six months into Volkman's tenure at Tri-State, the clinic moved. The new location was just a couple blocks from the first clinic, but it was a considerably bigger space, in a two-story brick building. Volkman would work there for almost two years.

The building at 1219 Findlay Street had a row of tall glass windows at the street level. And the facade of the building — at least when I first saw it, in 2010 — was a faded white, with grime between the cracks of the bricks. A small, sun-faded, semicircular blue awning hung over the main door. Next to the building was a tire shop with an outdoor, fenced-in yard containing stacks of black rubber tires. Across 13th Street was an empty lot, and across Findlay Street was a small, abandoned church.

Business boomed.

Shortly after arriving in Ohio, Volkman quickly distinguished himself as a high-volume purchaser of controlled substances. Between July 1 and December 31, 2003, Volkman's purchases of hydrocodone, which supplied the clinic's dispensary, surpassed not just any practitioner in the zip code but also every *pharmacy*. In 2004, the year after the move to Findlay Street, Volkman became the largest physician-purchaser of oxycodone in the United States.

During this time, the clinic was seeing an average of twenty-five patients per day. And there were reports of crowds outside the clinic and dozens of cars parked in the surrounding streets. A detective from the county sheriff's office would later say he had "never seen that outside of a doctor's office, where groups of people would hang out."

Because of this influx of patients, long wait times were common. "We had to spend most of the day there," one patient recalled during the trial.

"We might be in there from 9:00 in the morning till 9:00 at night." Another patient testified that the waiting room was sometimes so crowded that a clinic employee would tell people, "Get an F'ing seat or you're dismissed."

A video taken in January 2004 by a patient who aided the DEA's investigation by carrying a hidden camera in her purse for one office visit shows the clinic waiting room abuzz at around 6:30 P.M. when the patient arrives. As she waits for her turn with Volkman, employees mill around, sometimes grabbing files from behind the front desk. For the next hour, as the woman waits, patients — and, in some cases, the children accompanying them — walk back and forth in front of the camera, occasionally chatting and laughing with one another. In the background, a phone rings, and the front door of the clinic chimes when someone enters or exits. Volkman occasionally emerges from a hallway to talk to his staff or call the name of a patient, and then retreats out of sight.

The patients in the video appear to be between their midthirties and midfifties. Most are dressed casually, in jeans, sweatshirts, and sneakers, with many of the men wearing baseball hats. Only one patient in the video, a man hobbling with a cane, appears to be visibly in pain.

According to DEA estimates, with the clinic open five days a week and seeing twenty-five patients per day, each of whom paid $125 per visit, the clinic was bringing in around $3,125 per day in cash. This added up to $15,625 per week and $62,500 per month. And once the dispensary was established, investigators estimated that the on-site pharmacy brought in an additional $8,400 in weekly revenue. All told, according to DEA estimates, Tri-State Healthcare was hauling in around $95,000 for each month it operated with Paul Volkman as its sole physician.

The clinic was also deadly.

Starting in October 2003 and continuing through March 2004, patients from Tri-State died at a pace of approximately one per month.

On October 21, a forty-year-old patient named Charles Jordan died from what the Kentucky State Medical Examiner's Office determined to be "acute opioid toxicity." Jordan had been going to Volkman monthly since April, when the doctor arrived in Ohio. His niece, Machelle, told me that her uncle "was a normal, thriving person until the drugs got a hold of him." She described Volkman to me as a "pill doctor, period."

November brought the deaths of Danny Coffee, age forty-seven, and Jeff Reed, thirty-seven. They died three days apart.

January brought the death of thirty-two-year-old Mary Catherine Carver. Carver saw Volkman a total of five times, starting in September 2003. Like many of Volkman's patients, she had a history of injuries. She had been in multiple car accidents and had once taken a nasty fall into an open manhole at a local gas station. But she also had a history of drug abuse. During at least one visit to Tri-State, her unkempt appearance and erratic behavior prompted Alice Huffman to later testify, "She seemed . . . to have an addiction problem." As with other patients, Volkman prescribed her a regimen of opioids, benzodiazepines, and muscle relaxers.

During the testimony of Mary's husband, Stoney, he described how, on January 10, 2004, he woke up from his nap around 5:00 P.M. and saw Mary seated on the couch in a leaned-over posture with her head resting on the coffee table. She didn't appear to be breathing. In a panic, Stoney called his sister-in-law, who was a nurse, to ask her about how to perform CPR. He followed her instructions and began attempting to revive her. It was too late. An autopsy concluded that Mary had died from lethal intoxication due to the combined effects of oxycodone and hydrocodone.

February brought the death of a thirty-two-year-old father and union pipefitter from Ashland, Kentucky, named James Estep. James's wife, Angie, told me that he wasn't the kind of person whom you'd expect to have a drug problem. He was an athletic guy who played football and baseball in high school. He was outgoing. He drove a red Camaro that he washed frequently. He kept his hair neatly trimmed. He was a hardworking man who was proud of his job. "If he could work a job where he was working seven days a week, that's the jobs he wanted," she told me.

Angie said that she was alarmed by the size of the pill bottles that James brought home from Volkman's pain clinic. She remembered arguments with James about whether the clinic was legitimate. She said she told him, "You're gonna die from this stuff. You can't take this."

In response, he reminded her of the doctor's credentials. She also recalled him telling her, "I work every day. Do you think a drug addict makes $2,000 a week?"

James continued to visit Volkman's clinic for monthly appointments. Then, on the morning of February 11, 2004, James's ten-year-old daughter, Megan, came downstairs before school and saw her father motionless on the couch. He had a plate of food in his lap. He looked pale. A few minutes later, Megan's mom came downstairs and said, "OK, James. We're gonna go." There was no response. She started shaking him and yelling his name.

The funeral director later told Angie that there was no need to perform an autopsy to confirm something that they already knew: James had taken too many pills.

March brought the death of Kristi Ross, a thirty-nine-year-old mother of three who lived in Scioto County. When I asked her younger brother, Jeff, if she suffered from much physical pain, he was skeptical. He didn't believe that she had any serious physical conditions beyond asthma. He thought she simply liked taking pills because they made her less shy. "She'd get on her pills and she could actually talk to people," he told me. "It . . . gave her confidence."

Kristi first saw Volkman in April 2003 shortly after he began working at Tri-State, and she returned for monthly visits. Volkman's notes from these visits indicated that she suffered from lower back pain, hypertension, poor sleep, and the stress of a failing marriage. One of his notes read: "going thru divorce — husband trying to take daughter." Like many of Volkman's patients, she was prescribed a combination of narcotic pain relievers, anti-anxiety medications, and muscle relaxers.

On the day after her March 8, 2003, visit to Volkman, Kristi was found unresponsive at her mother's apartment and taken to Southern Ohio Medical Center, in Portsmouth, where she was pronounced dead.

A Portsmouth police investigator would later testify about the number of pills found in Kristi's purse, including three prescription bottles containing seventy-six hydrocodone, twenty-six Roxicodone, twenty-six Xanax tablets, and 103 carisoprodol. A toxicology analysis found the presence of opioids, muscle relaxers, and two separate tranquilizers in her system.

The section of her death certificate recording her cause of death would later read "drug overdosage." A few lines down, in a space for additional details, the author of the document added: "chronic pain — being treated at a local pain-management clinic."

GAMBLING

I don't know much about Denise Huffman's life during this time when Tri-State was in full swing. She was reluctant to speak with me for this project, and so were other members of her family and social circle. Even after reading her testimony from civil and criminal proceedings related to Tri-State, her personal life remains mostly obscured.

But there is at least one fact that I can report with confidence: She liked to gamble.

Over years of conversations with Volkman, he mentioned Denise's gambling multiple times. And more than once, he cited it as a reason for his eventual departure from Tri-State. In one email, he said, "I left [Tri-State] because Denise gambled away my paycheck." Later, he wrote that on the day of his September 2005 departure from Tri-State, a Friday, "Huffman did not show up to pay [me my] weekly $5000 check, choosing instead to remain at a casino in Kentucky." Later, when I asked specifically about this, he told me: "I don't know any details about Denise's gambling habits, but [I can] confirm that she spent every possible day at the casino."

Volkman was eager to paint Denise as the corrupt and deceitful half of their partnership, to make himself seem more honest and upstanding. And because of this motive, and his general unreliability as a narrator, I might otherwise dismiss his comments. But Denise's gambling was noted numerous other times in my reporting.

Volkman's description of Denise's frequent trips to the casino was echoed by a former acquaintance of the family from the time she owned Tri-State. (My source seemed eager to move on from this era of their life and requested anonymity, which I agreed to.) This person told me that Denise "lived" at the casino during this period and spent "every minute [she] could get there." During these trips, the source said that she "spent money like it was going out of style" and that her favorite game was the slot machines. This person went along a few times on these gambling trips but told me they couldn't afford to keep up with the amounts that Denise was spending.

Allegations of gambling would make their way into the criminal trial record as well, when a defense witness named Ida Renee Ames, who had worked at Tri-State and, later, for Volkman's post-Tri-State clinics, described "Denise stuffing money in bags and going to the track and sitting [there] for a week at a time." At another point in her testimony, she said that she found it a "bit suspicious . . . that [Denise] spends months in a seat at the betting track." Ames also testified that she had seen employees from the racetrack-casino that Denise frequented receive treatment at Tri-State for no charge.

Gambling also came up during Denise's sentencing hearing, in 2012, during a discussion about the money the clinic was bringing in at its peak. At one point during the proceedings, the judge asked Denise's attorney, "Is it true that your client has a gambling problem, or had?"

Her lawyer replied, "Not to the extent that she would go through that kind of money."

It wasn't exactly a firm denial.

When I asked Denise about gambling in our brief Facebook-message correspondence after her release from prison, her answer was characteristically vague.

"My husband and I went before and after Tri-State closed," she told me. "It had nothing to do with my earnings." To this, she added, in an apparent reference to the federal government, "The gov was aware of everything I did unlike Volkman."

I'm not sure exactly what she meant by the "gov" being "aware of everything [she] did." And I couldn't get her to clarify. Shortly after this exchange, she declined to answer any further questions and unfriended me on Facebook.

At one point in my research, I stumbled on what appeared to be a paper trail of Denise's gambling. I found it in six pages of bank statements from a small business checking account for Tri-State that were submitted as part of a wrongful-death lawsuit filed against Volkman and Huffman in Scioto County by the mother of a deceased patient. The transcript of that brief civil trial in 2008 indicated that the bank records were requested by the plaintiff's attorney, who wanted the jury to see the amounts of money flowing into and out of the clinic at the height of its business. The bank account was controlled by Denise Huffman.

Those pages of bank statements offer far from a complete picture. They include statements from just four months from 2003 (August through November) and two months from 2005 (February and March), which leaves more than twenty months of the Paul-Denise partnership missing, including the entirety of 2004.

But even in this limited time frame, there are transactions that appear to be gambling related. Included among orders to pharmaceutical supply companies are six ATM withdrawals for $500 — in August 2003, February 2005, and March 2005 — from the address of a greyhound track and casino in Cross Lanes, West Virginia, about a hundred miles southeast of Portsmouth. This appears to be the "betting track" that the trial witness and others were describing. The bank records also show ATM withdrawals and purchases totaling $1,984 from a casino and resort in southern Indiana, as well as another $1,000 in withdrawals from a nearby town where another casino was located.

In other words, bank statements from just a fraction of Volkman's tenure at Tri-State show someone with access to the clinic's credit card making regular withdrawals of hundreds of dollars at nearby casinos. And if it was Denise, the owner of the clinic at the time of these statements, it would certainly refute her claim that such trips had "nothing to do with [her] earnings." Whoever was making these cash withdrawals was taking money directly from the account that held the pain clinic's revenues.

DWIGHT

There were many reasons why a person might have gone to a southern Ohio pain clinic in the early 2000s. And Dwight Parsons had a lot of them.

Did he have pain? He did. He'd been in multiple car accidents. He had arthritis in his hands and knees. He had back problems.

Did he like the cash he could make from selling pills? Yes, he did.

Did he also enjoy how pills made him feel? This was also true. His stepson, Brad, told me that Dwight "liked to party" and sometimes used pills recreationally.

Brad even mentioned a fourth reason behind Dwight's regular visits to local pain clinics. His dad was an outgoing guy — a "Mr. Social" type, in Brad's words. And after Dwight had gone to the pain clinic, it seemed to his stepson like he was able to access a part of his personality that had begun to slip away. The drugs helped to take away his pain, and they might also have made him feel a bit high, Brad said. The pills would also attract a crowd of people, to whom he was either selling or giving them. All these factors combined to lift Dwight's mood and help him to feel like his old self.

"It was just like this perfect storm," Brad told me. "And he was the epicenter."

Dwight Parsons was born in 1957 in Ashland, Kentucky. He was the second youngest of six children. His father was a World War II Army veteran, a retired laborer for CSX railroad, and a co-owner of Parsons Mowers & Tillers, a small-engine mechanic shop in the town of Raceland, Kentucky.

Dwight was six foot two, weighed over 350 pounds, and went by the tongue-in-cheek nickname "Tiny." He had long hair, a big beard, and a tattoo of the outline of the state of Kentucky on the back of one of his hands. Because he worked as a car mechanic, his hands were often greasy and his knuckles were chafed.

Brad told me that his dad was the kind of guy whom you might see from a distance and think, "That's a mean motherfucker." But it was a false impression, he said. Because Dwight was actually a sweetheart.

Brad's first memory of his stepdad was when he was a little boy and Dwight helped him put on his socks and shoes. When he did this, Dwight took the time to adjust the seam on his sock so that it fit Brad's little foot properly. Brad remembered this small act. To him, it said, "Hey, this guy . . . cares about me."

As Brad grew up, his appreciation for Dwight deepened. He saw that his stepdad was a generous guy who was quick to give a ride or a meal to someone who needed it. And even if Dwight had grizzled biker pals with nicknames like "Hitman" and "Frankenstein," he also had Black friends and gay friends at a time and place where such relationships weren't the norm.

Dwight was passionate about engines. He loved muscle cars and hot rods. He would sometimes park his motorcycle in the living room instead of leaving it outside in the elements. The film *American Graffiti*, about early-1960s teenage car culture in California, was one of his favorites.

He also adored music, especially classic rock. Dwight played drums and guitar and sang with what Brad described as a "huge, wonderful voice." One day you might hear him play Cream's "Sunshine of Your Love"; another time, he would grab an acoustic guitar and belt out a version of Elvis Costello's ballad "Alison." He once encouraged Brad to learn to play the famous opening guitar riff from Blue Oyster Cult's "Don't Fear the Reaper."

Dwight had been a longtime patient at Tri-State Healthcare before the clinic moved to Ohio. He saw Paul Volkman during the doctor's first month at the clinic, in April 2003. At the time of this first appointment, Dwight reported chronic back and neck pain, headaches, hip pain, and knee pain. He returned to the clinic monthly for more than a year, tallying seventeen visits in total. Like many Volkman patients, he received prescriptions for opioid painkillers, an anti-anxiety sedative, and a muscle relaxer.

At Volkman's trial, a medical expert for the prosecution discussed a daily medication regimen that Volkman or someone else at the clinic had written for Dwight, which advised taking pills a total of seven times, at two-hour intervals, over the course of the day. The total daily pill count that Volkman had prescribed was thirty-one: fourteen Norcos, seven oxycodone, four Xanax, five Somas, and one Disalcid.

The expert who testified was alarmed by this schedule, and he compared the patient's body on such a regimen to a traffic-clogged highway, with more and more drugs coming in, and previously ingested drugs taking various times to be fully absorbed. Such a regimen carried "an unpredictable pattern of absorption and metabolism," the witness said, which made it hard to gauge when the drugs would have their cumulative peak effect. A regimen like this increased the chance of adverse side effects such as a depressed breathing rate or a person stopping breathing altogether. To prescribe powerful medications in such a way "dramatically compounds their risk," he said.

Dwight's stepson, Brad, remembered how terrible Dwight looked in August 2004, after he'd been seeing Volkman for more than a year. Dwight was sweaty and pale, and his eyes were red. He looked miserable — so bad that, on the night of August 11, 2004, hours after his most recent visit to Volkman, Brad told Dwight that he thought he needed to go to the hospital. Dwight got angry and talked Brad out of calling an ambulance.

That evening, while they were hanging out, Dwight was sitting at his favorite spot at a restaurant-booth-style table in his apartment. Brad was seated on a nearby couch, where he eventually dozed off. When Brad woke up a few hours later, he saw that Dwight had slid out of the booth and onto the floor. He was lying facedown. Horrified, Brad jumped up and tried to roll him over. He couldn't; Dwight was too big. He checked for a pulse and found nothing.

Brad said he remembered running to the neighbors' apartment to use their phone to call 911, but what happened after is blurry. He remembered the EMTs taking Dwight out of the apartment. He remembered a woman who lived nearby telling him, "Oh, Brad, honey, I'm so sorry."

Following a toxicological analysis, Dwight's death certificate listed the immediate cause of his death as "acute oxycodone toxicity."

He was forty-seven.

THE CLEVELAND CLINIC

There are few hospitals in the United States more celebrated than the Cleveland Clinic. By the early 2000s, the institution was internationally known.

Located on a campus of more than 125 acres, the complex was a city-within-a-city, featuring hotels, a conference center, and a top-ranked children's hospital, plus individual buildings for various specialties including cancer, heart care, breast care, and palliative care. New surgical and diagnostic techniques had been launched at the site. Kings from Jordan and Saudi Arabia had traveled there for treatment. The clinic had performed more than one thousand heart transplants and two thousand kidney transplants. With tens of thousands of employees, it was one of the largest employers in the state of Ohio.

Situated near the shores of Lake Erie, the Cleveland Clinic was 235 miles from Portsmouth. And so, despite the hospital's impeccable reputation, it was a bit strange that Paul Volkman referred his patients there. Why not pick something closer? In Cincinnati? Columbus? Lexington?

Testimony at Volkman's trial indicated that he referred several patients to the clinic. He sent one patient to Cleveland for treatment for fibroids (tumors that grow in the walls of the uterus). In another instance, when a patient had persistent ankle pain after a car accident, he referred him to the clinic's department of orthopedic surgery. In response, the doctor thanked Volkman for the referral, diagnosed the patient with an ankle sprain, and stated that he believed the risks of surgery outweighed any benefits.

Alice Huffman, in her trial testimony, described the clinic as Volkman's "favorite referral place." And Volkman never disputed this. During one court proceeding, he explained that he considered it the "best hospital in the country." At other times, his lawyers referred to these referrals as an indication that his practice was legitimate and that he had his patients' best interests in mind.

I've never quite figured out with certainty what was going on with Volkman and the Cleveland Clinic. But I have arrived at two reasons why he would send his patients on lengthy, costly, and — if we take Volkman at his word, that his Tri-State patients were suffering from various excruciating ailments — painful trips across the state.

One reason is that, just as he became shunned by pharmacists in Southern Ohio, his name was similarly radioactive with local physicians. Volkman himself has acknowledged that during his time in southern Ohio, he didn't have patient-admitting privileges at any local hospitals. And at one point during his trial, a witness mentioned how a staffer at a local hospital had said, "We don't do tests for Doctor Volkman, but if you want to obtain an order from another physician we will reschedule your test." It's possible that he referred patients to a hospital four hours away, by car, because local doctors and hospitals wouldn't do business with him.

Another reason for Volkman's interest in the Cleveland Clinic is that he wanted to work there. In April 2005, two years after he started working in Portsmouth, Volkman sent a copy of his CV to the clinic's pain-management department along with an email asking about a job. The email, which was submitted as evidence during his trial, begins, "I have been working in southern ohio [*sic*] for the past 2 years in Portsmouth, at Tristate [*sic*] Healthcare."

He continued:

> I have enjoyed the practice, consisting of medical pain management and learned a lot about the care of chronic pain patients, most of whom are poor hillbillies. This past December we began much more intensive monitoring of the patients including frequent drug screens with Mayo Clinic confirmations. This program revealed that about half of our patients were selling their pills instead of taking them, and they were summarily dismissed. Unfortunately, that leaves me with about a half time job. I am writing to explore any opportunities for me as a medical pain management specialist at the Cleveland Clinic or one of its outreach centers. Thank you for your consideration.

A couple of things jumped out at me when I read this email.

One was that, despite his patchwork history of locum tenens jobs, despite his record of malpractice lawsuits and his inability to obtain insurance, despite the fact that he was now working at a cash-only clinic with a heavily fortified dispensary, despite the fact that local pharmacists refused to fill his scripts, and despite the number of his pain patients who had died, Volkman saw himself as a viable candidate for one of the world's most prestigious medical facilities. The email is a snapshot of a man who, despite significant evidence to the contrary, viewed himself as a world-class physician. At the same time, it also shows that he viewed "most" of his patients as "poor hillbillies" and felt no qualms about saying so to a prospective employer.

I also read this email, as I read everything that he said and wrote, in the context of his ongoing claims of innocence. Volkman's claims of unjust prosecution often require extraordinary leaps of credulity on the listener's part, and this email is no exception.

Here he is saying that it took him until December 2004 — more than a year and a half after his arrival in Portsmouth — to figure out that "about half" of his patients were selling their pills. And if we apply this "about half" description to his own previous estimate of having "about 700" over-all patients,* it means he's claiming to have recently "summarily dismissed" around 350 patients for selling their pills. Even if we cut that number in half, he's still talking about dismissing more than 150 patients who, he said, successfully duped him about their true intentions for more than a year.

Remarkably, the clinic didn't reject Volkman's application outright. In response, an education coordinator (whose name is redacted in the document I obtained) thanked him for his interest and stated that they wanted to set up an interview with Volkman for the following month. "Please send me the possible days of your visit and we will arrange for some meetings with [redacted] the department's chair and some of our staff," the person wrote.

And this is, unfortunately, all I know about this application process.

The clinic declined to offer a comment when I reached out, and the email exchange submitted at trial includes just these two emails. If Volkman's interview with the Cleveland Clinic took place, it doesn't appear to have been successful. He remained at Tri-State through May 2005 and beyond.

STEVEN

Steven Hieneman was born on June 1, 1971, in the city of Ironton, Ohio, about thirty miles east of Portsmouth. He grew up in Greenup County, Kentucky.

Steven was an only child whose mother, Paula, was nineteen years old when he was born. She raised him as a single mother, and, in testimony in both civil and criminal cases against Volkman, spoke about how close she was with her son.

As she told it, Paula and Steven's bond was forged by the challenges of his childhood. He was born with a cleft palate — a condition that his mother suspected traced back to his father's exposure to Agent Orange

---

* This number comes from an email he wrote in October 2003.

while deployed in Vietnam — and underwent corrective surgery at three months old. As he grew older, he had difficulties with both reading and speaking. He also struggled with attention deficit disorder and what Paula described as "obsessive disorders where he would get sort of stuck on something and he couldn't let go of it until he got it done." She said that Steven also had "very, very, very low self-esteem" and that he would experience highs and lows in his behavior. He was later diagnosed with bipolar disorder.

During Steven's upbringing, Paula enrolled her son in speech therapy and, at times, also tutored him herself. She would later say that she was proud of the C's and D's on his report card because she knew how hard he had worked and struggled to get them. After leaving school following the eleventh grade, Steven moved to Florida and worked in convenience stores. In time, he worked his way up to a managerial position and completed his GED.

Around the age of twenty-five, he began to struggle with substance abuse and mental health issues. On one occasion, he tried to cut one of his wrists. Twice he was admitted to psychiatric facilities. In a third instance, after an overdose of prescription medication, he was hospitalized and placed on a ventilator.

Paula would later say that, during Steven's manic phases, he would binge on drugs and alcohol. But then, she said, he'd go six months where he wouldn't take a pill or touch alcohol and he would be "the perfect gentleman."

In early 2002, when Steven was thirty years old and living in Florida, he suffered an injury that changed the course of his life. That day, he had apparently been mixing drugs and alcohol and was found by a police officer. At some point afterward, Steven had an altercation with a paramedic.

I heard two different versions of what happened next. In one version, Steven's arm was injured when the EMT twisted it behind his back. In another, he was shoved to the ground and injured the wrist while breaking his fall. Whatever exactly happened, the incident resulted in a serious arm injury. Hospital records from soon after the incident include the note, "This gentleman got beat up very badly."

The aftermath of Steven's wrist injury was grueling. In the months afterward, he consistently reported pain and an inability to fully move his wrist or fingers, which remained in a clenched position. He had two surgeries, in which pins were first implanted in the hand, then removed. He also underwent physical therapy and nerve-block treatments and received Botox injections in his hand. One of his medical records notes that he also underwent "shock treatment through the arm and shoulder region." He was eventually diagnosed with reflex sympathetic dystrophy (RSD) syndrome, a painful condition characterized by burning, swelling, and extreme sensitivity to touch.

The injury also seems to have had a significant psychological effect. In August 2002, four months after the run-in with the EMT, he was admitted to a hospital in Ashland, Kentucky, for an apparent overdose. Hospital intake records indicate that he was found on his front porch "lethargic and stuporous," and a family member called emergency services. He was taken to a hospital where he was admitted to the intensive care unit. His records indicate that family members told the staff that he had the potential for self-destructive behavior.

In conversations with hospital staff during that stay, Steven was awake but uncooperative. His speech was slow and slurred. He said, according to notes, that "he has been taking OxyContin, Vicodin, Xanax, along with alcohol and some other medications" but denied that any of this was recreational. He admitted a past addiction to OxyContin, among other issues with substance abuse. He described a history of suicide attempts, overdoses, and admissions to psychiatric units in two states. "He stated he was not trying to get high he just tried to take the pain away," the notes read.

Two weeks prior to this hospitalization, he had been in a separate intensive care unit in South Carolina, for undisclosed reasons, and left after five days. Afterward, he told staff at the Ashland hospital that "he packed his clothes within five minutes and decided to move and had been to three states before he ended up here." He remained in the hospital for four more days, during which he attended group and individual therapy and received a new regimen of medications. He was ultimately discharged with instructions to "see his psychiatrist for further follow up and treatment."

Following his discharge from the hospital in Ashland in the summer of 2002, Steven received care for the wrist injury at a pain clinic affiliated with a local hospital. Notes from monthly visits in October and November 2002 show that he continued to struggle with pain and a lack of use of the fingers of his right hand, for which he underwent physical therapy. During these months he received prescriptions for hydrocodone, a fentanyl patch, and a muscle relaxant to address cramping in the injured hand. Records from that clinic note his past history of bipolar disorder but make no mention of his recent overdoses. One note from November mentions that, as a condition of his ongoing treatment at the hospital pain clinic, he had signed an agreement attesting that he would not obtain narcotics from other physicians.

In December 2002, Steven was dismissed from the hospital clinic for breaches of that narcotics agreement. The letter notifying him stated that he had been self-adjusting his doses and requesting pain medication early and that he had also refused to participate in routine blood and urine tests to screen for illicit substances and monitor compliance with his prescribed regimen. "Based on our policy, we are going to be discharging you immediately with no further pain medication prescribed and no further follow-ups to be scheduled," the letter said.

The next month, in January 2003, he became a patient at Tri-State Healthcare.

Four months later, when Tri-State moved to Portsmouth, Steven was among the many patients to visit Volkman during the doctor's first month at the clinic. In Volkman's summary notes, which he dictated after Steven's first visit, he noted a "history of bipolar disorder" and listed other psychological symptoms, including difficulty concentrating, irritability, fatigue, trouble sleeping, and excessive worry. But he said that those latter symptoms were "related to . . . the physical stressors presented by [his] medical conditions."

Under a section titled "Family History," Volkman noted, "Patient states he has smoked pot and taken cocaine in the past but denies having any abuse of narcotics." The summary included no mention of any prior suicide attempt or overdose, and Volkman later claimed to me that he had no knowledge of the suicide attempts. The notes acknowledged that Steven was previously treated at another pain clinic but did not mention his expulsion for noncompliance.

In a section titled "Management Plan," the first entry reads: "Use of chronic opioid therapy with objectives of improved sleep, reducing and controlling pain intensity, improving mobility, improvement of concentration ability, [and] improvement of daily functioning." A few entries below, Volkman mentioned his plan to add Valium to Hieneman's existing regimen of pain medications.

Steven walked away from his first visit to Volkman with prescriptions for 120 Percocet tablets and forty Valium.

———

Steven's visits to Tri-State were a cause of great concern for his mother, Paula, who believed that the medication her son was receiving there had the potential to kill him. In her later testimony, she recalled one conversation in which she told her son that she would rather kill the people who ran the clinic than watch him die from pills he was prescribed.

In addition to these conversations with Steven, Paula also made several calls directly to Tri-State. In one of these calls, she spoke with Alice. At another point, she reached Denise, whom she warned that Steven's prescriptions were enough to kill him. She also told Denise that she didn't want the doctor to see Steven again. In response, Denise reportedly told Paula that Steven was a "big boy" who could make up his own mind. To this, Paula responded to Denise that if Tri-State treated her son again, that she would go there personally, pull Denise out of the clinic, and "burn you like the little white witch you are there right out . . . in the middle of the street."

Paula was not finished.

One morning, she drove to the clinic to try to intercept Volkman on his way into work. She would later say that when she saw him coming, she got out of the car and tried to tell him about the danger she believed her son was in. Steven had heart problems, she said, and she pleaded with the doctor to stop seeing him. "You're going to kill him," she said.

She recalled that Volkman didn't stop to listen to her. His only response, as she recalled, was to say, "Get away from me, you crazy woman," before disappearing inside the building.

"That was the only opportunity I ever had to talk to Dr. Volkman," she would later testify.

Steven continued to see Volkman for months despite his mother's concerns. The doctor's notes from his visits indicate that Steven reported pain in his wrist, arm, and shoulder, as well as muscle spasms. A note from August 2003 shows that he was advised to take the following daily regimen of medications:

- One 5/325-milligram tablet of Percocet six times per day.
- One 5-milligram oxycodone tablet six times per day.
- One 10-milligram tablet of the opioid painkiller Demerol three times per day.
- One 500-milligram tablet of the nonsteroidal anti-inflammatory pain medication Disalcid three times per day.

• And one 10-milligram tablet of the sedative Valium three times per day.

In Volkman's notes from November, he wrote that Steven's pain symptoms were "well tolerated with meds." Steven's visits continued until early 2004, when he was dismissed from the clinic for not showing up for a pill count.

Steven was somehow re-accepted at the clinic thirteen months later, in February 2005. His records from that day make no note of the gap in his care, the reasons for his prior dismissal, or the conditions of his return. Once again, the doctor made a note of the patient's ailments and symptoms as if nothing out of the ordinary had occurred: "RSD, Clenched Fist Syndrome . . . Neck + Shoulder pain . . . Low back pain at times."

Steven left that day with prescriptions for Percocet, Valium, and Disalcid. For unclear reasons, he did not return in March.

Steven's last visit to Volkman took place on April 19, 2005. Volkman's notes from that visit indicate that the patient's pain level remained at a 7 out of 10, and the spasms in his legs were "very bad." Steven also reported that he had recently tripped over a concrete drain-off while at a park near his home and fell into a nearby car, breaking off the mirror and injuring his leg and arm. He left the clinic with prescriptions for 30 two-milligram tablets of Xanax, 360 fifteen-milligram tablets of oxycodone, and 120 ten-milligram tablets of Valium.

Paula Eastley later testified that she spoke with Steven five times on the phone that day. During one call, she told him that she was having the windows of her house cleaned for spring. In a call later in the evening, he told her that the spaghetti he had cooked for dinner had given him an upset stomach. During her courtroom testimony, when she was asked if it seemed like her son was under the influence of pills, she said that he sounded "straight as he could be."

According to Steven's partner, Jon Kiser, that night they were in bed watching the movie *Somewhere in Time*. Steven's feet were in Jon's lap, and the dog was in the bed next to him. They both fell asleep. Then, at some point, Jon woke up and moved Steven's feet off his lap so he could go to the bathroom. Steven's feet were cold.

Jon told me that he was initially "scared shitless," but he said that his instincts as a nurse soon kicked in and he dialed 911 and started performing

CPR. But he could tell from the stiffness of Steven's jaw that he was already gone.

Later that day, Steven's body was transported to the Kentucky medical examiner's main laboratory in Frankfort, where an autopsy was performed. The doctor began with an external examination, noting Steven's height of six feet; his scars, tattoos, and bruises; the "gray/tan" color of his eyes, his "short reddish mustache," his short "blonde/reddish" hair with bits of gray, and the "faint pierce hole" in his left earlobe. After making a Y-shaped incision in his abdomen, she examined and weighed the lungs, liver, spleen, kidneys, brain, and thyroid. She closely examined his heart and recorded the "significant" degree of blockage in key arteries: One was 30 percent blocked, two others were 60 and 70 percent blocked, respectively. Her findings were summarized in a report that also included the results of a toxicological analysis on Steven's blood and urine. Those tests identified the presence of oxycodone, alprazolam, and diazepam.

The doctor found that Steven's primary cause of death was the acute combined effects of the medications in his system, with a contributory cause of heart disease. In the section of his death certificate asking how his fatal injury occurred, the coroner wrote, "Drug Overdose."

He was thirty-three years old.

THE RAID

Paul Volkman's apartment in Portsmouth was considerably less glamorous than his home back in Chicago. He rented an apartment in a two-story house on Center Street, a quiet, brick-paved street about two miles from downtown. A search warrant later described the house as "a beige two story wood frame structure" with a gray shingle roof and "the numbers 1310 painted on the steps leading up to the front door."

On the morning of June 7, 2005, at around ten fifteen, three DEA agents walked to the front door of the house and knocked. There was no response.

The agents saw lights on inside and heard a TV playing, so they proceeded to the back door, where they knocked again. When Volkman opened the door, an agent explained to him that a search warrant was being executed at the pain clinic. The agents were interested in interviewing him at home, to avoid the commotion at the office. Volkman declined, but he later drove to the office and agreed to an interview there.

Trial testimony and evidence would later paint a vivid picture of what happened at the clinic that day. A representative from the Ohio State Board of Medicine who accompanied the DEA on the raid testified that she noticed several odd things about the clinic. Some medical records were stored in a stove in a kitchen area. Urine-specimen cups with urine in them sat on the floor. Miscellaneous pills were found in drawers. In the clinic's exam rooms, she saw no thermometers for taking patients' temperatures. She also noted the absence of a light box for viewing X-rays.

At some point during the day's raid, a video recording was made to capture the appearance of the building's interior. Portions of the grainy twenty-eight-minute video were later shown during the trial.

The video begins upstairs, in the nonpublic portion of the clinic, in what appears to be some kind of nursery or daycare space, filled with toys, stuffed animals, and high chairs. As the camera pans past the adjoining kitchen, viewers see an overflowing trash can, a sink containing dirty dishes, and a rifle propped against a wall.

From there, the camera operator moves to an office — presumably Volkman's — with two white coats hanging in a closet and a chess set sitting on an upper shelf of the desk. Down the hall, another office is cluttered with binders, folders, and stacks of paper. On the floor, wedged between various bags and a shoebox, is a second rifle.

Downstairs, on the clinic's main floor, the camera-holder walks through an administrative area with filing cabinets, corkboards on the wall, and tall shelves containing hundreds of folders for patient records. There are also examination rooms that have sinks, scales, exam tables, and physical exam equipment (an otoscope, an ophthalmoscope). Posters on the wall read LOW BACK AND SCIATIC PAIN and WHIPLASH INJURIES OF THE HEAD AND NECK.

Down the hall from these exam rooms, in the back section of the first floor, is the dispensary. The entrance is a two-part door that, when closed, has a solid wood lower portion and a top portion protected by metal bars, with an open space through which money and pills could be passed. Beyond this doorway is a cramped, narrow space with fake-wood paneling on the walls. The camera pans past drawers filled with empty prescription bottles, an ashtray with numerous cigarette butts, and a dispenser with ribbons of stickers for placing on pill bottles that read TAKE WITH FOOD and KEEP OUT OF REACH OF CHILDREN.

Much of the counter space in the pharmacy is occupied by what appears to be an assembly-line operation. The camera pans past stacks of prefilled bottles of pills that are hand-labeled with a marker: 90 LORCET, 90 VALIUM, 120 SOMA, 30 XANAX. In one corner of the dispensary is a cash register with pricing guides — based on the medication, dosage, and pill counts — taped to the walls above it. The camera lingers on the sheets so that certain entries are legible: 120 Xanax cost $30, while 180 cost $38. In another column 150 thirty-milligram oxycodone pills are priced at $270, while 200 pills are $360.

Within arm's reach of the cash register is a large wooden club propped against an emergency exit. On the other side stands a tall heavy-duty safe with its door ajar, revealing a handgun on a shelf inside.

During the day's raid, agents conducted interviews with Denise, Alice, and Paul. And excerpts from these conversations would later be typed into affidavits and recounted from witness stands.

During Denise's interview, she confirmed that the clinic accepted only cash. Alice, in her session, told investigators that the clinic's security staff was necessary due to the value of the medications stocked by the dispensary, but also as a precaution against disruptions from patients who became unruly after being dismissed.

Volkman met in an examination room with three agents from the DEA and two representatives of the Ohio Medical Board. At the outset, one of the DEA agents told him that he didn't have to speak to them; he was not under arrest, he was told, and he could leave at any time. His response, after looking around the room, was, reportedly, "It doesn't look like I'm not under arrest." And yet he said that he was curious to hear what the DEA had to say, so he stayed.

During the ensuing conversation — and in the absence of an attorney — Volkman spoke about a number of topics. He discussed his background, including his education and experiences in pediatrics and ER medicine. He spoke about the two modes of treatment the clinic offered: prescribed medication and free yoga classes. He spoke about the methods he used to monitor patient compliance, including pill counts and urine screenings. He claimed that such measures ensured that there were no addicts among the clinic's patients.

At one point in the conversation, he acknowledged that he didn't consult with other physicians in the area. And during Volkman's trial, a DEA agent who participated in the interview recalled what the doctor said about his lack of malpractice insurance. "He said he didn't need it, that his patients needed him and they wouldn't sue him," the agent testified.

The interviews with principal players of Tri-State Healthcare that day offered a preview of the finger-pointing that would intensify when the clinic came under further scrutiny.

During Denise's interview, she acknowledged that she ordered the pills for the dispensary but said that Paul directed her on what to order. She also stated that the clinic had never had problems with local pharmacies before Volkman's arrival.

Alice said that she was uncomfortable with the scripts Paul was writing and felt they were excessive. And she mentioned two instances when patients may have died after taking meds he prescribed. She admitted that she was generally responsible for filling the prescriptions at the dispensary, which constituted a violation of Ohio laws requiring that Paul sign off on every pill that was dispensed. She also acknowledged that there were no inventory records of the medications dispensed, which was also required by law. She stated that decisions about which patients got dismissed were made by Paul.

Volkman, for his part, attempted to toss responsibility back on Denise. He said she owned the clinic and played a deciding role in who became patients at Tri-State because she knew many of them personally. He also said that if the results of a patient's urine screen raised concerns, it was Denise who had the final say about whether the patient stayed or went. The dispensary, he continued, was entirely the Huffmans' responsibility; though, when pressed, he said that he could personally account for every pill that had gone out the door. At one point, he also attempted to push some responsibility onto the Ohio Board of Pharmacy, which, he said, having inspected and okayed the on-site pharmacy, was at fault if anything didn't look right.

Later that day, once the agents had dispersed, the Cincinnati DEA office received a phone call from Volkman, who asked to speak to the agent in charge. Instead, one of the agents who had interviewed him earlier in the day returned the doctor's call. When Volkman asked whether he was allowed to remain in business, the agent explained that there were no current restrictions on his DEA registration. When Volkman then asked if there were criminal charges pending against him, the agent said that he couldn't answer that, but he suggested that Volkman could try calling the US attorney's office.

THE END OF THE PARTNERSHIP

There is little doubt that Paul's relationship with the Huffmans deteriorated after the DEA raid. But as with many aspects of their partnership, there are conflicting accounts about what happened and who was to blame.

Paul told me that, after the raid, Denise became upset that the clinic's client base was shrinking. Throughout his time at Tri-State, he said, he continued to dismiss patients who didn't abide by his conditions for treatment. And he has also suggested that patients may have been spooked by the DEA's visit and decided not to return. "In either case, in her mind, [I] was clearly to blame," he said.

Notably, in this version of the story, he's the Good Guy who was standing up for the integrity of the clinic, while she is more interested in herding people through its doors. As he once told me, "She was pissed off that I was testing all these people and kicking out all of her patients."

Volkman has also said that, by the late summer of 2005, he had lost trust in Denise. He believed that she was skimming pills from the dispensary and using them in a quid pro quo scheme with an acquaintance at the racetrack-casino that she frequented. According to Volkman, Denise would give pills to an accomplice, and, in return, "the guy would either tell her which machines were going to win and when, or have some way of controlling that from the back room" so that the machines dished out winnings in her favor. He said she "won" thousands of dollars this way. He called it "basically a money-laundering operation."

Volkman also told me that he was increasingly fed up with Denise's unpredictability. In one instance, he said that he traveled to Portsmouth with the expectation of a regular workweek, only to find that she had closed the clinic for the week without telling him.

He reached his breaking point one Friday when she didn't return from the casino in time to give him his paycheck. This was the reason he finally chose to quit the clinic.

Alice Huffman told me that, over the time that Volkman worked at Tri-State, her initial impression of him changed. She said she first glimpsed a more unpleasant side to him when pharmacists called to ask questions or express concern about his prescriptions. In those calls, she said, he "would rudely remind them that he was a doctor and he meant to prescribe it that way and their job was to fill it."

She saw other changes during Volkman's tenure. As the months passed,

Volkman spent less time with patients, began prescribing more pills, grew more hurried and careless with his documentation of patient visits, and seemed less concerned with monitoring the dispensary. He was increasingly rude in conversations with the staff, she said. And, she said, "He was always asking Mom for more money and was doing less work."

In this tale, Volkman's portrait of culpability is flipped. As Alice told it, the Huffmans were the honest and upright clinic operators who hired an initially promising physician who then, for unclear reasons, went bad.

Denise, meanwhile, has said that she grew tired of Volkman's arrogance. In one sworn deposition, she referred to his behavior in his final months at the clinic as "erratic" and "rude" and said that he was prone to "little fits" and "temper tantrums." She has also said, during separate testimony, that he became increasingly unmanageable. "Dr. Volkman did what Dr. Volkman wanted to do," she said. In her version of the story, which she delivered under oath in federal court, she said that Paul didn't leave Tri-State on his own; he was fired.

During a lawsuit related to Tri-State in Scioto County Court in 2008, an attorney for Denise offered a bit more detail on how and why this firing supposedly happened. According to this account, Denise was unaware of any problems at the clinic until the DEA raid in June 2005, and, afterward, she made efforts to get the clinic into good legal standing. This included, in September 2005, complying with a DEA request to examine additional pharmacy logs from the clinic. And as her attorney framed it, during her visit to the DEA's office in Cincinnati, she had some sort of wake-up call about the physician she had employed for almost two and a half years.

"She didn't even wait until she got back from Cincinnati," her attorney told the jury. "She got on the telephone; called her daughter who was the office manager [and] told her to fire Dr. Volkman."

Whatever the exact circumstances, in early September 2005, Volkman parted ways with Tri-State Healthcare. His last day was Friday, September 9.

But there would be one more noteworthy incident before Denise and Paul's partnership completely ended. It happened on the evening of Volkman's departure, when he returned to the clinic after business hours to gather patient files and prescription pads, which he planned to use at his next clinic location. This late-night visit was recorded by the clinic's internal security-camera system, and edited footage was later posted to a local online message board called Moe's Forum.

The video, as posted, is a little more than eight minutes long. And it's composed of somewhat grainy footage from two security cameras inside the Tri-State clinic. One camera is positioned in an upper corner of the waiting room. Another is positioned near the ceiling of a small office abutting the clinic's entry area.

The video begins with the empty waiting room at night when Volkman arrives, wearing khakis and a tucked-in orange golf shirt that fits rather snugly around his midsection. Shortly after entering, he walks to the room's windows that face the street and twists a rod to close the vertical slatted blinds. He repeats this action twice until all the blinds facing Findlay Street are closed.

Over the course of the video, Volkman moves between the waiting area and the office. At times he speaks on the phone (though, without sound, it's unclear who he's speaking to or what he's saying). The primary purpose of his visit seems to be obtaining stacks of file folders — apparently containing patient records — which he places in plastic grocery bags that he has brought. Over the course of the video, he fills at least half a dozen bags with folders. At one point, he gets down on his knees and rummages under the desk in the office and returns with a box of what appear to be prescription pads, which he inspects, and then also carries into the other room to take with him.

About halfway through the soundless footage a large guy wearing sneakers, jean shorts, and a cutoff T-shirt arrives on the scene. This, apparently, is Alice's then husband, Chad, who was working as a security guard for the clinic at the time. In the footage, Chad makes phone calls and then, a bit later, two police officers arrive, and the four of them — Volkman, Chad, and the two police officers — engage in a conversation. The footage remains soundless.

Nothing appears to result from this conversation. The police officers don't handcuff Volkman or otherwise stop him. As the video ends, he picks up two of the bags containing files and exits the building, leaving the security guard and police behind.

The website where the video was posted, Moe's Forum, was a place where citizens gathered, often under pseudonyms, to swap observations and juicy tidbits about Portsmouth and Scioto County. At one point I spoke to the operator of that site, who was a local blues musician named Joe Ferguson. He explained that the local news outlets' narrow focus and general unwillingness to report critically on law enforcement left a lot of room for stories to be told. As a result, he said you could often learn more about what was *really* going on locally from his site. The Volkman video was an example of this.

Ferguson was given the footage by the Huffmans, and he told me that he found the clip doubly newsworthy. Not only did it show a doctor's sketchy late-night visit to a local pain clinic from which he had recently been fired, but it was also, to Ferguson's eyes, a case study in local corruption. He thought it showed two police officers who were called to the scene of an unfolding break-in and did nothing to stop it.

When I spoke to him in 2010, Ferguson was still proud of obtaining and posting the video, which caused a good bit of buzz on the site. He told me that Volkman's nighttime visit to Tri-State had gone entirely unmentioned by local news outlets. "But Moe's Forum reported it," he said.

When I asked Volkman about the incident, he didn't deny that it was him in the video, or that he had gone to the clinic late that night, drawn the blinds, placed patient files in bags, and, at one point, spoken with a police officer. And as usual, he offered no acknowledgment of how bizarre or unflattering the whole situation appeared. Instead he framed it as an example of his attempts to best serve his patients who might otherwise have been disrupted by his departure from Tri-State.

He told me that after he made the decision to leave Tri-State, his attorney advised him that the medical records belonged to him and that he ought to retrieve them to ensure continuing care of his patients, which, in Volkman's words, was "required by Ohio law." In Volkman's telling, the lawyer further advised him that any dispute over ownership of patient records would be a civil matter, not a criminal one, and thus the local police had no authority to interfere. This, he said, explained why the officers in the video took no action to stop him.

He also described closing the blinds as a prudent safety measure. "I pulled the blinds because I was alone in an office in a crime-ridden area at midnight," he said.

SCOTTIE

Scottie Lin James had dark hair and a dazzling smile. At Portsmouth High School, she had been a cheerleader and honor-roll student.

Scottie had two sisters, Terrie and Jakkie, who were five and eight years younger than her, respectively. Their dad wasn't around when they grew up, and when their mom died in 1993, Scottie took on a surrogate mother role. "She finished raising us," Jakkie told me.

In the years after her mother's death, Scottie got married, gave birth to a daughter, got divorced, and later had a second daughter in 1999. She worked as a telemarketer and as an aide in a nursing home. "She always made sure we had everything," Jakkie said.

One of her jobs was at the office of Dr. John Lilly, the Portsmouth-based pill mill doctor who was famous for the lines of patients outside his office on Chillicothe Street. Jakkie told me that Scottie helped Lilly with paperwork and patient files and was paid for her work in prescriptions.

To hear Jakkie tell it, at that time, pain clinics were simply an established part of Scioto County's economy. People would go to the doctor and get pills to sell, take, or both. And sometimes people who didn't do drugs would be "sponsored" by other people who would pay for their visit and then take a cut of the pills they were prescribed.

Jakkie told me that the pain clinics functioned on an unspoken understanding among everyone involved. "You went in there and literally would sit next to your uncles or aunts that you ain't seen in years," she said. "And you just know to keep your mouth shut." Everybody knew why they were there.

Jakkie remembered looking forward to her own eighteenth birthday, when she could become a patient of Dr. Lilly and start selling pills.

"I was ready for the money," she told me.

Jakkie and others described Scottie as kind, generous, and charismatic. She always had a big bright smile. "Everybody loved her," Jakkie said.

Scottie was also a drug user. By the time that Dr. Volkman arrived in town, she had been taking pills for years. Medical records indicate that Scottie first visited Volkman at his office on Gay Street in September 2003 with complaints of severe pain due to a recent diagnosis of ovarian cancer. At that first visit, she received prescriptions for oxycodone, Xanax, an antihistamine, and a pain-relieving patch with the powerful narcotic fentanyl. Within a few weeks of that appointment, however, phone calls from Tri-State to Scottie's doctors revealed that she had no history of a cancer diagnosis, and she was dismissed from the practice for falsifying her symptoms.

But when Volkman split from the Huffmans two years later, it offered a chance for Scottie to try visiting the doctor once again. And when Scottie went to Volkman's new clinic in Portsmouth, in September 2005, the doctor saw her and wrote prescriptions for Soma, Xanax, Percocet, and oxycodone. She returned ten days later for a second appointment and another round of Percocet and oxycodone prescriptions.

By this time, the fall of 2005, Jakkie was used to seeing her sister use drugs. But after one of Scottie's trips to Volkman, she said that Scottie was higher than Jakkie had ever seen her. Scottie's head was tilted back, and she was making a disturbing gurgling sound. Jakkie called her other sister, Terrie, and together they tended to Scottie, alternating hot and cold compresses and trying to wake her up. When they discussed going to the hospital, Scottie made sounds of objection, so they didn't go. Jakkie later described this incident as an overdose.

Scottie eventually sobered up and asked Jakkie to use her phone to score more drugs. An argument ensued. Eventually, Jakkie relented, but as soon as Scottie's call ended, Jakkie said she called the person her sister had just spoken with to tell them about Scottie's recent overdose and to urge them not to give her anything. She remembered telling them, "If you sell her anything and she dies, it's going to be on you." She said she made five or six of these calls.

Jakkie knew Scottie was intent on getting drugs and feared for her sister's life, given the events she had just witnessed. Jakkie begged her not to go anywhere, and when Scottie left the house, Jakkie walked with her, pleading, on the streets of Portsmouth.

"Please, Scottie," she remembered telling her. "I don't want to lose another mother. Please don't leave."

She remembered her sister replying, "I'll be OK, sissy. I'll see you tomorrow."

On September 29, 2005, Portsmouth police received a call about a possible overdose at a house on the city's East End. Upon arriving, officers found Scottie James lying motionless on the bathroom floor. Scottie's family members told officers that she had gone to Volkman's new office earlier in the week and received prescriptions for oxycodone, Xanax, and Soma. A search warrant from the Portsmouth police provides more detail about the investigation:

The family members advised that Scottie James was in fact a known drug user and that all of the prescription medication that she got from Dr. Volkman was already gone. The family members advised that they took a pill bottle away from Scottie earlier in the week and Officers of the Portsmouth Police Department later recovered and impounded the bottle. The bottle was empty and written to Scottie James for (135) Roxicet 5mg tablets, which is Oxycodone. The prescription was written by Dr. Paul Volkman for (9) tablets per day which would be a (15) day supply. The prescription was filled at East Main Street Pharmacy in Columbus, Ohio on September 27, 2005, which was two days before her death.

Among the items the police collected from the scene of Scottie's death was an appointment card instructing her to return to Volkman's office on October 7.

A toxicology analysis performed after her death identified the presence of numerous drugs, including oxycodone, benzodiazepine, and a metabolite of cocaine.

Jakkie believed medications from Volkman were the cause of Scottie's first overdose — the one that Jakkie and Terrie witnessed. She believed that, later, after Scottie left, she smoked crack and then took more of the pills Volkman had prescribed, to "come down" from the high.

She died just days after her thirtieth birthday.

THE HOUSE ON CENTER STREET

During his time in Portsmouth, Paul Volkman rented an apartment on the first floor of a house in a quiet, residential part of town. The address was 1310 Center Street.

"Center Street" is, in fact, not at the center of anything in Portsmouth. The one-block street is located about a mile and a half from the downtown business district, and the street itself is only about two hundred yards long. Like some of Portsmouth's less-trafficked streets, it remains paved with red brick, which makes it a throwback to the days when all the city's streets were paved that way. Car tires rolling on those bricks made a moist, rubbery rumbling sound. During Volkman's trial, a former investigator with the Portsmouth police described it as "a low-income area of our town" with quite a few vacant houses.

At one point, in 2003, Volkman wrote to a friend that when he was in Portsmouth he "essentially never go[es] out except to and from the clinic." So for the first two and a half years that he had commuted to town, the Center Street house was simply a modest place where Volkman slept when he was in town.

But in the days after his split from Denise Huffman, this changed. For a few weeks — in the most bizarre chapter of his tenure in pain management — Volkman attempted to run a pain clinic out of this house.

In the days following his split from Tri-State, he outfitted the apartment with phones, fax machines, and filing cabinets. He transformed the living room into a waiting room, complete with folding chairs. The kitchen was turned into a business office; a first-floor bedroom was converted into an exam room. He would later say that the house's interior was arranged in "quite a respectable manner regardless of how the neighborhood and the outside of the house looked."

The house never had any kind of sign indicating that it was now a medical facility. Although, later, prosecutors did submit as evidence a handwritten note that was affixed to the front porch. The page read: PLEASE USE BACK YARD TO WAIT.

Like many aspects of Volkman's case, the exact nature of what happened at 1310 Center Street is disputed in legal filings, trial testimony, and elsewhere. But all parties involved seem to agree on some basic facts.

By Volkman's own admission, the Center Street clinic was, like Tri-State Healthcare, a cash-only operation with office visit fees of around $150. And by his own account, at around eight o'clock on the first morning of operation — Monday, September 12, 2005 — there was a crowd of more than a hundred people on hand to fill out patient-intake paperwork.

The clinic's first day of business also marked the start of a series of complaints to Portsmouth police. According to law enforcement documents, the first call that police received was from a neighbor who was alarmed by a jump in the number of cars parked on the street. Two days later, another call described the house as a "pill mill." On September 26, two weeks after the clinic opened, yet another tip informed police that, at ten thirty that morning, there were seventeen people on the front porch waiting to see the doctor. One resident of Center Street later told the *Portsmouth Daily Times*, "A lot of neighbors are mad around here."

One of those neighbors was Sammie Ishmael, who lived directly next door to Volkman's house. She later described to me the dramatic changes that took place on Center Street after the clinic opened. As she told it, cars with license plates from Kentucky and West Virginia started appearing on the street. Crowds of people moved in and out of the house, spilling out into the backyard, the front porch, and the sidewalk in front of her house. One day she saw a van sitting in front of her house, filled with people. It was hot that day, and a passenger door of the car was open; inside, a woman was knitting. On other days, she returned home to find clusters of cigarette butts and greasy fast-food wrappers strewn across her front yard and walkway.

Ishmael told me that people came to the clinic at all hours of the day. And because there was no sign on the house identifying it as a clinic, some visitors mistakenly came to her house. She told me that she had knocks on her door at 5:00 and 6:00 A.M. from patients asking to see the doctor. She said that these people had slurred speech and dazed eyes.

After a few weeks, she was livid. She had complained constantly to the police but had seen no major changes to the operation next door. She had also tried speaking with Volkman. During one conversation, he had told her that the house was his new office and that he was in the process of obtaining a license to operate there.

Years later — and still clearly incredulous about the exchange — she recalled what she said in response.

"No, you aren't in [the] process to get your license there," she told him. "You need to take your doctor's office and take it to Chicago and put it in *your* neighborhood."

Inside the house, the clinic hummed with activity.

According to Volkman, he was seeing "about 35" patients there a day, with business starting about 8:00 A.M. and often continuing until 10:00 or 11:00 P.M. And based on his own numbers — thirty-five patients per day, paying $150 per visit — he was bringing in approximately $5,250 per day, which added up to over $25,000 per week. Without the Huffmans running the operation, the clinic's profits now went directly to him.

But despite the brisk business, Volkman had a problem: Leaving Tri-State meant leaving the on-site dispensary, which meant that he was once again reliant on pharmacies to fill his prescriptions. And given how many local pharmacists had previously refused to fill his scripts, there was no obvious solution.

Legal records indicate that at this time one of Volkman's patients, identified only by the initials D.S. in the records, helped to solve it. This patient apparently searched online for pharmacies in the area and made phone calls asking if they would fill scripts for oxycodone, hydrocodone, Xanax, and Soma in the dosages Volkman was prescribing. An unknown number of pharmacies said no; they told the caller that they either didn't have the meds in stock or weren't comfortable with the prescriptions. But one pharmacist agreed to the terms. His name was Harold Eugene Fletcher, and his store was ninety miles away, in Columbus.

Fletcher declined to speak with me for this project, so what I know about him is limited to what I could learn from various legal records. I know that he graduated from the Ohio State University's School of Pharmacy in 1991 and that he was licensed by the Ohio Board of Pharmacy the following year. I know that for six years he worked as a pharmacist at retail drug chains and in a hospital-based pharmacy; in 1998, he purchased a pharmacy practice in a Columbus building that included a medical office and dental practice. The business was called East Main Street Pharmacy.

Given the distance between Volkman's clinic and the pharmacy, some coordination was required between the two businesses. According to Volkman's former security guard, a call was made from Volkman's clinic "just about every day" to inform the pharmacist of the time when the doctor saw his last patient so that Fletcher knew when to expect his last customer. On some days, the pharmacist reportedly kept his shop open until midnight.

But such accommodations were apparently worth the trouble. Because in the weeks following his connection with Volkman, Fletcher saw a sharp influx of business and revenue. Records later discussed in DEA administrative proceedings show that his purchases of oxycodone and hydrocodone skyrocketed from 2004 to 2005 — specifically after September 2005, when his informal partnership with Volkman began. In 2004, East Main Street Pharmacy was the three hundredth largest purchaser of oxycodone in the state of Ohio. The following year, it jumped to the eleventh spot.

There were other noteworthy aspects of Fletcher's new influx of customers. According to DEA documents, "nearly ninety-nine percent" of the people who filled Volkman's prescriptions at his pharmacy didn't live in Columbus, and more than 85 percent of those patients paid for their prescriptions in cash, which was more than seven times higher than the national average of cash-paying customers.

And around the time when Fletcher welcomed his new rush of business, an employee at Commerce National Bank noticed a spike in his deposits and placed him on a "watch list" for suspicious activity. Other records indicate that during the month his partnership with Volkman began, the pharmacist made cash deposits on consecutive days of $9,000; $9,000; $9,750; and $9,900. He would continue to make similar deposits over the following months. In October, Fletcher even called the bank to ask about the legally required threshold for filing a deposit disclosure form and whether he could avoid that by making deposits into two separate accounts.*

Later, when DEA investigators asked about the due diligence he had performed to ensure that the doctor sending him so many customers was legitimate, Fletcher said that he had called Volkman, who told him about the MRI paperwork his patients produced in order to be seen and the blood tests the doctor ordered to ensure patient compliance. However, Fletcher admitted that Volkman's patients sometimes asked him to sell them extra pills (requests he said he declined); he was also aware that other pharmacies closer to Portsmouth had refused to fill Volkman's scripts. Fletcher apparently declined to call any of those pharmacists to hear their reasons because, as he told investigators, "I don't communicate with other pharmacists."

A former Volkman patient would later tell authorities that, during one trip to fill the doctor's prescription at East Main, she was so high that her speech was slurred, her walk was unsteady, her head was hanging down, and she was "probably drooling." And yet, when Fletcher was asked by investigators whether he believed that Volkman's patients were addicted, he responded that it was "hard to say." In those interviews with DEA agents, he maintained that decisions about the types and amounts of medications to prescribe belonged to a doctor and that it was "not his job to question a physician."

Volkman, it seems, had found a perfect partner: one who filled his prescriptions, didn't ask too many questions, and even kept his shop open to accommodate the unusual travel time between physician and pharmacist. Among the records from Center Street submitted in Volkman's trial was a printed page of directions from Mapquest.com. According to those

---

* Federal law requires reporting cash deposits of more than $10,000. Intentionally structuring deposits to avoid such reporting is a crime.

directions, the estimated drive time between Center Street and Fletcher's pharmacy was an hour and fifty-seven minutes.

Back on Center Street, Portsmouth police monitored Volkman's operation closely. According to a search warrant produced by the department, within days of the clinic opening, local officers sent in a patient wearing a wire who waited five hours before being called to see the doctor. During that visit, Volkman asked about previous injuries and surgeries, as well as the medications the patient had previously been prescribed. His physical exam consisted of checking the patient's reflexes and asking them to bend down to touch their toes. This visit resulted in the doctor writing prescriptions for 180 fifteen-milligram oxycodone pills, 180 ten-milligram Lorcets, 120 three hundred fifty-milligram Somas, and 90 two-milligram Xanax tablets. The patient was given a note with the name, address, and phone number of East Main Street Pharmacy, in Columbus.

Two days later, Portsmouth police sent in a second patient cooperating with their investigation. This time, documents indicated that there was a shorter wait, no physical exam, and Volkman wrote prescriptions for 270 thirty-milligram oxycodone pills, 270 five-milligram Percocets, 120 three hundred fifty-milligram Somas, and 60 two-milligram Xanax pills. According to police notes, Volkman instructed the patient to come back four days later, when he would give her more prescriptions.

And it wasn't just police who were following events on Center Street. In the weeks after their falling-out, Denise Huffman expressed her shock and outrage in comments on a local online chat board.* Whether Huffman's outrage was genuine or feigned to make herself look innocent by comparison is unclear. But in one comment she called Volkman "Dr. Doom," and, in another, she wrote, "Seriously I can't believe what I'm seeing . . . How can someone act one way and turn out to be this bad?"

In another comment, she asked what was taking the DEA so long to shut him down. "Wonder what they are waiting on," she wrote. "Corpses on his front porch?"

At Volkman's trial, numerous witnesses would help to paint a picture of what took place inside the Center Street house. But the testimony of two witnesses, a former patient and his mother, stood out.

---

* Screenshots of these comments were eventually included in the Portsmouth police's search warrant for the Center Street house.

Danny Colley was in recovery from a drug addiction but had recently relapsed at the time that Volkman's Center Street clinic opened. And on the witness stand he described the toll that drugs had taken on his life. Pills had taken "everything imaginable" from him, he said: his kids, his relationship with his mother, his ability to work. On drugs, he said he had become a "complete monster" who didn't care about himself or anyone else.

When the prosecutor asked him why he had gone to see Volkman at the house-turned-clinic, his answer was blunt: "'Cause that's where the medication was."

He went on to explain that he had heard about Volkman through the network of people who sold and used drugs. He did not have an appointment to see the doctor; he just showed up. He didn't have any medical records with him that day.

During his testimony, when he was asked to describe what he looked like at the time, he said that he was "dirty" and "sweaty." He said that he was frequently dope-sick at the time, and, as a result, he could barely talk. "I was a drug addict," he said.

Nevertheless, he was given an appointment to see the doctor. And Colley testified that, during the visit, he told the doctor that he had previously undergone spinal surgery, which was true, and he also told the doctor that he was a previous patient, which was not true. He testified that Volkman instructed him to bend over, and perhaps the doctor ran a hand up Colley's back. "He just acted like he knew me, so I went along with it," Colley testified.

Colley walked out that day with prescriptions for oxycodone, hydrocodone, Xanax, and Soma.

When Danny's mother, Diana, found out that her son was going to a local pain clinic, she was extremely worried. Danny had recently gotten clean and was living in transitional housing at the time. And it was painfully clear to her that he had relapsed. He couldn't focus. He would nod off mid-conversation.

Diana Colley is not someone you want to tick off.

She's tall and solidly built. By her own description, she was "raised up really hard" in a particularly gritty part of Portsmouth. She had previously worked as an assistant manager at a Walmart for a decade. And in the fall of 2005, she owned and operated a bar in downtown Portsmouth and also worked as a prison guard at the state penitentiary in Lucasville, fifteen miles north.

Eventually, she found out where her son was getting his drugs. And as she described from the witness stand at Volkman's trial, one day she decided to pay the doctor on Center Street a visit.

The house was crowded when she got there, with around twenty people sitting or standing on the front porch. Once she walked inside, she saw more people sitting on folding chairs in the living-room-turned-waiting-room. There was a woman who appeared to be some kind of nurse or receptionist, and when Diana asked to speak with the doctor, the woman responded that the doctor was currently with a patient. Soon thereafter, Diana grabbed the woman by the throat and, as she described from the witness stand, "kind of convinced her" to tell her where the doctor was.

The woman pointed toward Volkman's exam room.

Diana proceeded to the room and opened the door into what appeared to be a converted bedroom. Volkman was sitting at a desk and talking to a patient.

Interrupting the conversation, Diana told the doctor her son's name and explained that he was an addict who had recently gotten clean. He was now strung out again, and she pleaded with him not to write him anymore prescriptions.

His response, as she would later recall, was strikingly calm. "I'll take it under consideration," he told her.

Diana wasn't satisfied with the answer.

She swept the papers off his desk for emphasis and told the doctor that she had a .38 pistol in her car. "If you write another prescription in my son's name, I will blow your brains out," she told him.

Diana Colley's fears were not unreasonable.

By this point, since Volkman's arrival in southern Ohio, investigators had identified, or would soon identify, at least eight patients who had died within days of visiting him and filling his prescriptions. Many of those patients were under the age of forty. And the pattern continued on Center Street.

First was the death of Scottie Lin James, who died on September 29 after seeing the doctor at the house. And on the day after James's death, a patient named Bryan Brigner made a visit to Volkman's clinic.

Brigner was a thirty-nine-year-old father of four. He was a tall, lanky guy who kept his hair long, wore a Dale Earnhardt baseball hat, and always kept a pack of Marlboros in the breast pocket of his T-shirt. His daughter told me, "He just loved his kids more than anything."

A carpenter by trade, Brigner had worked in various demanding physical jobs, including construction, logging, and shifts at a local cabinet factory. But he had been collecting disability for six years, due to a series of injuries and ailments. In 1995, he was in a car wreck where he broke his nose and injured his back. In 2001, he was in another car accident where he injured his back and sustained nerve damage. His medical records also mentioned a number of additional on-the-job injuries and a series of MRI tests and X-rays he had undergone in an effort to pinpoint the exact source of his pain.

Brigner had seen Volkman twice on Findlay Street before the doctor left Tri-State, and during those visits, he had complained of pain in his neck, side, and lower back. In response, he had received prescriptions for Lortab, Valium, oxycodone, and Soma. His third visit to the doctor was on Center Street. That day he received prescriptions for two opioids (oxycodone and hydrocodone), a muscle relaxer (Soma), and a sedative (Valium). His daily medication regimen, as laid out in Volkman's notes, recommended that he take eight 30-milligram oxycodone pills over the course of the day, in addition to eight Lortabs, three 10-milligram Valiums, and three Somas.

Less than forty-eight hours after his last visit to the doctor, Brigner died at home in his apartment in West Portsmouth. After both an autopsy and toxicological analysis were performed, his death certificate recorded his cause of death as "Cardiopulmonary Arrest" due to "Drug Intoxication."

On October 4, 2005, a local judge signed a seventy-page search warrant for the house on Center Street. The document, prepared by Portsmouth police, noted that Volkman was seeing between thirty and fifty patients a day at the house, often until late in the evening. It also stated that no pharmacies in Scioto County would fill Volkman's prescriptions. Officers wrote, "Many patients appear to be very young, possibly late teens, early twenties . . . [a]nd display no signs of injuries or malformations." Elsewhere the warrant noted: "Toddlers have been observed in office in presence of above-described patients and can be heard on a recording made by a confidential informant who was seen as a patient."

On that day, WSAZ Channel 3 reporter Randy Yohe was at the TV station's office in Huntington, West Virginia, when he got a call from a law enforcement source about the impending raid of the house on Center Street. Knowing this would be a worthwhile story, he hustled into a car, hopped on Route 52, and headed west toward Portsmouth, about an hour away. When he arrived on Center Street, he found that the house had been cordoned off with yellow crime-scene tape. Portsmouth police officers had backed a truck up to the house and were wheeling away boxes from inside. Yohe saw patients being handcuffed and questioned. The police chief and the assistant county prosecutor were both on the scene.

Police made a thorough inventory of what they found in the house that day. They collected medical files from the top of the desk and the floor in Volkman's makeshift office. They took his briefcase from the trunk of his black Subaru sedan. They combed through filing cabinets in the kitchen that were stocked with more than four hundred patient files. They counted the cash they found in a Sentry safe in a kitchen drawer; it amounted to $3,212.14. They wrote in one note that they had found "1 Blue pill labeled 4356, 20 MG found in hallway between [living room] and kitchen."

Outside the house, one officer tallied the out-of-county cars that were parked on the block at the time of the raid. There were thirteen from Kentucky, four from Ohio, and one from West Virginia. "Most traffic bypassed the street due to the police vehicles in the street, and still the traffic was heavier than normal for a residential street," the officer wrote.

On the day after the raid, a story ran in the *Portsmouth Daily Times* with the headline: "Dr. Volkman Again Target of Police Raid." In the article, one Center Street resident described recently seeing license plates from Indiana and Michigan among the cars on the street. "It was just a racket down there. I didn't know what was going on, but I'm glad it's taken care of," he said. The article estimated that fifty people were inside the house when police arrived.

Portsmouth police chief Charles Horner told the *Times* that it was "very strange and highly unusual for law enforcement to come across something like this."

Assistant Scioto County prosecutor Pat Apel, who was also interviewed, confirmed that his office was investigating Volkman. But he spoke about the challenge of bringing a successful criminal case against a doctor. "To prosecute a case that involves a physician and prescribing drugs you have to show it was not a bona fide treatment of a patient," he said. "That has to do with what the subjective intent of the doctor is . . . That's pretty difficult."

Accompanying the article was a picture taken from the backyard of 1310 Center during the raid. Six people were pictured, sitting on folding metal chairs, looking dejected. They appeared to be in their thirties, forties, and fifties. A few were smoking cigarettes. A uniformed police officer stood behind them, his hands clasped behind his back, his eyes obscured by dark sunglasses.

Volkman was not arrested that day, although he was temporarily handcuffed. As part of the raid, he received a legal notice that the house could no longer be used as a clinic. But for the time being, he was not charged with any crime.

And even after two raids of his offices by law enforcement, he was determined to continue working. According to his own remarks about this time, when the Center Street raid occurred he had already signed a multi-year lease and placed a $10,000 down payment on an office in downtown Portsmouth. But that plan was no good now. He needed to leave town.

He had a new clinic up and running within days.

NAKED TRUTHS

The *Portsmouth Daily Times* story on the raid at Volkman's house ran on the same day as an installment of a four-day series in the paper called "Naked Truths." The focus of the articles was prostitution: how it was rampant in the city, how it cut across class lines, how sometimes ten women were seen soliciting in a particular place at one time, and how a local judge had seen a woman who appeared to be a prostitute working one block from the high school. But it was also a series about prescription drugs. One of the articles was headlined "Process Starts with Addiction." Another was "More Drugs, More Prostitution."

In those articles, interviewees described the inextricable ties between the city's problems of prostitution and drugs. The program director for a local women's residential drug and alcohol treatment center told the paper, "I know almost all of those women out there, and they were all drug addicts first." She said that in cities like Las Vegas or New York, it was possible that sex work might be a conscious career choice, but in Portsmouth it was not.

A Portsmouth police lieutenant told the paper that he had no illusions about the source of the problem: "It's the drugs."

The police chief, who was also interviewed, agreed. "Drug use is far greater today than it may have been 20 or 30 years ago," he said.

A municipal judge told the paper that most women he had seen in his courtroom for prostitution-related charges were also addicted to drugs.

The county coroner, who spoke about an alarming spike in drug-related deaths in recent years, was similarly certain of the cause. "The greatest tragedy for me is to see a beautiful young person lying there for no good reason," he said.

Volkman was not mentioned by name in the articles — no local doctors were. But the medications Volkman prescribed in high volume certainly made an appearance.

In one article discussing a rash of recent deaths, the coroner said that opiates were the most common drug found in the decedents' system, followed by benzodiazepines such as Valium and Xanax.

"Something we frequently see is two or three of these drugs in the system with alcohol, not an overdose of one drug in their system," he said.

In another article, the *Times* reporter spoke with a local woman described as "the mother of a 38-year-old prostitute" and who was referred to by the pseudonym "Katie." Katie's daughter had previously had a job and been enrolled at Shawnee State University but started taking Xanax after the death of a boyfriend.

Her addiction escalated from there. And as the article noted, "Katie became frustrated as her daughter frequented 'pill mills,' the common name for clinics or offices that have doctors with reputations for liberally prescribing medication."

ERNEST

Melissa Ratcliff said that it was love at first sight.

It was the late 1980s in Grayson, Kentucky, a town of around thirty-five hundred located forty miles south of Portsmouth. Melissa was a senior in high school, and on some nights she and her friends would hang out at the Kmart parking lot. On any given night, there could be dozens of cars and a large crowd of teenagers.

Melissa was there with some friends one night when she saw an old, bright-yellow 1970s-style van pull up. The car had been souped up with big racing tires. It was "hideous," she said. But when the window rolled down, she saw a handsome man a few years older than her behind the steering wheel. He had dark eyes, dark hair, and a mustache. He looked at her and said, "Hey, beautiful. What are you doing?"

His name was Ernest Ratcliff. And despite the goofy van, she felt an

instant attraction to him. She would later say that she knew from that
first moment that they were going to be together. She broke up with her
boyfriend the next day and soon started going out with Ernest.

Ernest was born in Ashland, Kentucky, the youngest of three sons. He grew
up in Willard, Kentucky, a tiny town set deep in the rolling hillside of Carter
County. For work, he followed in his father's footsteps and became a boilermaker, which meant that he performed repair work on pipes and metal boil-
ers in various industrial settings. Melissa told me that he was a skilled welder
who could pass any kind of welding test his employer asked him to perform.

Ernest was a charismatic and generous guy. He loved to hunt for
grouse and pheasant. He adored Christmas. He took Melissa to her first
rock concert to see the hair-metal band Cinderella at the Big Sandy Super
Arena in Huntington, West Virginia. They enjoyed going on canoeing trips
together. "He was just a fun-loving, bighearted person," Melissa told me.
She sometimes referred to this younger version of him, the one she fell in
love with, as the "Old Ernest," due to the changes he would later undergo.

Ernest and Melissa were married in June 1997 at the Stinson Church of
Christ in Grayson. He wore a tuxedo with a white bow tie. She wore a white
maxi dress with puffy sleeves, a pearl necklace, and a sequined headpiece.

As Melissa remembered it, for at least a few years afterward they had a
great life. Ernest was busy flying around the country for temporary jobs
and making good money. And she was working as a receptionist at the
local health department in Grayson. Together, they were earning more
than $100,000 a year. They had money to buy clothes and to eat out at
restaurants. Melissa could afford to buy her first brand-new car: a fully
loaded 1999 beige Honda Accord LX.

There is little question that Ernest had dealt with a lot of physical pain.
In high school, he had suffered a nasty football injury when an opposing
player slammed into his lower back and fractured more than one of his
vertebrae. Doctors warned him to avoid manual labor, but he did it anyway.

His career as a boilermaker was prone to on-the-job injuries. Once
he pulled a muscle in his back so badly that when he got home, Melissa
remembered that he had to be helped to the porch of their house. Another
time, he was on the job when a large heating unit slid off a pallet and
crushed his knee and lower leg against a guardrail. His leg turned black
from his knee to his toes, but the doctors insisted nothing was broken.

In the early 2000s, Ernest underwent a surgery on his back in Lexington, which required him to wear a brace during recuperation. Melissa believed that the surgery was a success and said that he didn't seem to be in as much pain afterward.

But as was the case with Volkman patients who had legitimate pain issues, Ernest also struggled with addiction. Melissa told me that he had always had a compulsive personality. His first drug of choice was alcohol; then he moved on to cocaine, which he eventually began injecting. Over time, she watched him transform into someone else. He looked awful. He lost weight. He developed sores on his arms from the IV drug use.

As Ernest's drug use progressed, he also stopped working as much. Melissa recalled instances when she came home from work to find the house a mess. Ernest would get spurts of energy and frantically start cleaning or working on a project and then get distracted and not finish the task, leaving things messier. Other times he was so zonked that he would fall asleep with a lit cigarette in his hand. Melissa told me that if you ever walk into someone's house and see burn holes in a ring on the floor around the recliner or the toilet, it's a sure sign that someone there is taking hard drugs.

At some point in the late 1990s or early 2000s, Ernest shifted his drug use to pain pills. This was a practical choice: Cocaine had become harder to access, while pain pills had become cheaper and easier to obtain due to the rise of pain clinics. One such clinic was in New Philadelphia, Ohio, which was a four-hour drive away from where Melissa and Ernest lived. When Ernest heard about it, he and Melissa started making the trip.

It was a cash-only clinic, where patients paid a flat rate of around $200 or $250 to see the doctor and walked away with prescriptions for pain pills and muscle relaxers. Melissa and Ernest would both go in to see the doctor, then Ernest would keep one of the prescriptions for himself and sell the other one. Melissa said that she was prescribed pills even though there was obviously nothing wrong with her.

At some point, the clinic in New Philadelphia was raided and shut down by authorities. But before long Ernest heard about another doctor with a similar approach: a cash fee to get in the door, a low bar for getting prescriptions, and a high likelihood of walking away with scripts for a lot of pills. His name was Paul Volkman.

Going to Volkman required a significant amount of up-front cash for the office visit fee and, later, the pills that were prescribed. Ernest found an investor in his mother, who agreed to help him with the costs. He had apparently convinced her that his addiction was under control and that he could obtain from the doctor significant amounts of pills, which he would then sell for a handsome profit and pay her back with money to spare.

His expectations were based on Volkman's reputation. Melissa told me that during the doctor's tenure in Portsmouth it seemed like most of the Tri-State area was going to him. "Everyone knew about Doctor Volkman," she told me. "If you wanted to get a shit-ton of pills, that's where you [would] go."

Because a trip to Volkman was likely to bring a financial windfall, as well as an abundance of pills, Ernest was excited about his visit to the doctor. And after he cobbled together the money to pay for it, Melissa said that he approached the trip as if it would be "the end of all his worries."

Ernest's first and only visit to Volkman took place on Friday, October 21, 2005. It was about a two-hour drive from Willard to Chillicothe, the town forty-five miles north of Portsmouth where Volkman moved after Center Street. Ernest and a friend left early in the morning before Melissa had woken up to go to work.

For unclear reasons, there are no existing records of Ernest's visit with Volkman. Volkman would claim that Ernest's file was among those stolen from him by a disgruntled security guard who broke into his office after he was fired. And as a result, unlike many other patients who were discussed during Volkman's trial, I have no paper records to indicate what was said before or during his appointment.

In writings after his trial, Volkman said that Ernest complained of severe back pain that had not been fixed by a back surgery and said that he "spent a lot of time with Ratcliff" evaluating his problems and advising him how he ought to take his medication "for maximum safety and efficacy." He also ordered a hospital-administered urine drug screening for Ratcliff to complete in two weeks, to ensure his compliance with the prescribed regimen. He claimed that Ratcliff did not tell him that he was taking methadone, which was crucial information, because, as Volkman explained, "methadone is quite dangerous even when taken alone, due to the high risk of overdose and respiratory depression, and even more deadly in combination with oxycodone, Xanax, alcohol and many other drugs."

Whatever the exact conversation that took place in Volkman's clinic that day, the prescriptions themselves were preserved and were presented as trial evidence. From those slips, we know that on October 21, 2005, after his first visit to Volkman, Ernest received prescriptions for four medications: 240 thirty-milligram tablets of oxycodone, 90 tablets of the muscle relaxer Soma, 240 tablets of Lortab (hydrocodone), and 90 tablets of the sedative Xanax. It was a total of 660 pills.

He was advised to fill those scripts at the pharmacy that Volkman was using at the time: East Main Street Pharmacy in Columbus, which was fifty miles north of Volkman's clinic. However, by the time Ernest left Volkman's office, the pharmacy was already closed, which meant he would have to drive home to Kentucky and make the 150-mile trek to Columbus the next day.

We know what happened next thanks to Melissa Ratcliff, who was present for what would turn out to be the final hours of her husband's life. She testified about these events at trial and elaborated on that testimony during multiple conversations with me.

Melissa didn't want to go to Columbus on the day after Ernest's visit to the pain clinic. But she reluctantly drove. She estimated that she and Ernest took around $700 in cash with them for the trip. Most of it was for the pills he planned to buy, but some would cover gas and food.

On the drive up, Ernest was excited to finally get the pills, but Melissa said that he was also tired from the "the hype and the worry" involved in the whole process. And he was apologetic. By this point she and Ernest had been broke for quite a while, and she said he spent some of the drive to Columbus explaining that they were now going to have money to "do what we need to do and . . . get the things that I needed to get."

What stuck out in Melissa's mind about the trip, aside from the distance they traveled, was Ernest's paranoia. During his visit the day prior, Volkman had apparently given him detailed instructions about handling the pills he prescribed. He had advised Ernest to purchase a safe that could be bolted to the floor for storage of the pills and told him to be careful when going to the pharmacy, because it was being watched and there might be someone who would try to snatch his pills on the way to the car. Ernest was so nervous about the visit that Melissa remembered becoming nervous herself.

They arrived at the pharmacy and sat in the car for a few minutes. Eventually, Ernest got out and went inside the pharmacy. He emerged a bit later hiding a bag of pills under his jacket. Soon they were on the road back to Kentucky.

At Volkman's trial, Melissa testified that during the drive home, Ernest swallowed one pill from each of the medications he had been prescribed. Then, a little while later, he crushed and snorted a couple more pills. At some point on the ride back, they stopped at KFC for a meal, where Ernest ate a heaping plate of food. Back in the car Ernest fell asleep, which struck Melissa as odd, because usually pain pills made him hyperactive. He slept for most of the rest of the drive, until they got to their highway exit in Grayson.

When they got back to town, there was a frenzy of activity. First, Ernest wanted to go to Kmart to buy some things with the leftover money his mother had given him for the doctor's visit. On his way out of the store, he ran into someone he knew, whom he proudly invited to come take a look at his haul from the pharmacist. Melissa believed that he gave this person some pills before they left.

From there they went to the house of a friend who was, in Melissa's recollection, "known to be a guy that peddled pills pretty quickly for people." Ernest dropped off the bottle of Lorcet for the guy to sell, and Ernest and the man snorted a pill each. Then Ernest and Melissa left.

Once they were home, it wasn't long before the friend who had driven Ernest to Volkman's clinic the previous day dropped by to collect his end of the agreed-upon payment, which Melissa said was "a couple pills." Then, afterward, another friend and her boyfriend stopped by and Ernest snorted some pills with them, too. They bought some Somas from him and left.

Then it was off to Louisa, a town forty miles away, where Ernest had made a deal with someone to sell the bulk of his recently obtained pills for a few thousand dollars. By this time he was "kind of hyper and agitated and not thinking real clear," Melissa said, and, for a portion of the drive, a Kentucky state trooper was following them, which triggered new waves of paranoia for both of them. Melissa remembered thinking, "Well, maybe all the rumors were true: Dr. Volkman's being watched and we were being followed." But it was a false alarm; the cruiser eventually pulled off the road.

Soon Ernest started digging around in the car for the bag of pills before he realized that he had accidentally left them back at home. At this point, Melissa was furious from all the running around she had done for Ernest. She declared that they were going home and she wouldn't be driving him anywhere else.

That night they went to sleep in separate beds, which they had done since Ernest's back surgery. Ernest slept on a bed in the living room so he could be closer to the bathroom, kitchen, TV, and phone. And Melissa slept in the bedroom in the back end of the trailer, which was located past the kitchen and through a hallway.

———

Ernest was a loud snorer. He snored throughout the night of October 22, and in the morning Melissa got up to check on him. She recalled that he seemed okay; he opened his eyes and looked at her, so she went back to bed.

Later, at around 6:30 or 7:00 A.M., she was woken up by the sound of a car honking in the driveway. It was the friend from Louisa whom they had planned to visit the previous day.

Melissa remembered getting up and asking, "Ernest, who is this guy?"

She checked on him again, his eyes opened, and he made a noise that indicated he wanted to be left alone. So she went back to bed and, before doing so, turned on the electric furnace in the hallway. It was loud.

An hour or two later, the guy from Louisa was back in the driveway and honking again, and this made Melissa mad. She got out of bed, threw on a robe, and walked out to the kitchen. That's when she saw Ernest.

He wasn't snoring anymore.

His lips were blue.

Melissa panicked. She said she thought, "This can't be happening."

She called 911, and while she was on the phone, she tried to perform CPR on her husband. But she couldn't move him off the bed to do it properly. His body was warm to the touch, but he wasn't moving.

When the ambulance was on its way, the friend returned to the driveway and continued to honk, unaware of what was happening inside. Melissa went outside and screamed at him to leave.

The ambulance eventually arrived, and the EMTs filed into the trailer. But there was nothing they could do. Ernest had been dead for hours. On his death certificate, the cause was listed as "Multi-Drug Intoxication."

CHILLICOTHE

In 1803, when Ohio became the seventeenth state in the Union, the town of Chillicothe was designated its capital. It held the distinction until 1810, when the capital moved to Zanesville for two years before moving back to Chillicothe until 1816, at which point it permanently relocated to Columbus. Nowadays, when you drive through town, a sign painted on a water tower announces that you are passing through OHIO'S FIRST CAPITAL.

The city saw another surge in relevance after the United States entered

World War I, when it was selected as the site of a training facility named Camp Sherman. In short order, more than thirteen hundred buildings were constructed, including barracks, offices, a library, a hospital, and multiple theaters. Thousands of soldiers passed through en route to the front lines. For a short time, the town's population swelled to sixty thousand.

But the camp was dismantled after the war ended. And by the mid-2000s, Chillicothe was, like Portsmouth, a quiet place long past its heyday. It was home to a satellite campus of Ohio University, a paper mill, two state prisons, and around twenty thousand residents.

The raid on his house on Center Street changed Volkman's thinking about moving his clinic to downtown Portsmouth, as he'd planned. He was no longer interested in staying in town, and he would later say that an attorney advised him to find a new location for his clinic at least two counties away from Portsmouth.

Chillicothe fit that bill.

Volkman scoped out at least one prospective location for the clinic that didn't work out. His security guard at the time would later say that they were interested in a building in the town of Waverly, fifteen miles south of Chillicothe. But when the landlord learned about the doctor's plans for a pain clinic, he wasn't interested in that kind of tenant.

Within days, Volkman found another viable location in a single-story building along US Route 23 on the outskirts of Chillicothe. The building had the look of a prefabricated home, which would prompt it to be referred to at various points in Volkman's case as a "double-wide." The building had a large dirt parking area with room for dozens of cars. And it was located next to a wooded area at the base of a hill, far from any immediate neighbors. It was, as Volkman later described it, "an ideal site."

On Friday, October 7, just three days after the Center Street raid, Volkman signed a three-year, $2,500-per-month lease for the property. Over the weekend, he and his staff bought used furniture for the office, set up a phone system, and hired a carpenter to construct an alcove for the receptionists.

On Monday, October 10, the clinic still didn't have exam tables in the rooms where Volkman planned to see patients. (In fact, it never would.) But that week, the doctor was once again open for business. According to a former employee, the clinic brought in $9,000 in cash on its first day.

———

Not long after the Chillicothe clinic opened, a local pharmacist named John Brauner received a call from Volkman. Brauner had been a pharmacist for more than twenty-five years, including two decades at chain drugstores. He had been hired to work for a family-owned pharmacy in Chillicothe the previous year. He would later testify that he was accustomed to filling prescriptions for a few dozen local doctors, with the occasional script coming from Ohio State, in Columbus, or the University of Cincinnati.

On the phone, Volkman told the pharmacist that he was starting a practice nearby and was looking for a pharmacy to fill his prescriptions. He said that he was treating pain patients who had fallen through the cracks of the medical system, and he would be prescribing large doses of narcotics. He assured Brauner that his prescriptions were backed by X-rays and CT scans and that his patients were routinely screened for drugs. He was calling to ask: Would Brauner be willing to fill his prescriptions?

Brauner had never gotten a call like this from a doctor, and he chose to proceed cautiously. He declined to give Volkman a blanket yes or no and explained that he would have to look at each individual prescription before making a decision, as he was legally required to do.

The next day, three Volkman patients showed up at the pharmacy with prescriptions, and they immediately stood out from the shop's usual clientele. One patient was from Portsmouth, forty-five miles away. Another was from Greenup, Kentucky, more than sixty miles away. A third was from Olive Hill, Kentucky, a hundred miles away. The distances were unusual.

A second unusual aspect of these new customers was their willingness to pay in cash. Brauner would later explain that the neighborhood where he worked was "somewhat impoverished," and "most everyone" paid for their scripts with either an insurance card or a state Medicaid card. In the rare event that his customers did pay a portion of their costs with cash, they were usually interested in the amount of those costs. These new patients seemed relatively unconcerned with the prices, which made their purchases stick out even more.

Brauner also said the amounts of narcotics that the doctor was prescribing struck him as "unsafe."

Brauner filled the prescriptions. But when five more Volkman patients came the following day fitting a similar profile — high doses of controlled substances, traveling from long distances, willing to pay cash — he made a phone call to Volkman to share his concerns about the doctor's prescribed doses of oxycodone. Brauner said he wouldn't be filling any scripts at that dosage, and Volkman said that he would consider lowering them.

Then the next day, according to Brauner's eventual trial testimony, a Volkman patient arrived with prescriptions for the same high dosages that had prompted the pharmacist's concerned call the previous day. By this time, Brauner had spoken with the owner of his pharmacy about his concerns with this new crop of patients, and they had mutually decided that, going forward, the business would only fill prescriptions for customers from Ross County, where the pharmacy was located.

Brauner called Volkman and told him about the decision, explaining that the decision was based on the high doses, and the fact that these patients came from, as he testified, "a geographic area . . . well past what we had decided to focus on." Volkman expressed concern about his patients' ability to get their scripts filled, but Brauner held firm.

The following week, when Volkman patients continued to show up at the pharmacy and Brauner asked them why, they told him that his shop was listed by Volkman's clinic as a place to have their scripts filled. The pharmacist told them they were misinformed and called the clinic to ask that it remove his pharmacy from the list.

Having struck out with at least one local pharmacist, Volkman resumed sending his patients to East Main Pharmacy in Columbus. From Chillicothe, the commute was shorter than it had been from Center Street; it was now fifty-six miles, down from ninety-four. But it was still a lengthy drive.

During subsequent interviews with DEA diversion investigators, Harold Eugene Fletcher told them that he didn't find the long distances that his customers traveled suspicious, nor did he find their prescribed medications or cash payments worrisome. He also stated that he had spoken with Volkman and been assured that the doctor conducted blood tests to monitor his patients' compliance and also sent patients out for MRI testing to confirm their complaints of pain.

But Fletcher apparently did little to follow up on this early phone call. A Volkman employee would later state that Fletcher occasionally asked to speak with the doctor, but the majority of the calls concerned how late the pharmacy should stay open that day in order to fill Dr. Volkman's prescriptions. Mostly, Fletcher downplayed his responsibilities when it came to filling Volkman's scripts, saying to investigators that it was "not his job to question a physician."

DEA records illustrate the rewards for Fletcher's lack of curiosity about Volkman. During a five-month period that began in the fall of 2005 and extended into early 2006, three-quarters of all controlled-substance prescriptions he filled came from Volkman, at an average rate of dozens per day. In the three weeks of October 2005 after Volkman moved to Chillicothe, Fletcher made seventeen cash deposits at local banks, totaling more than $150,000. An employee at Commerce National Bank would later describe phone calls Fletcher made in October 2005 during which he asked specific questions about the amounts of cash deposits that would necessitate additional paperwork. The employee said that "it was really a big red flag when he started asking questions about dollar amounts" and that she ultimately reported these calls to her bank's compliance officer.

An expert later hired by the DEA to review Volkman's prescriptions filled by Fletcher would be harshly critical of the pharmacist's activities. In sworn testimony, Donald Sullivan, a longtime professor of pharmacy at Ohio Northern University who had worked in numerous retail pharmacies in central Ohio, emphasized that, according to both state and federal law, pharmacists are bound by "corresponding responsibility." This means that they have an equal amount of legal responsibility as doctors to ensure that prescriptions they fill are legal, safe, and appropriate. As Sullivan testified, "The argument that 'Just because a physician wrote the prescription, I can legally fill it' is no excuse."

After reviewing hundreds of prescriptions written by Volkman and filled by Fletcher, Sullivan found flaws in numerous aspects of Fletcher's (and, by extension, Volkman's) conduct. He described the distances many of the patients were driving to have their scripts filled by Fletcher as "extremely unusual and very suspicious." When discussing Volkman's prescribing of hydrocodone, he described the lack of individualization across patients to be "clinically impossible," and, elsewhere, observed that most of Volkman's scripts for benzodiazepines exceeded the FDA's maximum approved daily dosage. He expressed alarm that 75 percent of the Volkman patients whose prescriptions he reviewed received the same combination of medications: an anti-anxiety agent, a muscle relaxer, and two narcotic painkillers. He also said that he had previously only seen a doctor prescribe two Schedule II narcotic painkillers for cancer and hospice patients.

In his summary of Fletcher's activities during this time, Sullivan said that the prescriptions the pharmacist filled appeared to be "textbook examples of drug abuse and/or drug diversion" and that Volkman's clinics seemed to be "nothing more than a controlled substance prescription mill for patients who are diverting and abusing narcotic drugs." He also said that in all his years of work and teaching, he had "never seen such an abuse of controlled substances dispensing by one pharmacy."

A DEA diversion investigator would later estimate that, all told, Fletcher's profits from filling Volkman's prescriptions between September 2005 and February 2006 amounted to "almost $500,000."

While Volkman's business in Chillicothe flourished, the DEA's investigation pressed on.

On a Wednesday in mid-December 2005, a DEA agent watched the office for four and a half hours in the middle of the day and reported seeing approximately twenty-five patients walk in. He noted cars parked from eastern Kentucky and one from a hundred miles away, in Nitro, West Virginia.

The agency also conducted interviews with the doctor's former employees. On December 1, the agency interviewed a man who had worked for Volkman as an armed security guard for six weeks from mid-September to late October, at both the Center Street and Chillicothe clinics. The guard, who was paid $15 per hour by Volkman, had a license to carry a gun and was specifically instructed to have the gun visible at work.

The guard said that he saw patients come to the clinic as early as 7:00 A.M. and as late as 2:00 A.M. He didn't believe Volkman asked medical questions during visits; instead, he believed the doctor made "small talk" as he wrote scripts for narcotics. He said that he had seen people whom he knew to be addicted obtain narcotics prescriptions from Volkman, and he believed that some died days after receiving those scripts.

The former guard also told investigators that at the end of each day at the clinic, he watched staffers count the day's cash proceeds, which usually totaled between $4,000 and $7,000. Volkman kept around $5,000 in cash for himself each week as a salary. He recalled that, over an eight-day period in October after the Chillicothe clinic opened, Volkman instructed him to transport cash from the clinic to a bank in Chillicothe and deposit it. During this period, he said, he had personally carried and deposited "tens of thousands of dollars in cash."

A month later, the DEA interviewed another former employee who had been a nurse assistant at both the Center Street and Chillicothe locations. She told authorities that working for Volkman was unusual for many reasons. She said that she heard about the job when an acquaintance reached out and asked her if she needed a job. There was no job application and no interview, and Volkman did not ask her for any references. When she was hired, she never filled out federal or state tax forms or other paperwork, and she was never given an official job description. She further explained that she was paid each week via personal check, though this changed after the move to Chillicothe, when taxes began to be deducted from her paychecks.

During her interview, she told investigators that Volkman's patients were required to fill out about twenty pages of paperwork before seeing him, but she said they generally didn't complain because they knew the paperwork was a necessary step to get the drugs they sought. She said that some patients waited hours to see the doctor. She described the clinic as a "script mill" and estimated that 95 percent of Dr. Volkman's patients were drug abusers or drug dealers.

Volkman's patients continued to die.

Ernest Ratcliff died in late October after a visit to Volkman's new clinic in Chillicothe. The following month, on the morning of Saturday, November 19, 2005, a detective from the Portsmouth Police Department responded to a call at a house on the east side of town. When he pulled up to the address, he saw a woman outside the house crying. He made his way inside and saw a man named Mark Reeder lying motionless on the bed.

Reeder was a hefty guy with brown hair and a brown goatee. He had grown up in Portsmouth. He went by the nickname "Bluto" after the burly character from Popeye to whom he bore a resemblance. The mother of one of his close friends said he was "like a big Teddy bear."

In his intake paperwork for Dr. Volkman, Reeder had described himself as a self-employed subcontractor working for a construction company.* Reeder had visited Volkman at the Center Street clinic in late September, complaining of severe pain in his knees, ankles, and lower back. Volkman's notes from that visit indicate that Reeder said that he worked six-to-eight-hour days four or five days per week and was able to function much better with medication. He left that day with four prescriptions — for Xanax, Soma, Norco, and oxycodone; a total of nine hundred pills — plus a script for MRI scans of his knees, ankles, and spine. He returned to visit Volkman in Chillicothe the following month.

---

* Mark's sister-in-law, Kimberly, told me that his actual profession was selling drugs. "Mark . . . never worked a job, because he dealt drugs," she said.

When the Portsmouth detective arrived at Reeder's house that morning in November, he took photos at the scene, including close-ups of Mark's face that showed, as he later described from the witness stand, "a brownish-gray fluid, coming from his mouth." He said Reeder's shirt was wet from a combination of the fluid from his mouth and water thrown on him by his girlfriend in a failed effort to wake him up.

Toxicology reports later identified the presence of all four medications that Volkman had prescribed in his system. He was thirty-four years old.

ORDER TO SHOW CAUSE

Volkman would later describe his time in Chillicothe in surprisingly positive terms. To hear him tell it, despite everything that had happened in the preceding two years — the patient deaths, a falling-out with his former employer, run-ins with distressed and furious family members of patients, multiple raids by law enforcement — things were actually going quite well.

He would later write that he was "quite pleased" with the office and his staff in Chillicothe, and he also said that he found working with patients gratifying. During one of our in-person interviews, Volkman told me, with no trace of self-consciousness, that he was on track to make an annual salary of $1.5 million at his final clinic. It was, he said, "the first time in my life that I made what I thought was decent money." He added, "I was, I felt, serving a desperately poor . . . underserved part of the population, giving them very good service, and making a very good living at the same time." He saw it as a win-win situation.

Operations at his fourth clinic location seemed to him to be going so well that, in addition to seeing patients, he began working on an ambitious project. Nearly three decades after walking away from the world of academic medicine, he was once again interested in publishing research.

Volkman would later explain to me that, while working in pain management, he was frustrated at the lack of diagnostic tools at his disposal. There was no blood test that could assess patients' pain levels. Nor were there any wires you could hook up to them that would confirm or measure their suffering. Various imaging tests — MRIs, ultrasounds, X-rays — were of little use for this purpose. This meant that, even in the twenty-first century, to determine a patient's pain level, clinicians had to rely on questionnaires, interviews, and surveys that used 1-to-10 scales or cartoonish drawings of smiling and frowning faces. Such a reliance on self-reported symptoms would be frustrating in any specialty. But it was especially fraught in pain management because of the abuse potential and high black-market value of the medications involved. Patients had a lot of incentives to be dishonest with a doctor who could prescribe them opioids.

Volkman said that he had tried his best to ensure patient compliance through pill counts, blood tests, and urine tests. The idea was that by performing such analyses of their blood or urine, he could see whether they were taking the meds he prescribed. But he told me that when he began working in pain management he was surprised at how inaccurate those tests were. Beyond offering a binary yes or no answer, even the best tests, like the ones he was sending off to the Mayo Clinic, were still frustratingly inexact. "A person could be either taking all of his medicine or half of his medicine and I wouldn't be able to tell," he once said.

Volkman, with a PhD in pharmacology, believed he could design a better test.

He later explained that he wanted to design a urine test for pain patients that would not just confirm the presence of a particular substance but also would tell a clinician how *much* of that substance was present. Such data would be invaluable for helping doctors to see through the diagnostic fog and identify real patients from those with ulterior motives, he said.

To bring this dream to fruition, he would need to partner with a scientist at a university who could help translate his concept into a working prototype. And he told me that he had found a willing partner in a toxicologist at the University of Utah who had confirmed that he could measure the metabolites Volkman was interested in tracking, and do so at an affordable price.

Volkman had high hopes for this research. During one of our in-person interviews, he told me, matter-of-factly, that he planned to have the results published in the *New England Journal of Medicine*, one of the medical world's premier journals. And this claim even made it into one of his legal filings, in 2009, when his lawyer wrote: "The long-term view was to publish the eventual findings in the most widely-read and prestigious American medical journal, *The New England Journal of Medicine*."

In an echo of his belief that he had discovered a paradigm-shifting treatment for strokes in the late 1970s (an outcome that he said never materialized due to his lab director's refusal to sign off on the paper), he believed that his forthcoming discovery of a more accurate urine test for pain patients would have been a medical breakthrough. "Thousands and thousands of doctors would start prescribing pain medicine because they would be able to effectively monitor whether their patients were taking it and they would be able to effectively defend themselves against any bogus charges," he told me. He said that the discovery would "radically, radically" change the field.

When I contacted the University of Utah toxicologist with whom Volkman claimed to have been working, he confirmed that the doctor had contacted him about a potential testing regimen and that he had begun working on a method of analysis to test those samples. But he said the project never made it past the preliminary stages. "A little later, I was suspicious of Dr. Volker [sic] because he said the project was not monitored by an institutional review board," he told me, via email. Shortly thereafter, the toxicologist backed out of the collaboration. In his email, the toxicologist noted that he did not analyze any samples from Volkman's research subjects, and the university received no payment from Volkman.

Volkman's big idea had apparently never gotten far off the ground. But I don't think it's far-fetched to interpret his ambitious plans as an attempt at achieving some of the glory he felt had been previously denied to him in the world of research. In other words: In addition to having finally achieved the kind of income he felt he was owed, Volkman seems to have been seeking *academic* redemption as well.

The incident also reveals how detached he was from the grim reality of his situation. At no point in describing his plans to publish in the *New England Journal of Medicine* did Volkman acknowledge the hurdles posed by his lack of academic affiliation, the fact that he hadn't published in three decades, or that he was working out of a cash-only pain clinic on the side of a highway in southern Ohio.

In an autobiographical narrative that he wrote from prison, Volkman said that he was working on this research project at his desk at the Chillicothe clinic in February 2006 when "all hell broke loose." As he described it: "Helicopters hovered above. The parking lot was filled with SUVs . . . The SWAT team stormed the office, guns drawn."

Later, at Volkman's trial, a nurse who was working at the clinic corroborated much of this description. "There was helicopters flying over, camera crews," she said. "There was guns in everybody's faces at the office, including patients and staff."

The raid, which took place on February 10, 2006, marked the third time law enforcement officers had entered one of Volkman's offices in southern Ohio. Once again, Volkman was not arrested. But he did receive a regulatory knockout punch: a thirteen-page document informing him that his DEA registration was immediately suspended.

All prescribers of controlled substances in the United States must have a DEA number by which the agency can track their prescribing activity. Some doctors don't use their DEA numbers very often; my father, for instance, rarely prescribes opioids or other controlled substances in his endocrinology practice. But as a high-volume prescriber of opioids and other controlled substances, Volkman was using his DEA registration dozens of times every day. The number appeared on each of the prescriptions he wrote.

To continue prescribing controlled substances, a doctor or other distributor must remain in good standing with the DEA. And if the agency is concerned enough about a particular registrant's activity, it can suspend or permanently revoke that doctor's registration. Before taking such a measure, however, the agency issues a document explaining its reasons for taking the action. This is called an Order to Show Cause.

In the pages of Volkman's February 2006 order, the agency laid out its case for the action. The report pointed to a series of concerning aspects about Volkman's southern Ohio clinics, including the fact that they only accepted cash, they employed "bodyguards stationed within the clinic," and patients had quick visits yet walked away with large prescriptions. Some of the agency's concerns were based on conversations with Volkman himself, who had stated on the day of the Tri-State raid in June 2005 that he did not coordinate patient care with other doctors.

The order further reported that Volkman was the number one physician-purchaser of oxycodone in the nation in 2004, with a number of pills purchased (438,000) more than ninety times the national physician average; and that, in 2003, he had ranked second in the country for his purchases of the narcotic. For both years, he was the top physician-purchaser of oxycodone *and* hydrocodone in Ohio.

The order went on to state that, following the July 2005 raid, the Cincinnati DEA office had attempted an audit of the controlled substances moving through the dispensary, but this had initially not been possible due to the clinic's failure to maintain proper records (which was itself a breach of the law). The agency eventually determined that Volkman "could not account for more than 850,000 dosage units of controlled substances that were ordered and dispensed under your DEA registration."

Most pressingly, the document cited eleven (unnamed) patients who had died from apparent overdoses of medications Volkman had prescribed. All but one of the deceased patients were younger than forty years old, and six were thirty-five or younger. The majority of them had died within days of their last visit to the doctor. It was, the order said, an "alarmingly high rate of deaths involving patients of Dr. Volkman for whom he had prescribed multiple prescriptions for large quantities of potentially lethal combinations of controlled substances shortly before their deaths."

Considering all these facts, the deputy administrator of the DEA stated her "preliminary finding" that Volkman was responsible for the illegitimate diversion of large quantities of controlled substances and that, in the interest of public safety, his registration needed to be suspended. The document noted that he would remain prohibited from prescribing until a final ruling could be made.

LOSING BATTLES

Volkman would later use the words *saddened*, *devastated*, and *crushed* to describe how he felt after the raid of his last pain clinic in Ohio. And I have little reason to doubt that he felt this way. Though, to be clear, the basis for his sadness was not the deaths of so many of his patients, for which he accepted no responsibility then or afterward. He was "devastated" by the injustice he felt he had sustained with the loss of his DEA registration.

Back in Chicago, he apparently made various attempts to find work. He said that he called "lots of different people, in different kinds of jobs," but had no luck. He described the revocation of his DEA registration as a "huge black mark" against him. As he later explained it, "Why would anybody hire somebody who has any kind of question in his background when you can very easily hire somebody else that has no problems [and] no questions?"

Meanwhile, his family was increasingly concerned about what had happened in Ohio. Volkman's daughter, Jane, told me that her mother had already been worried, and when the raid occurred, it was a confirmation of her fears. Jane said the news "terrified" her mother and that she, too, was "traumatized" by it.

She also said that the raid prompted her to ask her dad new questions about the clinic. In response, he insisted that the DEA was overstepping its bounds, and that any issues with his practice were for the state medical board to consider, not a federal agency. He also pointed to his drug-testing regimen as an indication of his efforts to ensure patients were taking the pills as directed.

In the weeks after the raid on his office in Chillicothe, the distance between Volkman's Chicago life and his Ohio clinics began to collapse.

Around the time that armed agents swarmed into his Chillicothe office, authorities had also seized the contents of two Volkman-associated bank accounts. One, which was registered in Paul's name, contained $24,442.25, while another, in Nancy's name, contained $10,525.52.

The grounds for this action was a provision in the Controlled Substances Act stating that all funds gained from the illicit sale of controlled substances, or traceable to such sales, are subject to forfeiture to the federal government. In support of its seizure, the DEA later filed a twenty-five-page affidavit describing Volkman's activities in southern Ohio. "Based on my training and experience," wrote the agent who signed the document, "I believe that all of these deposits are traceable to illicit prescription mill activities."

Volkman was outraged. And in March, the month after the raid, he fired off a letter in protest. "In no instance did the medicine prescribed fall outside the bounds of normal, accepted, medical practice," he wrote. In the letter, he acknowledged that "in approximately ten instances," his patients had "expired from apparent overdoses." This was noteworthy phrasing considering the fact that, later, at trial, he and his attorneys would adamantly dispute that many of those same patients had died from overdoses.

But in the letter, Volkman said that he was not to blame for such "apparent overdoses" because they were "most likely self-inflicted in chronic pain patients well known to have a high risk of suicide." He was not to blame if patients took their medications in ways other than how he directed, he argued. He added that the seizure of his bank accounts and the suspension of his DEA registration imposed a "severe hardship upon me and my family and [are] not justified by any realistic presumption of criminal activity on my part."

Paul's letter was accompanied by a similar letter from his wife, which, based on my review, seems to be her only direct comment in the expansive legal record of Paul's case. Nancy's letter also adopted a defiant tone, defending what she referred to as "my husband's legitimate practice of pain management medicine" and stating that some of the seized funds deposited in her account came from her salary payments from the Chicago Board of Education and "clearly have no conceivable relationship to any criminal drug enterprise."

A few months later, an Ohio-based lawyer working for Volkman filed a motion to dismiss the asset-forfeiture case. In that document, he called the government's complaint laying out its case for seizing the assets "an unbelievable litany of unverified, unsworn hearsay recitations, hearsay lay opinion, and inflammatory, factually-unsupported innuendo."

The motion, and Volkman's entire fight to recoup his seized assets, failed. But that legal filing includes a memorable distillation of how Volkman and his sympathizers viewed his activities in southern Ohio.

"This is not a story about drug dealing thugs or smugglers," the lawyer wrote. "Rather, it is a story of an accomplished, experienced, competent physician working in a rural under-served area trying to help manage the pain of his patients."

The dispute over seized assets was just one of the legal battles Volkman faced after the close of his last clinic. The DEA's Order to Show Cause had included notice of his right to contest the suspension of his registration, either in writing or in a hearing. And he intended to do so.

Volkman was advised by at least two people not to do this. His daughter told me that she believed his arguments that the DEA had overstepped its statutory bounds were a "dead end" not worth pursuing. And Kevin Byers, the lawyer who was representing him at this time, told me that he advised Volkman to save his energy and money for the criminal case that was likely in the works. Volkman's response to him, as Byers recalled, was "I don't care. They haven't indicted me yet. Let 'em try. We'll beat this, then we'll beat that." Thus, Volkman's DEA-registration case proceeded to a hearing, which took place over six days in late 2006 and early 2007, in front of an administrative law judge in Columbus.

Much to my frustration, I never gained access to the transcripts of that proceeding, which, according to Volkman, totaled fifteen hundred pages. But two lengthy published rulings on the case include considerable detail about the evidence and testimony presented.

The hearing included testimony from the widow of Jeffrey Reed, who testified that her husband was addicted to drugs at the time he was a

Volkman patient and that he was receiving prescriptions for large amounts of three different kinds of medication (opioids, tranquilizers, muscle relaxers), sometimes totaling more than six hundred pills per month.

The government's case also included an agent from the Ohio State Board of Pharmacy who described the number of complaints about the doctor he had received from pharmacists, which began as soon as Volkman arrived at Tri-State. During his own visits to Tri-State the agent had taken note of the clinic's noncompliance with the strict regulations for maintaining an on-site dispensary, and other unusual aspects about the clinic, including the weapons kept in the dispensary (a Glock handgun, a nightstick, a long wooden club). He had also noted that both Denise and Alice were being prescribed narcotics by Volkman and appeared to be "over medicated." It was "not your normal doctor's office," he said. After his second visit, he believed it was a "prescription mill."

Some of the most extensive testimony came from a chronic pain physician the DEA had asked to review medical charts, as well as other documents, including autopsy and toxicology reports, for six of Volkman's patients who had died while under his care. The doctor identified repeated inadequacies in Volkman's charts, including a lack of diagnostic testing or past medical records, a lack of proper patient histories or physical exams, strikingly similar methods of treatment across patients, few instances of treating symptoms with noncontrolled-substance medicines or other methods, and little follow-up about the efficacy or side effects of his prescribed medications. "Each one of these deaths was preventable," the witness testified.

For his defense, Volkman called three former employees who spoke favorably about his methods. However, this testimony seems to have carried relatively little weight, since two of them had only worked for him after his rift with the Huffmans, which represented less than a quarter of his time in Ohio. Another witness testified that she only worked at Tri-State "a few hours now and then" answering phones, pulling charts, and occasionally conducting intake interviews with patients.

This left Volkman to testify on his own behalf. During his testimony, Volkman claimed that he didn't think to ask Denise about her background and training, or lack thereof, when he first took the job, and only learned that he should have done so when an attorney told him about it "two years later." He claimed that "virtually all" of his patients had previously seen neurologists or neurosurgeons, and that that most had histories of surgery and "extensive" injections that had done little to ease their pain. He also said that an evaluation of these medical histories — which included reviewing charts tracking prior treatments, X-rays, MRIs, lab tests, and treatment from other doctors — was a key part of his patient-intake process. He claimed that he thoroughly documented his diagnoses in his charts, in addition to noting any adverse effects patients experienced from his prescribed medications.

During his testimony, Volkman cited various measures that he claimed kept his patients on their agreed-upon regimens, including narcotics contracts, pill counts, blood and urine testing, examining patients for signs of intravenous or nasal drug use, and dismissing patients who didn't comply. He also defended the combinations of pills that he so frequently prescribed. He said that the muscle relaxer carisoprodol was necessary for the painful muscle spasms that "almost all" of his patients experienced in their legs, and the benzodiazepines were similarly essential to help them sleep. And he claimed that the two opioids — a stronger and longer-acting one, such as oxycodone, prescribed alongside a shorter-acting one, like hydrocodone, for "breakthrough" pain — were "perfectly appropriate" for the issues his patients reported.

At one point he said, "As far as I was concerned — as far as my knowledge of Ohio law, Federal law, standards of care of pain management, and anything else I could find — I had done nothing wrong." He added that he believed that he had been "following absolutely prescribed procedures . . . in every respect."

He lost.

In a decision from June 2007, the administrative judge recommended that Volkman's registration be revoked and any future applications be denied because his continued registration would not be in the public's interest. The judge cited a litany of reasons in her decision, including Volkman's inability to account for more than a million controlled-substance tablets from the dispensary, the fact that he "prescribed the same combinations of controlled substances to a majority of his patients," and that his treatment had "directly contributed" to the apparent drug-related deaths of "at least" sixteen patients. His staunch refusal to acknowledge any problems with this conduct had also factored into her decision, she said.

Volkman appealed the decision twice, and twice the verdict was upheld: first by the DEA's deputy administrator, in 2008, and again by the Sixth Circuit US Court of Appeals in 2009.

His career prescribing controlled substances was over.

INDICTED

Independent accounts of Volkman's arrest are hard to obtain.

His wife, Nancy, was home at the time that it happened. But she had passed away by the time I began working on this project. When I asked his daughter, Jane, who was also home, she would say little more than, "It was horrible when they came." The entry on the online court docket for Volkman's case reads simply "ARREST of defendant Paul H. Volkman," with the date May 21, 2007. My attempts to get info from the agency that carried out the arrest, the US Marshals, were unsuccessful.

As a result, I am mostly left with Volkman's account, which he returned to repeatedly over the years I spoke with him. And from his telling and retelling, I have a sense of what happened — or at least how the event exists in his mind.

He said that it started with an early-morning bang on the door of his Lake Shore Drive apartment. Waiting for him on the other side of that door, he said, was "a SWAT team of about sixteen DEA agents wearing flak jackets and masks, [with] guns drawn." At some point thereafter, they handcuffed him, shackled his legs, "dragged him away from his terrified and disoriented wife," and led him to the elevator, at which point, as he described it, "everyone . . . in the lobby saw me marched out with chains on my legs and handcuffs." From there he was ushered into one of "six or seven SUVs parked in front of the building."

In the absence of additional detail, I am left to reverse-engineer this scene from other available facts. I know, for instance, that the arrest took place at a building described by one promotional video as one of the city's "most gracious rental addresses," with a lobby that, according to another ad, has "marble floors, gilded ceiling, and crystal chandeliers." Records indicate that the weather that morning in Chicago was around fifty-five degrees, and the sun had risen at 5:25 A.M. The arrest took place on a Monday, which means that Lake Shore Drive was likely humming with commuter traffic, as well as walkers, joggers, and bicyclists on their morning workouts.

When scanning local media, I found no coverage of the arrest itself. Though, two days later, an article on page 7 of the Metro section of the *Chicago Tribune*, "Doctor Faces Federal Charges in 14 Fatal Overdoses," did describe the details of the indictment.

———

The indictment against Paul Volkman was thirty-five pages long. At the top of the first page were three names: Denise Huffman, Alice Huffman Ball, and Paul Volkman.

The indictment contained twenty-two counts. At its core, it was a case about drug dealing. With this document, federal prosecutors were alleging that, in their time together at Tri-State Healthcare, Denise Huffman, Alice Huffman, and Paul Volkman had participated in a conspiracy to illegally distribute dangerous prescription drugs. The indictment further alleged that, once Volkman parted ways with the Huffmans, he had continued his illegal drug dealing for five more months at two additional locations.

The indictment contained a few different types of charges that stemmed from this central allegation of drug dealing. Four of the charges were based on physical locations where drug dealing took place: the two Tri-State locations in Portsmouth (1200 Gay Street, 1219 Findlay Street); 1310 Center Street; and Volkman's final clinic in Chillicothe. In each instance, prosecutors were arguing that these addresses were not medical facilities, but, rather, as a prosecutor would later say in court about Tri-State Healthcare, "in essence . . . a crack house dealing OxyContin and oxycodone." Four more counts were related to the possession of a gun in furtherance of a drug-dealing offense, which was its own crime. Thirteen of the counts alleged illegal drug distribution to individual patients.

Each indictment tells a story. And this document, amid its legal jargon, told a remarkable tale. It was a story with three main characters. First was Denise, a woman with "no known medical education" who, the document noted, had worked in the medical office of Dr. David Procter ("an illicit pain clinic," as the indictment described), before starting her own clinic the following year in the same town of South Shore. This clinic was managed by her daughter, Alice, who also had "little or no known medical education or background." In early 2003, the mother-daughter duo hired a doctor who had an MD/PhD from the University of Chicago.

The indictment described this trio's clinic as fundamentally illegitimate. It frequently referred to the people who came to the clinic as "customers" instead of patients. And it said that the facility's aim was not to treat pain but "to satisfy the demand for the illegal distribution, sale, and consumption of controlled substances" for a wide geographic area that included southern Ohio and northern Kentucky, and parts of West Virginia and Tennessee. The motive of this illegal operation was "to make as much money as possible."

The indictment alleged that Volkman's customers, who purportedly suffered from severe pain, would nevertheless travel long distances to visit his clinics. It stated that the clinic accepted only cash, that it did not offer refunds even when customers had not seen the doctor, and that customers got only cursory physical exams before receiving prescriptions for large amounts of controlled substances. Over the course of customers' treatments, Volkman was alleged to have rapidly increased their medication levels in ways that were likely to cause addiction. In fact, the indictment alleged that addiction was central to the clinic's business model, since, once a person became addicted, it meant "customers would then return more frequently to Tri-State . . . thus insuring [*sic*] additional payments."

The indictment went on to portray Tri-State as a place where Volkman rarely, if ever, offered alternative, non-narcotic treatments or suggested physical therapy; where weapons including "firearms [and] ball bats" were kept on the premises to maintain order; and where, once pharmacies refused to fill the clinic's scripts, the co-conspirators opened an on-site dispensary through which a torrent of pills flowed. All of this took place, the document noted, at a time when street demand for oxycodone had "grown to epidemic proportions in parts of Ohio, Kentucky, and other parts of the United States."

And people died.

While Volkman wasn't formally charged with murder or manslaughter, he was charged with dealing prescription drugs with "death or serious bodily injury result[ing]." And in the pages of the indictment, he became a kind of serial killer. In the cases of Aaron Gillispie (Count 4), Charles Jordan (Count 5), Daniel Coffee (Count 6), Jeffrey Reed (Count 7), Mary Catherine Carver (Count 8), James Estep (Count 9), Kristi Ross (Count 10), Steve Hieneman (Count 11), Scottie Lin James (Count 17), Bryan Brigner (Count 18), Ernest Ratcliff (Count 20), Mark Reeder (Count 21), and William Wicker (Count 22),* prosecutors described a chilling pattern. Again and again, these people traveled to the clinic, met with the doctor, received a prescription, and then, often within days, took the medicine and died.

The indictment ended with a section estimating the amount of money that Volkman and the Huffmans had made from their scheme and that,

---

* Wicker's death, as well as his previous interactions with Volkman, were discussed in far less detail than the other twelve patients during Volkman's trial. I wasn't able to obtain much additional info through my own reporting. As a result, I have chosen not to discuss him in this book.

thus, the government was seeking to seize. Denise and Alice were each individually held liable for $3,087,500, while Volkman was responsible for $3,787,500.

If such funds were not readily available, the indictment stated, the United States would seek the forfeiture of equally valuable property in their possession.

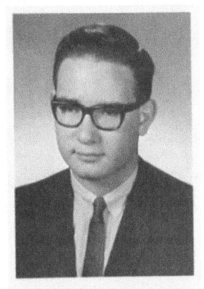
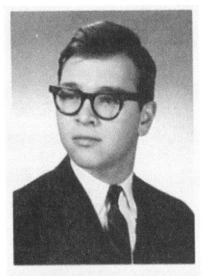

PAUL H. VOLKMAN
Washington, D.C.
Chemistry

CHARLES EIL
Yonkers, N.Y.
Chemistry-Philosophy
Honors

Paul Volkman and Charles Eil (the author's father) met in 1964 as undergraduates at the University of Rochester. *Courtesy of the University of Rochester*

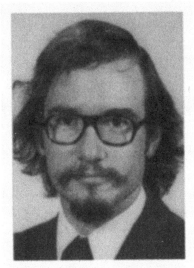
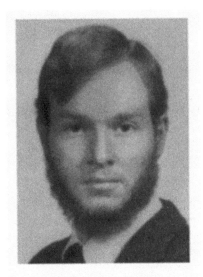

Paul H. Volkman   *Charles Eil*

After college, both Volkman and Eil attended the same federally funded MD/PhD program at the University of Chicago. They graduated in 1974. *UChicago Medicine Photographic Archive*

16. That ████████ went into cardiac arrest shortly after Respondent intubated her.

17. That ████████ was transported to Children's Memorial Hospital by the paramedics.

18. That ████████ was pronounced brain dead on December 4, 1987.

19. That ████████ was pronounced dead on December 5, 1987.

20. That performing intubations on children is very difficult.

21. That performing an intubation in an office without the proper equipment is extremely dangerous and reckless.

22. That Respondent's conduct was unprofessional and of a character likely to harm the public and caused actual harm to ████████.

23. The foregoing acts and/or omissions are grounds for revocation or suspension of a Certificate of Registration pursuant to Illinois Revised Statutes, (1987), Chapter 111, paragraph(s) 4400-22(5) as defined by 68 Illinois Administrative Code, Section 1285.240.

WHEREFORE, based on the foregoing allegations, the DEPARTMENT OF PROFESSIONAL REGULATION of the State of Illinois, by Richard P. Ryan, its Chief of Medical Prosecutions, prays that the

Following the death of pediatrics patient Amanda Frey in 1987, the Illinois Department of Professional Regulation filed a complaint against Volkman. *Illinois Department of Financial and Professional Regulation*

Volkman spent years as a locum tenens physician, taking temporary emergency room jobs in cities across the Midwest. This contract was included among court filings from a malpractice lawsuit in Central Illinois.

Macon County (Illinois) Clerk's Office

this contract. Such coverage shall be in the amount and form required by DEMS' hospital contracts.

5. **Compensation.** Doctor's sole compensation for services rendered under this contract shall be $ _130.00_ per hour for active duty, and $ _100.00_ per hour for call.

6. **Modification.** This contract may only be changed by a writing signed by both DEMS and Doctor.

Dated at Decatur, Illinois this _26_ th day of _DECEMBER_ 1994

DECATUR EMERGENCY MEDICAL SERVICES, S. C.

DOCTOR

LOCUM TENENS CONTRACT

This Contract entered into this _26_ th day of _DECEMBER_, 1994 at Decatur, Illinois, by and between DECATUR EMERGENCY MEDICAL SERVICES, S.C., an Illinois corporation (hereinafter referred to as "DEMS"), and _PAUL VOLKMAN_, M.D. (hereinafter "Doctor").

1. **Background.** DEMS provides the services of physicians licensed to practice medicine in the State of Illinois who specialize in the field of emergency room services. DEMS' workload is increasing, but in an irregular pattern. DEMS does not wish to hire another full-time physician at this time, but does desire to engage Doctor as a locum tenens to assist DEMS with its varying workload. Doctor wishes to work for DEMS on a part-time and interim basis.

2. **Term.** This Contract shall be effective on _DECEMBER 26_ 1994 and shall terminate upon the earlier of its three month anniversary, or upon the date on which either Doctor or DEMS gives written or oral notice of termination to the other.

3. **Work Duties.** Doctor will make himself/herself available to perform duties as required from time to time by DEMS, and as agreed to by Doctor. This will include taking call.

4. **Malpractice Insurance.** DEMS, at its sole expense, will provide Doctor with malpractice insurance coverage for the days that he/she works under

C-163

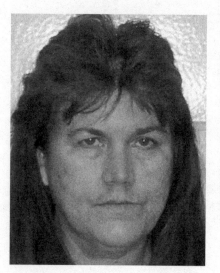
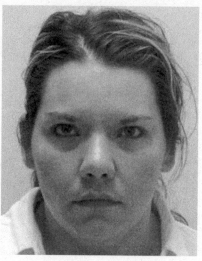

In 2001, Denise Huffman — who had no college education or medical training — opened Tri-State Healthcare in South Shore, Kentucky. The clinic later moved across the river to Portsmouth, Ohio. *US Marshals Service*

Denise Huffman's daughter, Alice, managed day-to-day operations of the Tri-State pain clinic. Both were indicted along with Volkman in 2007 and later pleaded guilty. *US Marshals Service*

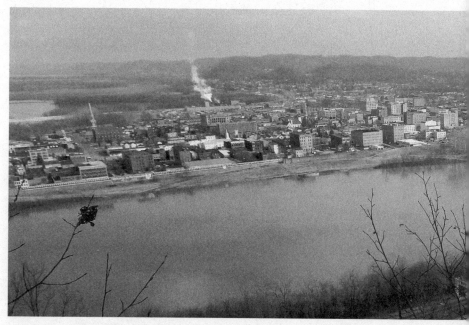

When Paul Volkman began working in Portsmouth in 2003, the town had already earned the nickname "The OxyContin Capital of the World." *John Kuntz/*The Plain Dealer. © 2011 The Plain Dealer. *All rights reserved. Reprinted with permission*

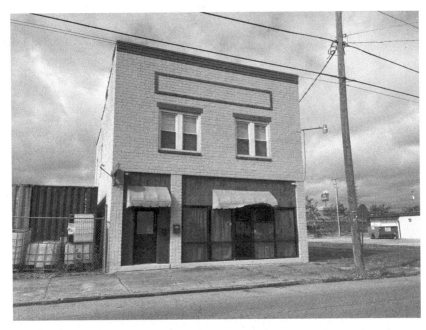

Most of Volkman's employment at Tri-State Healthcare took place in this building, at 1219 Findlay Street, in Portsmouth. Taken in 2022. *Courtesy of Philip Eil*

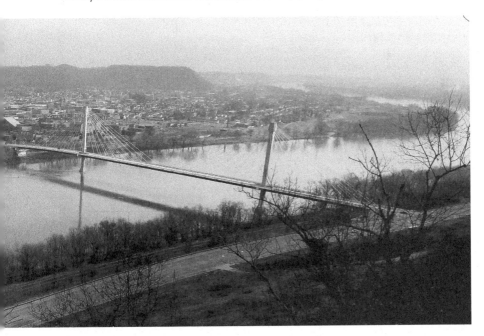

TERRY A. JOHNSON, D.O.

SCIOTO COUNTY CORONER

Courthouse, 602 Seventh Street, Portsmouth, Ohio 45662
Telephone ▆▆▆ (740) 355-0113

CORONER'S SUBPOENA

July 14, 2003

Paul H. Volkman, M.D.
1200 Gay Street
Portsmouth, Ohio 45662

Re: ███████████████████
    Date of Birth – █████████
    SS# ████

████████████ was pronounced dead on June 27, 2003. You are hereby ordered
to produce copies of any and all medical records on this patient by Friday,
July 25, 2003. You may bring the records to the Coroner's office in the Courthouse,
or you may mail them to: Terry A. Johnson, D.O., Scioto County Coroner, Courthouse,
602 7th Street, Portsmouth, Ohio 45662.

Thank you for your assistance.

Ordered by:

Terry A. Johnson, D.O.
SCIOTO COUNTY CORONER

By authority of the Ohio Revised Code Section 313.17.

AYNE WHEELER, M.D., J.D.   STEVEN W. CRAWFORD, M.D.   GEORGE PETTIT, M.D.
    Deputy Coroner   Deputy Coroner   Deputy Coroner

Within months of Volkman's arrival in Southern Ohio, Volkman received a coroner's subpoena
concerning the death of a patient. More deaths — and subpoenas — followed. *US Department of
Justice*

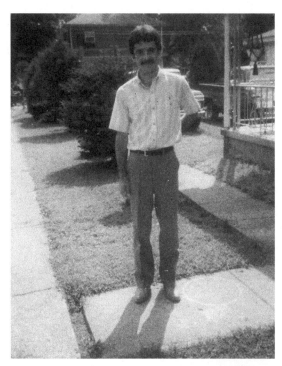

Volkman patient Daniel Coffee died in November 2003 at age 47. He was a father of three who was known for his playful sense of humor.
Courtesy of Carley Coffee

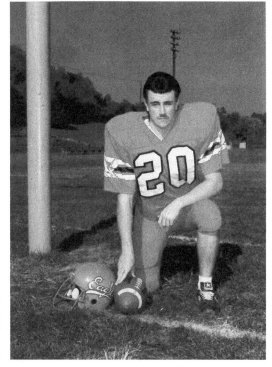

Volkman patient James Estep died in February 2004 at age 32. In high school, he was a multisport athlete.
Courtesy of Megan Rose Estep

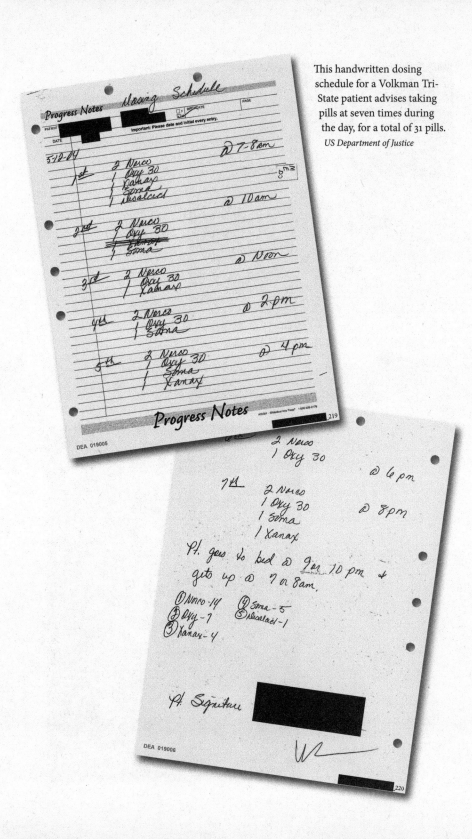

This handwritten dosing schedule for a Volkman Tri-State patient advises taking pills at seven times during the day, for a total of 31 pills.

US Department of Justice

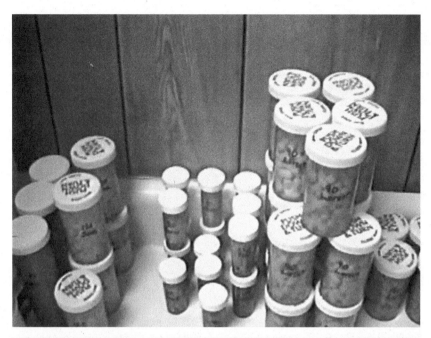
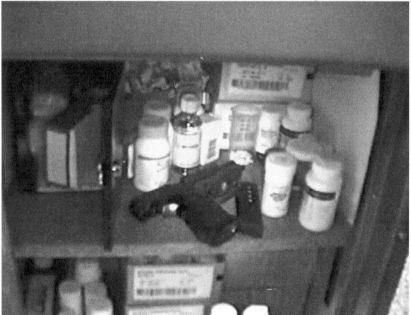

When DEA agents raided Tri-State Healthcare in June of 2005, they found stacks of prefilled bottles in the dispensary and multiple guns on the premises. *US Department of Justice*

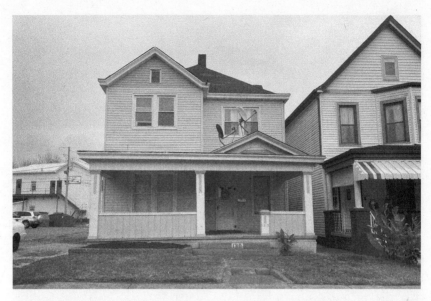

After leaving Tri-State Healthcare, Volkman ran a pain clinic out of this house, at 1310 Center Street, in Portsmouth. Within weeks, after numerous complaints from neighbors, the house was raided and the clinic was shut down. Taken in 2022. *Courtesy of Philip Eil*

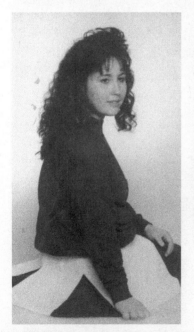

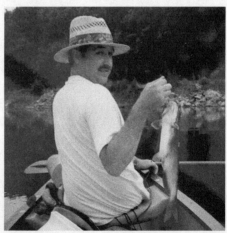

Volkman patient Ernest Ratcliff died in October 2005 at age 38. He loved to fish and hunt. *Courtesy of Melissa Flaugher-Ratcliff*

Volkman patient Scottie Lin James died in September 2005 at age 30. "Everybody loved her," said her sister Jakkie. *Courtesy of Jakkie Layne*

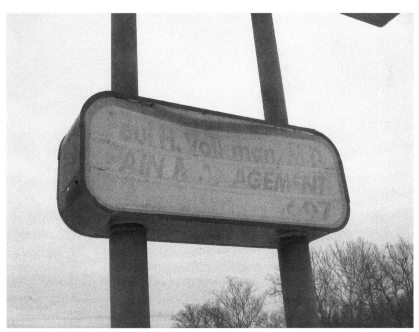

DEA # AV6952837   State Lic. #35-07-0722

PAUL VOLKMAN, M.D.
5565 US 23 · Chillicothe, OH 45601
Office (740) 663-4607 - Fax (740) 663-4625 - Cell (740) 357

Nº   2287

GOVERNMENT
EXHIBIT
1-16 b

Name

Address _____ Date 10-27-05

Oxycodone 15

240
two forty   #93h   8/day
Refill NR 1 2 3 4 5
severe LBP

☐ 1-24
☐ 25-49
☐ 50-74
☐ 75-100
☐ 101-150
☒ 151 and over

DEA 006957   Prescription is void if more than (1) prescription is written per blank

A Volkman prescription for oxycodone, written from his final office location, in Chillicothe, Ohio. *US Department of Justice*

In 2011, at the site of Volkman's Chillicothe clinic, traces of his practice were still visible. *Courtesy of Philip Eil*

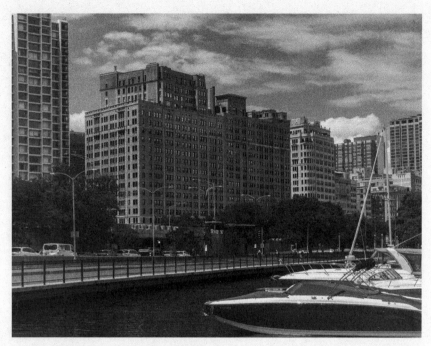

In 1999, one year after filing for bankruptcy protection, Volkman and his wife moved to an apartment at 3240 North Lake Shore Drive (center left), in Chicago. According to sworn testimony by Volkman's son, by 2007, rent was $4,500 per month. *Eric Allix Rogers*

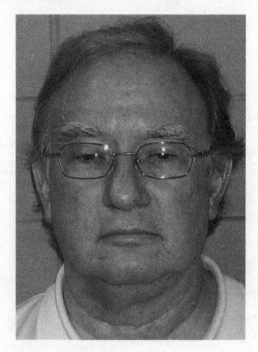

Throughout his case, Volkman maintained his innocence. At his sentencing in 2012, he said, "I have no regrets about my treatments and no apologies to make." *US Marshals Service*

In fact, I have every intention of appearing for any scheduled court date in my criminal case to vigorously contest the vicious, fabricated allegations with which the gov't has attacked me and my family. Your statement on 5/29/07 that my [pre-indictment] appearances for DEA hearings in Columbus bore no weight or relevance to my likelihood of appearing in Cincinnati when scheduled in essence meant that you considered it reasonable and appropriate to discount my entire life history as a law abiding, responsible physician and family man with no previous history of any violations of law and no history of any actions against him by any state medical board.

I respectfully request reconsideration of my continued incarceration at a second bond hearing to be scheduled as soon as possible.

Since, as I stated supra, I have not been able to have any access to advice of counsel, I am in no way waiving further consideration of any of the issues I have mentioned herein subsequent to any decision or action you may take

Respectfully

Paul H Volkman, MD, Ph.D.
Inmate 22435-424

After Volkman's arrest in 2007, he wrote a letter to the magistrate judge overseeing his detention. As this excerpt shows, he signed it with his credentials, as well as his current inmate identification number. *Public Access to Court Electronic Records (PACER)*

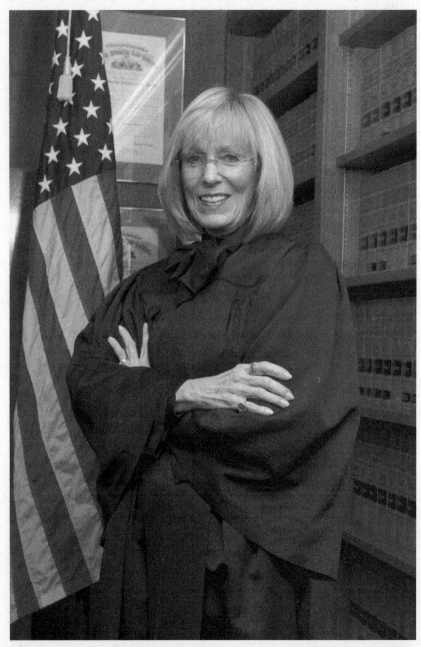

United States District Judge Sandra Beckwith presided over Volkman's criminal trial in 2011. At his sentencing hearing in 2012, she described him as "a truly dangerous man." *Courtesy of the University of Cincinnati*

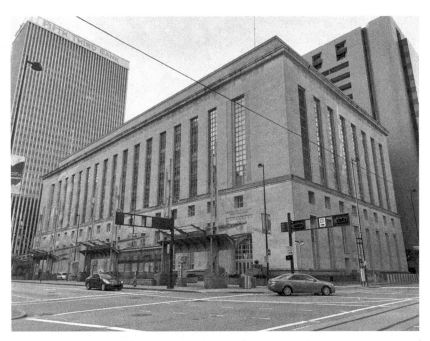

Volkman's criminal trial took place from March 1 to May 10, 2011, at the Potter Stewart US Courthouse in downtown Cincinnati. *Warren LeMay*

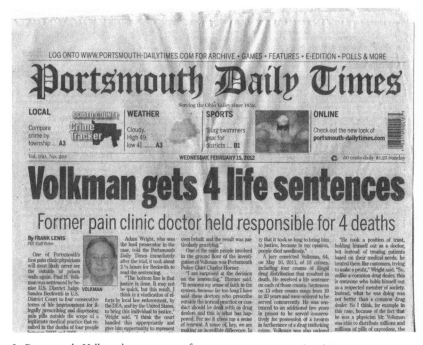

Portsmouth Daily Times

Serving the Ohio Valley since 1852.

LOCAL
SCIOTO COUNTY Crime Tracker
Compare crime by township ... A3

WEATHER
Cloudy.
High 49;
low 41 ...... A3

SPORTS
'Burg swimmers gear for districts ... B1

ONLINE
Check out the new look of portsmouth-dailytimes.com

Vol. 160, No. 218 WEDNESDAY, FEBRUARY 15, 2012 50 cents daily/$1.25 Sunday

Volkman gets 4 life sentences

Former pain clinic doctor held responsible for 4 deaths

By FRANK LEWIS
PDT Staff Writer

One of Portsmouth's first pain clinic physicians will most likely never see the outside of prison walls again. Paul H. Volkman was sentenced by Senior U.S. District Judge **VOLKMAN** Sandra Beckwith in U.S. District Court to four consecutive terms of life imprisonment for illegally prescribing and dispensing pain pills outside the scope of a legitimate medical practice that resulted in the deaths of four people between 2003 and 2005.

Adam Wright, who was the lead prosecutor in the case, told the Portsmouth Daily Times immediately after the trial, it took about 2½ hours for Beckwith to read the sentencing.

"The bottom line is that justice is done. It may not be quick, but this result, I think is a vindication of efforts by local law enforcement, by the DEA, and by the United States, to bring this individual to justice," Wright said. "I think the court handled this appropriately and gave him opportunity to represent

own behalf, and the result was particularly gratifying."

One of the main people involved in the ground floor of the investigation of Volkman was Portsmouth Police Chief Charles Horner.

"I am surprised at the decision on the sentencing," Horner said. "It restores my sense of faith in the system, because far too long I have said these doctors who prescribe outside the normal practice or conduct should be dealt with as drug dealers and this is what has happened. For me it gives me a sense of renewal. A sense of, hey, we are making an incredible difference. In

ty that it took so long to bring him to justice, because in my opinion, people died needlessly."

A jury convicted Volkman, 64, on May 10, 2011, of 18 crimes including four counts of illegal drug distribution that resulted in death. He received a life sentence on each of those counts. Sentences on 13 other counts range from 10 to 20 years and were ordered to be served concurrently. He was sentenced to an additional five years in prison to be served consecutively for possession of a firearm in furtherance of a drug trafficking crime. Volkman was also ordered

"He took a position of trust, holding himself out as a doctor, but instead of treating patients based on their medical needs, he treated them like customers, trying to make a profit," Wright said. "So, unlike a common drug dealer, this is someone who holds himself out as a respected member of society. Instead, what he was doing was not better than a common drug dealer. So I think, for example in this case, because of the fact that he was a physician Mr. Volkman was able to distribute millions and millions of pills of oxycodone, the

In Portsmouth, Volkman's sentence was front-page news. Portsmouth Daily Times

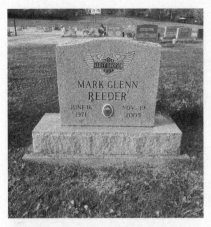

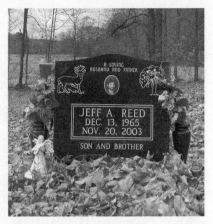

Volkman patient Mark Reeder is buried near Portsmouth, in the town of Friendship, Ohio. *Courtesy of Philip Eil*

Volkman patient Jeff Reed is buried in a small cemetery outside Greenup, Kentucky. *Courtesy of Philip Eil*

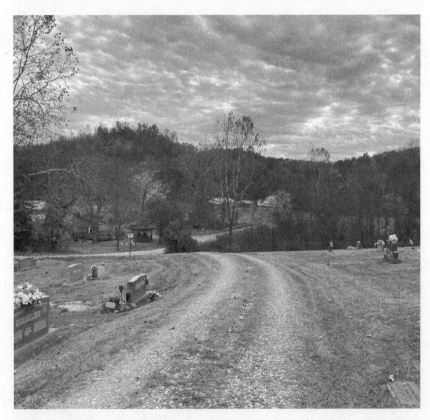

The view from Owl Creek Cemetery in Lucasville, Ohio — where Volkman patient Bryan Brigner is buried — is typical of Ohio's Appalachian region. *Courtesy of Philip Eil*

— PART THREE —
FACE-TO-FACE

THE PHONE CALL

One morning in June 2008, my father, Dr. Charles Eil, received a phone call at his office in Fall River, Massachusetts. It was Paul Volkman, calling to say that his wife, Nancy, had died. He wanted to know if my parents would come to the funeral.

In addition to calling my dad, Volkman made calls to classmates from the University of Rochester and at least three other colleagues from the University of Chicago. As he later explained to me, at the time — after his indictment and his wife's death — "I felt in large part that the life I had lived for 34 years was melting like a snowball on a warm day, soon to be gone without a trace." He felt a need to reach out to people who had known him in earlier, less complicated times.

Volkman's decision to call my dad that morning would prove pivotal in my life. It is, quite literally, the reason why this book exists. And I'll tell that story shortly. But first, I need to share a bit about who my dad was on the morning he heard from his long-lost former classmate.

Paul and Chas went in different directions after medical school.

Paul went to Duke briefly before returning to Chicago, where he soon left academic research, established a pediatrics office, and, later, supplemented his income by working in emergency rooms around the Midwest. My dad, meanwhile, embarked on a career in academic medicine — specifically, in the field of endocrinology.

Endocrinology — for those of you who didn't grow up hearing your father dictate insulin prescriptions over the phone — is a specialty of medicine that deals with hormones. While cardiologists are experts in the heart, pulmonologists focus on the lungs, gastroenterologists deal with the digestive system, and endocrinologists work with the pancreas, the thyroid, the pituitary gland, and other glands.

Endocrinology isn't particularly flashy or famous. Two endocrinologists won the Nobel Prize in 1923 for the discovery of insulin. And in the mid-1980s, endocrinologists were called to testify in the widely covered criminal trial of wealthy socialite Claus von Bülow, which involved a victim — Claus's wife, Sunny — who had been allegedly injected with insulin and fallen into a diabetic coma as a result. But generally, endocrinologists tend to stay out of headlines.

The practice of endocrinology doesn't involve a lot of procedures, and, because of this and other factors, it's not a particularly lucrative specialty. But if you, or someone you know, is one of the tens of millions of Americans with diabetes, then you may encounter an endocrinologist who is trained at treating the condition. Other reasons to consult an endocrinologist include osteoporosis, an over- or underactive thyroid, or issues with growth, metabolism, blood sugar, or sexual function. It's a particularly cerebral specialty. It's not uncommon to hear endocrinologists referred to as medical "detectives" who run tests, read the results, and try to figure out the source of a particular patient's distress.

My dad's first exposure to the field came in high school, when he participated in a four-week course in mammalian physiology as part of a kind of sleepaway camp for science. (Did I mention he was a bit nerdy?) Lectures were delivered by faculty members from the endocrine department of Cornell Medical School. Later, in medical school, he was fascinated by the way glands released chemicals that circulate through the body and carry messages between organs. He also liked that the field involved solving puzzle-like problems. A career in endocrinology promised a constant mental challenge.

My dad's post-med-school career started with an internship and residency at the University of Michigan, followed by fellowships at the National Institutes of Health, outside Washington, DC. In 1976, he enlisted in the US Public Health Service. And a few years later, he transferred to the US Navy, where he would remain — on active duty, then reserve status, rising in rank from lieutenant commander to commander to captain — until his retirement from the military in 1997.

But if you're picturing my dad performing gun-toting combat training, or even spending time on a battleship or in a submarine, think again. The navy, like other branches of the armed services, has its own doctors and hospitals. And my dad was one of them. I've heard him joke that, in decades of service in the navy, he never set foot on a boat.

It was during his early thirties, while working in a position at the Uniformed Services University of the Health Science outside Washington, DC, that he was set up on a blind date with a lawyer who worked at the Securities and Exchange Commission. Her name was Adele Geffen. As it turned out, she, too, had grown up in New York and she had also gone to the University of Chicago (as an undergrad). They had a rapport that I can still observe: She is funny, feisty, and outspoken, while he is more reserved, though quick to guffaw at her jokes. They're a good match.

As family lore has it, a pivotal moment took place early in their courtship when the two of them were walking to a concert in downtown Washington and came upon an elderly woman lying unconscious on the sidewalk, with her distressed husband nearby. My dad performed CPR on the woman and revived her before paramedics arrived. For a quiet and unassuming guy, it was a rare show of physical heroism. According to my mom, it made an impression.

My parents were married in July 1978 on a blazing-hot summer day in Washington. My oldest brother, Andrew, was born in January 1980. Then came Matt, in December 1982. And finally, I — the couple's third and youngest son — was born in April 1985.

One day in the mid-1980s, my dad was flipping through the *New England Journal of Medicine* and saw an intriguing job ad for a program director of the General Clinical Research Center at Brown University in Providence, Rhode Island. The job was affiliated with a local hospital, and it came with an appointment as a professor in Brown's medical school. It was an appealing prospect, and when he applied, he got it.

My parents didn't know anyone in Providence. But they found a house in a pleasant, tree-lined neighborhood, lined up a school for my older brothers, and my mom landed a job at a law firm downtown. In the summer of 1986, our family moved to Providence, the city I would come to know, and love, as my hometown.

My dad's position at Brown was, like many jobs in academic medicine, contingent on external funding. The university guaranteed only about half of his salary, and the rest was expected to come from grant funding.

For the first few years of the job, this wasn't a problem. Grant funding had been previously established when he arrived, and when the time came for reapplying, he succeeded.

But grant funding for medical research was then, as today, extremely competitive. In 1990, only around one in four applications to the National Institutes of Health received funding. And because the NIH was *the* predominant source of funding for academic research, if an application wasn't approved there, the applicant was left to scramble for elusive alternative options.

In my dad's case, when he applied for NIH funding for a second time, around five years after his arrival at Brown, he didn't get it. When his attempts to secure funding from non-NIH sources fell short as well, the chair of his division told him he was going to have to look elsewhere for a job.

At this point, my dad faced a tough choice. He could try to find a new academic job, but he didn't think the grant-funding prospects would be much better anywhere else. Even on the slim chance that he did secure funds, it would likely involve selling our house in Providence and uprooting the family once more. And such a move carried the strong possibility that, once again, the grant funding could dry up and he would be back in a similar position.

But there was another option: He could leave the academy and seek work in private practice — that is, he could put his PhD on the shelf and focus on the MD aspect of his training by treating patients for a living. In doing so, he would almost certainly earn a steady and comfortable income while avoiding the volatility of academic life.

I don't personally remember this period in our family's history. In 1991, when my dad left Brown, I was six years old. I know about it because I interviewed him numerous times for this project. And as both a journalist and as his son, I was particularly interested in this moment.

Learning about my dad's career in academia involved reconfiguring my sense of who my father was, professionally. Prior to this project, I knew him as a doctor who saw patients. I had perhaps seen the "PhD" on his business cards, but I didn't appreciate that he had been trained to conduct research, worked in that field for fifteen years, and then left the academy with great reluctance.

My dad is not particularly inclined to talk about his feelings. And yet when he spoke about his pivot to private practice, he told me that he was disappointed in himself and "depressed" about the whole situation. Leaving academia felt to him like a kind of admission of defeat. For a period, he saw a therapist about it. "I struggled with it," he told me.

As it turned out, the hardest part about leaving academia was the decision itself. The logistics of his new job fell into place rather quickly. While the job at Brown was winding down, my dad answered an ad from a clinic in Fall River, Massachusetts, seeking a general internist. By coincidence the doctor who conducted his interview was an endocrinologist who perked up when he heard about my dad's specialty. He needed a partner, and he promptly asked if my dad wanted to come work at his endocrinology office instead of taking the advertised job. My dad started working in Fall River on June 1, 1990.

It was a good fit. The commute from Fall River to Providence was less than half an hour, and my dad and his new partner, Howard, got along well. When it came to the duties of the office, they split the workload: They both saw the patients who came to the office for appointments, and they alternated seeing endocrinology patients in area hospitals for one- or two-week blocks at a time. In short order, my dad became a full partner and co-owner of the practice. And when his partner retired in 2001, he became the practice's sole owner.

It was around the time of my dad's shift to private practice that my memories start to kick in. So at this point in the story, I can share a bit from personal experience.

My dad is not a loud person, literally or figuratively. He is content to let others steer the conversation. He is not prone to argue, complain, or get angry. Even well into his seventies, he maintains a sunny, optimistic disposition.

He is extraordinarily steady and reliable. I would guess that, in thirty-some-odd years of working in private practice, he could count the number of days he's called in sick on two hands. And though my mother worked after we moved to Providence — first, as an attorney; then, later, after going back to graduate school, as a high school English teacher — my dad has remained our family's financial engine.

He is a man of habits and routines. Each morning he reads the newspaper at the kitchen table while drinking a cup of home-brewed coffee. In the evenings, after work, he'll often have a small glass of whiskey with ice. (It's never more than one drink. I don't think I've ever seen him drunk.) On workdays, his "uniform" consists generally of khakis, a button-down shirt, and a tie. On weekends, he'll wear an old pair of jeans and a sweatshirt.

When he's not working, you can find him reading, or watching football or golf on TV. For as long as I can remember he has also sang in choral groups, through either his synagogue, a local civic chorale, or both.

Some of my clearest childhood memories of him are from the mornings when he drove me to school on his way to work. He would hum along to the classical music on the radio and often ask me, or my brothers, if we knew who had composed a particular piece. I would never know; classical music wasn't really my thing. And he proudly would inform me that it was Bach or Strauss or Mozart or Schubert.

In 2008, when my dad received the call from Paul, endocrinologists were in high demand in the United States. Studies had shown that, for at least a decade, demand for their services had outpaced supply. And for a number of reasons, including rising rates of diabetes and the overall aging of the US population, which brought with it a higher need for endocrinological care, that demand was surging even higher as Baby Boomer doctors began to retire.

My dad's practice was no exception. In 2008, it had been more than five years since his partner, Howard, had retired, and he had not yet found a full-time replacement. As a result, my dad's days were completely booked with appointments, and he had a waitlist for new patients at least three months long. In addition to this office-based work, he was also personally handling the load of hospital-based patients that he and Howard had once split.

In terms of my dad's "business" (and medicine *is* a business), things were going well. If anything, things were going too well: He was over-worked, and had been that way for quite a while. On the morning that he received Paul's call, he had started the day by seeing patients at one of the local hospitals. When he got to his office, he was preparing for a full day of seeing appointments when the phone rang.

As my dad listened to the details about his classmate's wife's funeral, he wasn't sure if he would be able to attend. The memorial service was two days and a thousand miles away. If he abruptly missed work, the patients whose appointments he would have to cancel would fall to the back of a multi-month waiting list. He told Paul he would call him back and discussed the call with my mom later that night. She helped to dispel any indecision: They had to go; it was the right thing to do. Even if they couldn't attend the funeral, they would at least attend the shiva.

Nancy Volkman's memorial service took place on Friday, June 6, at a funeral chapel in Skokie, Illinois. Because she had been a beloved elementary school librarian, the room was filled with children, teachers, and parents from the school where she had worked.

During the service, a friend, Natalie Cohen, whom she had met as a little girl in Chicago, told stories of how as high school cheerleaders, they would often burst out laughing about how neither knew the rules of the games they were cheering for. Later, they had gone to the same college and then returned to Chicago, where they each started families. She described her friend as quick-witted and funny. In a draft of her prepared remarks, she described Paul as "caring, kind, loving and completely devoted."

The following morning, my parents flew to Chicago, where they were picked up at the airport by their friends, Dr. Oliver Cameron and his wife, Susan, who had also received an out-of-the-blue phone call from Paul. Oliver was also an MD/PhD graduate from the University of Chicago, and, afterward, he joined the psychiatry faculty at the University of Michigan, where he had stayed until retiring in 2003. Like my dad, Oliver had fallen out of touch with Paul within a few years of medical school. But the Camerons had remained close friends with my parents.

After taking Paul's phone call, Susan Cameron had, quite understandably, plugged Paul's name into an internet search engine to see what she could learn about him. In doing so, she had stumbled on coverage of Paul's criminal case and indictment. She was shocked. Now, at breakfast with my parents, she asked if they had heard about Paul's legal situation.

My parents had no idea what she was talking about. So she described what she had read online. My parents were also stunned. Compounding their shock was the fact that nobody at the table knew much about Paul's life after the University of Chicago.

After breakfast, the couples piled into the Camerons' car and drove to Paul's apartment.

If the story about Paul's criminal case had been hard to believe, his apartment reflected his new reality. He lived in a low brick building on a cul-de-sac on the west side of town. A short walk from the building's front door stood a guardrail, a chain-link fence, and a steep drop onto the whooshing cars and belching semi-trucks on Interstate 94. Planes flew low overhead on their descent to the nearby O'Hare International Airport.

The group walked up the stairs to the third floor and entered an apartment where guests were clustered in small groups. Paul stood in one of those groups, wearing athletic shorts. His gray hair was stringy and uncombed. To Susan Cameron, his disheveled appearance had an added poignancy. She remembered how, after she had first introduced Nancy to Paul, Nancy had spruced up Paul's appearance. She had encouraged him to shave his scraggly beard and dress in more appealing clothes. Now that she was gone, he seemed to have reverted to what she described as "the old Paul."

Paul greeted my parents and the Camerons and thanked them for their condolences. And as they chatted, he spoke freely and defiantly about his case. He said that he was the victim of an out-of-control government and that, in the Drug Enforcement Administration's zeal to win the War on Drugs, the agency had started going after innocent doctors. He explained that he planned to fight the charges against him. And he was hopeful that if Barack Obama was elected in the upcoming election, the new administration would sweep out the Bush-appointed US attorneys in the Department of Justice and dismiss the case.

That night, as a measure of sympathy, my parents and the Camerons took Paul out to dinner at a local restaurant and picked up the bill. Afterward, they again offered their condolences and said good-bye. The next morning, my parents flew home to Rhode Island.

THE QUERY LETTER

I know the exact day when I first heard Paul Volkman's name.

I was twenty-three years old, and I was on a trip to South Florida with my family to visit my ninety-nine-year-old great-aunt. There were five of us driving in a rented minivan one afternoon: my parents, my brother Andrew, my aunt Phyllis, and me. I don't remember where exactly we were driving, but at some point, the conversation in the car turned to my parents' recent trip to Chicago for Nancy Volkman's shiva. This was the first time I had heard about this trip, and it was *definitely* the first time I had heard about my dad's indicted former classmate. I immediately snapped to attention.

That night, I scribbled an entry into a diary. And given the odyssey that would follow, that piece of lined notebook paper has become a kind of memento. The date on the page is March 19, 2009. My handwriting is, as usual, barely legible. The entry is filled with factual errors: I misspelled Volkman's name, misstated the number of years that he and my dad were classmates, and incorrectly described the charges against him.

But the note captures my instant fascination with the story. As soon as

I heard about Paul Volkman, I was burning to know what had happened to him.

And beyond mere curiosity, I wanted to tell this story to the world.

As a longtime reader of true crime stories, I am keenly aware that these texts do not arrive in the world as fully formed objects. Fact-based crime narratives are produced by people who have distinct values, experiences, and blind spots. And I am also aware that authors can, despite their best attempts to be fair and impartial, leave their fingerprints on the stories they write. Because you've made it this far into this story, you deserve to hear a bit about me and my fingerprints.

Providence, my hometown, has a reputation for political corruption and organized crime. In fact, there is such a wealth of material here that the podcast *Crimetown* decided to spend its entire debut season telling stories from the city.

And yet, the part of the city where I grew up is quite safe and picturesque. The East Side of Providence is home to Brown University, the Rhode Island School of Design, and lots of big houses and carefully manicured lawns. I didn't hear gunshots growing up, nor was I accustomed to the sight of flashing red and blue police-cruiser lights. I grew up in a three-story house, with a spacious side yard on a tree-lined street. I went to the same nearby private school from pre-kindergarten through high school.

In other words, I spent my first eighteen years in a small and privileged bubble. And a large part of what drew me to the Volkman story was its sheer foreign-ness from the world in which I was raised.

At the same time, there were aspects of the story that were instantly familiar. I grew up around a lot of doctors. There was my dad, of course. There were also both of his parents (my grandparents), Lois and Harry. And I also had at least half a dozen friends or classmates in Providence whose parents were psychiatrists or cardiologists or allergists or gastroenterologists or men's health specialists or vascular surgeons. Most of these doctors were Jewish.

And when it came to Paul Volkman's general milieu — living in wealthy suburbs, paying for private school and costly bar mitzvah parties* — it sounded a lot like the world I knew. In fact, later, when I was slowly driving

---

* In 1988, to celebrate Adam's bar mitzvah, the Volkmans held a party at Cafe Spiaggia, the sibling restaurant of Chicago's Michelin-starred Spiaggia. Adam told me that the party must have cost "tens of thousands of dollars."

through the streets of Winnetka to get a feel for the neighborhood where the Volkmans lived, I remember thinking, "This looks just like where I grew up."

So when I first heard the bare outlines of Volkman's story, it was a collision of the foreign and the familiar.

This drew me in.

In college, I majored in English. I graduated in 2007 and without much of an idea of what to do next. I decided to follow my love of books to an entry-level job at a children's publishing house in New York City, which turned out to be a generic cubicle-based, spreadsheet-driven, nine-to-five job.

It wasn't a good fit.

With dismay, I saw my life stretching out ahead of me in an endless, colorless, tasteless chain of forgettable workdays and business-casual clothing. After a few months, as a break from the monotony, I signed up for a night class in nonfiction writing at a local college. And then everything changed.

In hindsight, I can see that my journalist's sensibilities had been with me for quite a while. I loved to read. I loved words and ideas. I loved talking to people. I loved hearing and telling stories. And during this night class in New York, at age twenty-two, my life's purpose suddenly clicked into focus: I wanted to be a journalist.

I soon began applying for newspaper internships and landed one at an alternative weekly paper in San Francisco called the *San Francisco Bay Guardian*. I quit my publishing job in early 2008 and spent the summer in California, learning the basics of the trade. I got my first reporter's notebook, conducted my first interviews, and published my first stories. The pieces were hardly earth-shattering: One was about a barbershop that doubled as a boxing gym, another was about a retro-themed diner in the neighborhood where I lived.

But I was hooked.

After the internship, I moved home to Providence to work as a substitute eighth-grade English teacher at my old school, filling in for a teacher who was on maternity leave. On the side, I started writing articles for a couple of small local papers. Over the next few months, I developed a portfolio of short, colorful human-interest stories published in local papers. One piece for the *Providence Phoenix*, the local alt-weekly, commemorated the one hundredth anniversary of a local pool hall. Another, for a local Jewish newspaper, the *Jewish Voice and Herald*, described a klezmer concert at a coffee shop.

By the time I learned about Paul Volkman in March 2009, I had published around ten stories.

Looking back, I marvel at the chutzpah that it took for me to decide, almost instantly, that I was going to write a book about my dad's indicted classmate. I was less than a year into my journalism career. I had never written about crime. I hadn't published anything longer than fifteen hundred words. All I knew was that it felt like every atom in my body was pulling me toward this story.

Since then, I've had plenty of time to think about the many factors behind that raw excitement.

Foremost was that I was, at the time, still riding the euphoric high of finding my life's calling. At that stage, the discovery of each new story idea brought a little spark of adrenaline and joy. And this Volkman story was a whopper.

It was also a story that, by necessity, would involve learning more about my dad. And because he had always been the quieter of my two parents, this appealed to me. At twenty-four years old, I still didn't feel like I understood what made him tick. Although I was aware that the project wouldn't be about him specifically, I knew that it would offer a chance to dig into the decade when his life and Paul's ran on parallel tracks. It would give me a chance to sit and talk with him about his life long before I was born.

It was also, quite obviously, a dark story, involving loss, grief, corruption, crime, and failure. And for my entire life up to this point, I had struggled with anxiety. For years, I had felt drawn to stories of things *going wrong*. (A friend of mine is deathly afraid of flying, and yet researches planes obsessively. This is something similar.) From very early on, this story spoke to me on a level that I wouldn't fully understand until I went through years of therapy.

I was further assured in my decision to pursue the project because, just two weeks before learning about Volkman, I had been accepted to a graduate writing program at Columbia University, in New York. In my application, I had described how inspired I was by the true crime book *In Cold Blood*. Now a major crime story had fallen into my lap. The timing seemed almost preordained.

––––––

When I returned to Rhode Island from the family trip to Florida, I set out to learn as much as I could about Volkman. I read the indictment, which had been released around two years earlier. I tracked down the *Columbus Dispatch* article that Susan Cameron had read, along with other coverage of the case. At one point, deep into a Google search on Volkman's name, I found a book called *America's Dumbest Doctors* that contained a short entry about Volkman's case titled "Physician Denied DEA License to Prescribe Medications After Deaths of 12 Patients." The cover over the book featured a slithering snake with a stethoscope for a tail.

Online, there was a fair amount of damning coverage of Volkman. But there was one notable exception. On a blog called *War on Doctors / Pain Crisis*, a physician and pain-patient advocate named Alex DeLuca came to Volkman's defense. DeLuca had apparently read the same articles I had, and he accused the mainstream media of a "one-sided prosecutorial view of the case." To correct outlets that had, to his eyes, breezed over or omitted key facts, he stressed Volkman's PhD in pharmacology, his certification by the American Academy of Pain Management, and his "extensive Clinical Pharmacology experience, and a quarter century of experience in Emergency Medicine, Family Practice and Pediatrics."

He reminded readers that Volkman had carefully monitored his patients through drug testing, ordered them to keep their medications locked in a safe, and frequently dismissed patients who reported their medicine stolen. He called the eye-popping pill counts mentioned in coverage of the case "trash" that lacked proper context.

"Dr. Volkman is a highly credentialed and experienced physician, a vocal critic of the DEA, who has been actively fighting them in courts for a year and a half," he wrote. "Isn't that part of the story, Associated Press?"

It was my first indication that this case could strike observers in radically different ways, depending on their views about medicine, law enforcement, opioids, and the treatment of chronic pain.

I added DeLuca's blog post to my files and kept digging.

As I searched for info about the Volkman case online, I continued to make progress in my journalism career. During the spring and summer of 2009, I passed a few early-career milestones. In late March, while covering the mayor of Jerusalem's visit to Harvard for *Jewish Voice*, I asked my first question at a press conference. In May, I published my first feature-length cover story: a *Jewish Voice* profile of a local engineer who had designed an easy-to-use circumcision device called the Accu-Circ that was intended for use in third-world countries. (Feel free to laugh about this; I certainly do.) In July, for the *Providence Business News*, I interviewed the superintendent of the Providence Public Schools, which marked my first one-on-one Q&A with a prominent public official. Then, in September, it was time to move to New York for the start of graduate school.

By the time I arrived in the city, I was fully committed to writing about Paul Volkman. I envisioned conducting at least a portion of the research during my graduate program, and, if things went as well, publishing a book sometime afterward. But the fate of the project seemed to hinge, at least somewhat, on whether Volkman would speak to me. The story would still be doable if he declined, but it would certainly be tougher. If he agreed to speak with me, though, it would be a clear sign from the universe to continue working on the project.

Whatever the case turned out to be, I was eager to learn.

And so, shortly after I had unpacked my bags and boxes in my new apartment, I typed out a carefully worded letter. This letter, like the diary entry from six months prior, has remained a relic from the early days of this project. It was dated September 4, 2009.

"Dear Dr. Volkman," I began. "My name is Philip Eil (son of Dr. Charles Eil) and I am a writing student at Columbia University."

I continued:

> Last spring, my father told me a little bit about your situation — the charges, indictment, etc. — and I became interested in the story. I started poking around online and found a number of documents pertaining to the case: newspaper articles, legal documents, blogs. None of the articles I found included your side of the story.
>
> I am interested in writing about this story, but before doing so, I would like to hear your version of the events. Would you be willing to be interviewed, at some length, for this purpose? I come to the story with no prejudice or preconceptions—simply as someone interested in understanding what really happened.
>
> If you would like to chat, I am happy to make arrangements about where, when, and how this can happen.

I was unsure of where Volkman lived, so I sent one copy of the letter to the apartment where my parents had seen him and another to an address for his daughter that I had found online.

About a week later, I was with a friend at a bar downtown when I received a phone call from an unknown number. When I walked out of the bar onto the noisy Manhattan sidewalk and opened my flip phone, I heard a sharp, slightly nasal voice on the other side. It was Paul Volkman, calling in response to my letter.

He said would be happy to talk to me, but he had one condition: I would have to agree to suspend any preconceptions that I had about the United States government. Without giving it much thought, I quickly agreed.

We spoke for a few minutes longer about the logistics of our meetings. I told him it made sense for us to meet in December, when I had a school break for the holidays, and I could drive out to Chicago to see him in person. That was fine with him. He even invited me to stay with him during my visit. I politely declined.

The call ended after a few minutes, but we continued the discussion over email. Two days after he called me, he wrote, "You sound like your Dad on the phone. Give my regards to him."

REMARRIED

I arrived in Chicago in December expecting to meet Volkman at the walk-up apartment where my parents had seen him for Nancy's shiva. Instead, via phone, he directed me to a tall, white apartment building on South Michigan Avenue, just a short distance from the Chicago Art Institute and the stretch of boutiques and high-rises known as the Magnificent Mile.

Inside the lobby, polished stone floors squeaked under my shoes as I checked in with a doorman who took my name and made a phone call to a man he called Mr. Volkman. After receiving a go-ahead to send me up, the doorman ushered me toward a bank of elevators, where he swiped a card over an electronic pad that beeped and allowed me to whoosh up toward the building's upper floors.

I would eventually learn the story behind Volkman's improbable move back to relatively posh surroundings. Within five months of his wife's death, he had gotten remarried, and, together with his new wife, they had moved to this upscale building in Chicago's South Loop.

How did a sixty-two-year-old man, facing a federal indictment and having just buried his spouse of thirty years, manage to get hitched so quickly?

This is what I learned from conversations with Paul, his daughter, and his second wife.

Shortly after Nancy's death in June 2008, Paul created an account on a Jewish dating website, JDate, where according to a description I later got from his daughter, he began "maniacally seeking companionship." It didn't take long for him to meet someone. Her name was Clara.* She lived in Chicago. They were around the same age. And she was a practicing clinical social worker.

Clara was born in Russia and lived in both Poland and Israel before immigrating to the United States, which explained her thick Eastern European accent. She had gone to college and graduate school in the Detroit area and practiced social work there for decades before moving to Chicago in the mid-2000s. When she arrived in the new city, she told me that she knew few people other than her two daughters and her sister. So she signed up for an account on JDate.

Paul was hardly effusive in his descriptions of Clara, which was consistent with his overall disinterest in describing things or people that he liked. He described her to me at different times as "a very nice lady," "a very nice and intelligent person," and "a very nice person" with whom he had a "nice relationship." They apparently spent their first dates going out to dinner, taking walks, and going to art fairs. And things got serious quickly. "We spent pretty much every day together for two months," Paul told me.

When I interviewed her in 2011, Clara admitted that Paul initially "didn't really seem like a big catch," which struck me as a rather extreme understatement. There was his pending criminal case, of course. But there was also the fact that his wife had recently passed away, and he sometimes cried when he spoke about her. On one of their first dates — in an incident that aligns with earlier accounts of his obliviousness about his appearance — she said that he wore an enormous yellow golf shirt that fit him "like a dress." He looked "awful," she said.

Her first trip to his apartment didn't help. She told me that, though the place seemed nicely decorated (for which credit must go to Nancy and her

---

* As a condition for speaking with me for this book, Clara asked that I not use her real name, and I agreed.

trusty interior decorator), she noticed that Paul's late wife's clothes were still hanging in closets, and, at one point, she opened a drawer and found a pair of Nancy's glasses. "It looked like his wife just stepped out," she told me. When she described Volkman to one of her daughters, the daughter advised her to steer clear of him. But she ignored the advice.

The reason, she explained, was that, despite the long list of things Paul didn't have going for him, she liked him. She thought he had a great sense of humor, and she found him "friendly," "warm," and "very straightforward and honest." Perhaps most important, unlike some of the other men she had dated during her time in Chicago, he lived in the city, not the suburbs. During our interview, she explained that her move to the city of Chicago from the Detroit suburbs was intentional. And when she began going on dates after arriving, she found men her age to be reluctant to meet her in the city. They complained about parking or would drive in for dinner and want to drive back at the end of the night. This was a "huge turnoff," she said.

Paul was different. He was willing to meet up with her in the city. So they did.

But even if Paul and Clara enjoyed each other's company, according to both of their accounts in separate interviews, practical factors pushed the relationship to move faster.

First was the fact that, within a few months of their meeting, Clara's lease was set to expire. She wanted to have a place where she could see patients at home, and Paul, as a longtime resident of her new city, offered to help her look for one. Paul was, as it turned out, keen to move from the apartment overlooking the interstate. And it wasn't long before they arrived at the idea that, by pooling their resources, they could afford a place they both liked. Clara later explained that the pair struck an agreement whereby they would try living together, and if it didn't work, they'd go their separate ways.

They found an apartment they both liked on Michigan Avenue, in a building that was completed just a few years prior. This where I would meet Volkman for our first interviews in December 2009. The apartment was spacious and attractive enough that Clara felt comfortable seeing her patients there. And with the help of Paul's Social Security checks — his only source of income — the two could afford it. They made the move.

But beyond their living situation, another factor prompted them to push the relationship even further: health insurance. Clara later explained to me that, when she met Paul, her insurance plan cost more than $500 per month and required her to travel back to Michigan to see an in-network provider. She was distressed about this. It wasn't a tenable situation, and, at some point, Paul pointed out that if they got married, Clara would gain access to the coverage he had through his late wife's Chicago-public-schools pension. And this seems to have been the real motivating factor behind the wedding.

Volkman described the marriage to me as a product of "financial convenience, combined with the fact that we liked each other." His daughter, meanwhile, later offered her own succinct take: "INSANE."

But how had Clara gotten past Paul's indictment?

The answer, I learned, was that he convinced her of his innocence.

When I spoke with her in 2011, she admitted that when she first heard about the case, it seemed clear that he had done "deliberate, terrible things." She was skeptical that the US government would charge someone with those kinds of crimes out of thin air. She also acknowledged that Paul was "very stubborn" and "arrogant" and said that he had made several foolish decisions that led him to his situation.

But on a fundamental level, she believed his story.

She said that, in response to her questions, he had given her lots of information, including showing her his patient charts. She said that he was "very up-front about all of it and he didn't hide anything."

It clearly worked.

During our conversation in 2011, her comments on the case echoed many of Paul's, sometimes word for word. She, too, believed that when his patients had died, it was because some of them were "very sick." She, too, used the word "hillbilly" when discussing the region where Paul was working. She, too, thought that press coverage of his case had been woefully unfair. "They present him like he's like a maniacal serial killer, almost," she said. She did not seem to have considered that perhaps Paul's version of the story was, itself, biased or unbalanced.

And when it came down to it, she did not think that Paul was a criminal. She explained that her mother was born in Russia and raised during the Stalin era, and she felt that Paul's case reminded her of the stories her mother told. His case struck her as a kind of "contriving and forcing and twisting things" to fit a certain picture that suited the aims of the government, she said.

She described the case as "like a Greek tragedy." Though, when she said it, she seemed to mean that a lot of the tragedy lay in what had *happened to* Paul, and not what he had done.

And so it came to pass that, in October 2008, just four months after Nancy Volkman's funeral, Paul and Clara flew to Las Vegas for a prepackaged vacation that included plane tickets, hotel reservations, and a rental car. Paul notified his bond officer about the trip, as he was legally obligated to do. They stayed at the Monte Carlo hotel and casino. And during their stay, the couple drove to a local government building where they paid a fee, filled out some forms, and coaxed two passing strangers to serve as their witnesses. And then — as public marriage records from Clark County, Nevada, confirm — they were married on October 28, 2008.

As Clara relayed these details to me during our conversation, I remarked that it didn't sound particularly romantic. "No, it wasn't," she said.

But the timing was fortuitous.

Back in Chicago, within a few weeks of her Vegas nuptials, Clara accidentally fell, broke her wrist, fractured her back, and wound up spending a few days in the hospital. The bill added up to more than $20,000. But a significant portion was covered by her new insurance from Nancy Volkman's retirement plan.

At this point in her story, I asked, "Did it ever feel weird to have that be the situation that you were receiving benefits from —"

"His ex?" she interrupted.

No, it wasn't weird, she said. Because, she explained, when you're married, whatever one person has, the other person shares.

CHICAGO

I was greeted at the apartment door by a short, pale, pudgy man with white eyebrows that tufted out from behind his eyeglasses. Paul Volkman was dressed casually in a black T-shirt tucked into jeans. He reached out to shake my hand and led me down a hallway into his apartment.

We turned a corner and the hall opened into an open kitchen, dining area, and living room. In one corner was a sliding glass door that led to a terrace. Lining the perimeter of the room was a series of floor-to-ceiling windows that, on a clearer day, would have offered wide views of the city. On this day — foggy, with frozen rain — I saw only the faint outlines of skyscrapers. When I peered down at the street level, the elevated trains looked like toys.

After our initial greetings, we settled into seats in the living room. I took out a pen, a notebook, and my digital voice recorder. When I asked if I could record, Volkman granted his permission.

"In your high school civics class, you might have heard about 'innocent until proven guilty'?" he said after I began recording. "If it was ever true, it hasn't been true for quite a while."

One of the first things that struck me about Volkman was just how unremarkable he was. He wasn't physically imposing, and his voice had a slightly nasal quality. As we sat together, he didn't shout or twitch or do anything that suggested he wasn't fully in control of himself. He was a middle-aged, paunchy Jewish guy with a forgettable face. If I had been introduced to him at a coffee shop or cocktail party without knowing about his case, I wouldn't have given him much of a thought.

In our conversations over the next few days, he spoke about his love for the impressionist collection at the Art Institute of Chicago. He told me about his two cats, Twinkletoes and Butch. He described how he played bridge several times a week and enjoyed online chess. He said that he watched the left-leaning news and commentary network MSNBC, and he spoke disparagingly of its right-wing counterpart, Fox News. When we talked about national politics, he expressed admiration for two of the most liberal US senators, Al Franken of Minnesota and Bernie Sanders of Vermont.

But once we got past the small talk, I started to see what made Volkman different from the average highly educated, liberal, city-dwelling retiree. It emerged as he shared the story of how he found himself, at age sixty-three, indicted, stripped of his DEA registration, and awaiting a trial that would determine whether he'd spend his remaining years in prison.

The mood of the story that Volkman told me about his life could be summed up in a single word: *dark*.

He told me that he hated his hometown of Washington, DC — partly because he found the swampy climate there "disgusting," but largely due to his utter lack of fondness for his family of origin. He described his parents as "terrible." He said that he hadn't talked to his brother, Alan, in six years, and if he saw him on the street, he'd walk right past. "Hopefully, he's dead," he said. "I can't stand the son of a bitch."

After describing his upbringing, Volkman moved on to what he viewed as his life's defining mistake: pursuing a career in medicine. "If I could re-run my life I would not be a doctor," he said. "It's just a terrible way to make a living."

His negative feelings about medicine seemed to cast a shadow over the institution where he had studied it. One afternoon, we drove down to the University of Chicago campus. And as we drove, he said, "I don't have any particularly warm feelings about this place."

He explained the school had probably more Nobel Prize winners per square inch than any institution in the world. And as he remembered it, students were considered lucky to "breathe the same air with all of these exalted people."

He believed that these attitudes were reflected in the lack of instruction about the practical aspects of a medical career. At one point, he told me, "I had a PhD from the University of Chicago, but that doesn't mean I knew shit about anything." He said that he wound up learning on his own to set up an office, how to bill patients, and other logistical aspects of being a doctor. If he hadn't, he said, "I would have starved very quickly."

To hear Volkman tell it, his career after medical school had been a series of disillusionments. It began during his residency at Duke when, as he told it, he noticed a pattern of the hospital performing unnecessary, and yet lucrative, exploratory abdominal surgeries on teenage girls. He said that when he spoke up about the practice, his concerns were ignored. "At that point, I realized that the prevailing principle in America is that 'Money talks and bullshit walks.'"

This experience was followed by his brief and unsuccessful stint in academic research back in Chicago, during which his lab director had refused to allow him to publish his "major paper with major implications" on the treatment of strokes.

More disappointments followed.

There was his realization that pediatrics "paid like shit" and wouldn't be able to sustain the standard of living he wanted to provide for his family. There was the time, a few years later, when he was blamed for the failed equipment that Chicago paramedics brought to his office, which, in his telling, both doomed his efforts to save the girl's life and led to an unfounded lawsuit and jury verdict against him. There were the ensuing instances when, after pivoting to locum tenens work in emergency rooms around the Midwest, he faced more baseless lawsuits and ultimately became uninsurable. Of those lawsuits, he said, "One was more ridiculous than the next."

To hear Volkman tell it, he was an honest, innocent guy who had tried to navigate a corrupt world and fallen victim to a long list of injustices along the way.

Our conversations during those first meetings were sprinkled with little comments about my dad, which gave the interviews a bit of warmth. As we drove around the University of Chicago's campus, Volkman pointed out one building, "where I had my lab and where Chas had his lab," and a gymnasium where he and my father had once played basketball. At another point, when discussing his diabetes, Volkman said, "I was taken care of by an endocrinologist, like your father." Such comments made it feel almost like I wasn't interviewing a stranger but, rather, some kind of long-lost uncle.

At other times, while Volkman narrated his story, I would occasionally ask questions for clarification. And when a portion of his story begged for a bit of commonsense pushback, I would give it.

But mostly I listened.

Partly this was simply my personality. I am, by nature, polite and nonconfrontational, especially if I'm just meeting someone.

And partly it was due to how recently I had arrived at the story. In December 2009, Volkman was one of the very first people I had interviewed. I hadn't yet dug into the stories of his malpractice cases. I hadn't yet spoken to his children or people from different stages of his life who might offer an alternative perspective. I hadn't been to Portsmouth. The criminal trial hadn't taken place, which meant that I hadn't read its forty-three-hundred-page transcript. It wasn't just that I was uninclined to push back strongly against his story at that point; I also didn't have the means to do so.

As it turned out, Volkman was quite comfortable in the role of the experienced expert, holding forth about his life and the lessons it contained. And so, quite quickly during those first meetings, we settled into roles resembling teacher and student. He was a gray-haired sixty-three-year-old man with two advanced degrees and two grown children, and who had

worked in medicine for decades, who had weathered lawsuits, the death of
his wife, and a criminal indictment. I was a twenty-four-year-old graduate
student with no kids, no marriage, and minimal real-world experience.

Eventually we arrived at his time in Ohio.

Before he got to the specifics of what happened in Ohio, Volkman wanted
to share some essential context.

The first piece was what he described as nearly a century of ill-advised
American drug and alcohol policies. These policies traced at least as far
back as the Harrison Act, from 1914, which criminalized the practice of
treating addicts with narcotic medication. As a result, tens of thousands of
doctors were thrown in prison. After this came Prohibition, in the 1930s,
which ushered in with it what he described as "great waves of organized
crime and mob violence," government corruption, and a rash of poison-
ings from people drinking bad batches of home-brewed spirits. Then in the
1970s came the War on Drugs, which, in Volkman's telling, was a "stupid"
and "self-destructive" policy, responsible for countless deaths from violent
turf wars that were an inevitable by-product of such prohibitive policies.
Volkman believed that substances like cocaine and heroin ought to be
legalized and regulated like alcohol and said that banning them was "the
dumbest thing you could possibly do."

In telling this story, he said that, at some point, the federal government
had broadened the goals of its drug war and embarked on a campaign
of "terrorizing" doctors, who were easy prey for prosecutors. In addition to the political benefits of successfully prosecuting doctors, which
allowed politicians and law enforcement to tout progress in their drug war,
Volkman claimed that there was also a major financial incentive at work.
He believed that there was a $500 billion black market for pain medica-
tion in the United States that the DEA controlled. And he said that the
investigations and prosecutions of pain doctors were designed to make
other doctors too scared to prescribe the medications that patients needed,
which, in turn, sent millions of legitimate pain patients into a black market
of street dealers who, he claimed, ultimately funneled money to the DEA.

As far-fetched and conspiratorial as it was, this scenario was apparently
a bedrock belief for Volkman: the notion that, due to his legitimate and
law-abiding prescribing of opioid painkillers, the DEA saw him as a threat
to its criminal enterprise. In his eyes, the federal agency tasked with enforc-
ing drug laws was not acting out of an interest in public safety or public

health; they were snuffing out a competitor who had taken too big of a bite from their black-market profits.* "You're talking about a massive web of corruption affecting the entire country," he said at one point. "It involves police. It involves prosecutors, local officials. I mean it goes straight up to the top, just as it did during the prohibition of alcohol."

Here again was his theme of the honest man — himself — battling sinister and corrupt external forces.

The second piece of context for his case related to pain. Chronic pain was incredibly widespread, he said, and it affected between thirty and fifty million people in the United States. "Anywhere you go — if you sit on the bus, there's probably five pain patients," he said.

This pain originated in all kinds of ways: illnesses, car accidents, sports injuries, aches and pains from physical labor. And it was a remarkably destructive force, he said. Not only was it miserable, but it also led to a number of hellish secondary symptoms. At one point, he ticked off the problems that stem just from a pain patient's lack of sleep, which include anxiety, headaches, and hypertension. He added that sleep-deprived pain patients were also perpetually sleepy, which made it dangerous to drive, which sometimes led to car accidents, which led to more pain.

In Volkman's telling, this problem of widespread chronic pain was connected to his first piece of context. He said that because of the government's prosecution of doctors, the DEA had spooked medical practitioners out of giving people the medicine they desperately needed. "Pain patients, in general, do not get . . . adequate pain medicine," he said. "Because a lot of doctors who would otherwise give them appropriate prescriptions are basically scared to death to do so."

He continued, "Why was I the number one prescriber of oxycodone? Because I was one of the few doctors who was either honest enough or dumb enough, depending on how you want to look at it, to actually prescribe real pain medicine to people who had pain."

————

* This theory echoed what Volkman had written in 2006, in a series of online comments in response to online coverage of a prominent pain doctor's drug-dealing trial in northern Virginia. In those comments, he wrote that the DEA was "a ruthless mob that runs the illegal drug business, taking a healthy cut of every street drug sale," and doctors and pharmacies that prescribe opioid medications "cut into the DEA's core business and are therefore attacked and put away, after bogus charges and sham show trials are held." In Volkman's telling, these prosecutions built on one another to achieve multiple DEA goals: They took DEA competitors out of the picture, and, in doing so, "scare[d] other doctors away from prescribing real pain medicine and interfering with the DEA's cash cow."

As Volkman walked me through his tale of what happened in Ohio, he addressed some of the red flags that had been mentioned in the indictment and the ensuing press coverage.

Why had he worked for a clinic owner with no medical background?

Volkman said that Denise Huffman was a long-suffering pain patient herself, and many of her family members were, too. Her husband had hip problems, and her son had "terrible" problems with his leg and a medical record "six inches thick." He believed that she had started the clinic, in part, to make sure her own family could get proper care. And he said that she had told him that a lot of other folks in the area were similarly undertreated. He viewed the clinic as a way for Denise to perform a civic duty while making a good living at the same time. And he saw nothing wrong with that.

Nor did he find fault with Tri-State's decision to accept only cash. One of the lessons he had learned from his time in pediatrics was the difficulty in getting reimbursed for patients who received public assistance. Payments would take months to process, he said, and forms could be sent back to the office due to something as small as a misplaced comma. If he were to treat those kinds of patients, "you could be busy all day in your office and go home with absolutely nothing at the end of the day," he said. He seemed to view the fulfillment of insurance claims in a similar light.

The lack of physical examinations at his clinics?

"What examination, exactly, could I do on you to find out that you're in pain?" he asked. There was none, he said. Just like there was also no test and no scar and no medical record that could definitively prove that a patient was in pain. He also said that exams were of little use for the kinds of patients who came to his pain clinic. These patients had been examined by primary care doctors and referred to neurologists and ortho-pedic surgeons before they came to him. Their prior gauntlets of medical treatment had been ineffective. He was, he said, a "tertiary" physician, the doctor to whom a patient was sent when everything else failed.

And what about the amounts of opioids he was prescribing?

In Volkman's telling, it was *not* prescribing opioids that was dangerous for pain patients, since high doses of over-the-counter anti-inflammatories were proven to cause gastrointestinal bleeding that led to thousands of deaths every year. Meanwhile, he believed that other non-narcotic meds that doctors prescribed for pain were virtually useless. As he saw it, any honest doctor would admit that "basically the only way to treat pain is with narcotics."

His story continued in this vein, in which he seemed to have an answer for every concerning aspect of his stint in pain management.

The crowds that were milling around outside of the Findlay Street clinic? They were patrons of the soup kitchen across the street.

The high levels of security at his clinics?

That was simple common sense, he said. He was working in a high-crime area and handling thousands of dollars in cash every day. "So, it was pretty clear to me that I needed to have a security guard," he said.

But the biggest red flags of all, of course, had been the deaths of his patients. And as I would hear, Volkman had detailed explanations for these, too. In each case, his answer moved the responsibility off his shoulders and placed it elsewhere.

He started by reminding me that if a patient came to him for chronic pain care, they likely had some serious illness or injury to begin with. As a pain physician, he had no more ability than any other doctor to keep patients alive if they suffered from a life-threatening illness like heart disease. And so, he said, the mere fact that several of his patients had died was not a sign of his criminality. What about cancer doctors? All of their patients die, but nobody thinks they're bad doctors. "It depends on the population you take care of," he said. He also said that, due to the punishing nature of their pain, his patients' risk of suicide was "100 times higher" than the general population's.

It was these factors, not overdoses, that explained many of his patients' deaths. In Volkman's telling, one patient died from cancer, and another died from complications due to morbid obesity. Two died from heart attacks, while three had committed suicide. He even believed that one had been choked to death by her husband. All such deaths were, quite obviously, not a reflection on him. Nor, he said, was it his fault if a patient died because they hadn't been taking the meds as prescribed and yet tried to pass a urine or blood screening by taking a bunch of pills at once. "I feel no sympathy for people like that," he said, "because they were trying to *use* me and they died in the process of trying to *use* me." He accentuated the word "use" as if to convey how repugnant he found the thought.

It was also not his fault, he argued, if a patient took the pills in ways other than how he had advised to take them. He recalled family members of his former patients who had testified at his DEA hearing that their relatives had died after snorting their medications or taking more than he had advised. Volkman said that these patients had signed forms that explicitly absolved him of responsibility for such outcomes. And he also claimed to have personally explained the dangers of the medications he prescribed.

"There's something called personal responsibility," he said. "If I give you a pill to take four times a day and you take fifteen of 'em all at once, that ain't my fault."

To Volkman, the accusations that he had caused patient deaths were an egregious misrepresentation of what he had been doing in Ohio. And perhaps the worst distortion of all was the so-called death waiver.

This waiver appeared midway through the indictment, in a portion titled "Ways, Manners, and Means of the Conspiracy." Tucked into this section were two paragraphs that read:

84. During the course and in furtherance of the conspiracy, VOLKMAN had a customer sign a "death waiver" and had him acknowledge that the customer was aware of the risk to the customer's life if that customer then took the medication.

85. During the course and in furtherance of the conspiracy, VOLKMAN would then prescribe an excessive amount of controlled substances to the "death waivered" customer.

Coverage of the indictment from the *Columbus Dispatch* and *Chicago Tribune* had mentioned the waiver in a way that suggested that everyone involved knew how dangerous the clinic's activities were, and the waiver was Volkman's attempt at protecting himself legally while doing little to curb the actual danger of his actions.

But during our interviews, Volkman claimed that the so-called death waiver was actually a note that appeared in the medical files of one of his particularly sick patients. This man was a former coal miner, and he was in awful shape when he came to Volkman: He had lung disease, chronic pain, and "a bunch of other things," Volkman said. Volkman treated the man for two years, he said, and then, in November 2005, the man got so sick that he was sent to a hospital and placed on a ventilator to assist his breathing.

During one of the patient's post-hospital visits to the pain clinic, Volkman said, he learned that the guy had been on a ventilator, and he knew that, for a patient with chronic lung disease, this meant that the man likely only had a few weeks to live. Volkman viewed his role in that situation as basically "try[ing] keep them comfortable and hold[ing] their hand" as the end neared.

And so Volkman recounted the conversation he had with him. "I said, 'Look, I'm sure I'm not going to tell you anything you don't know, but you're real near the end. And you don't have more than a week or two to live,'" he told me.

In Volkman's telling, the man acknowledged that he knew this to be true.

Volkman inhaled deeply and his lip began to tremble. He paused, then said, "It still bothers me," in a half-choking voice. He took off his glasses, wiped his eyes with his hands, and then, after another pause, continued.

"He said he wanted to make it to Christmas, so he could give his ten-year-old son his gifts," Volkman said. So Volkman said that he had explained to the man the potential side effects of the medication he was prescribing — mainly, that it could slow his respiration considerably and that, in his current state, this could be fatal.

According to Volkman, the patient replied, "I know that, but I'm willing to take the risk, because if I don't have pain medicine, I'd rather die right now anyway."

After hearing this, Volkman said that he wrote out a statement that essentially summarized his warning to the patient and the patient's accompanying acknowledgment of the risk, called a few nurses into the room as witnesses, and had the man sign it.

This, he said, was the infamous death waiver. What had been touted by the prosecutors as an example of a cash-hungry doctor's ruthless tactics was, in Volkman's telling, a compassionate move to extend a dying man's life, ease the pain of his final hours, and provide informed consent of the dangers of his treatment.

Overall, Volkman was unequivocal that he bore no responsibility for the deaths of any of his pain patients. And he refused to admit that he had even caused anyone harm. As he told me at one point, "I never found a single instance where, if a patient took the medicine as I prescribed it to them, [they] had any type of ill effect from it. Not even once. Not even a hint of it."

If it sounds like Volkman was asking me to believe a lot, he was.

These conversations were my first glimpse of what would become a familiar experience during the decade I spoke with him: listening to his

straight-faced accounts of elaborate scenarios in which he was an innocent and unfortunate victim, paired with his aggressive attacks against all
conflicting accounts and their sources.

And while I didn't walk away from this first series of interviews as a
dyed-in-the-wool believer in his cause, he did present an extraordinarily
detailed counter-reality to what I had read online. After listening to him
for ten hours, over two days, it was hard to remain completely defended
against his version of events. He wore a listener down with facts and statistics and expertise — or at least the appearance of these things.

This was perhaps the most tangible benefit of traveling to Chicago to
speak to Volkman before I conducted almost any other on-the-ground
reporting about his case. By hearing his story with fresh ears, I was able to
better understand the people I later met who accepted his story as truth.

This list of Volkman believers and defenders included Clara, who would
tell me that her husband was perhaps guilty of stupidity and arrogance, but
certainly not drug dealing.

It also included his ninety-two-year-old former therapist who, after
waiving doctor-patient confidentiality for Volkman, told me he viewed
the man as "obviously a brilliant guy" who had "a great compassion for
people" and "great concern about people suffering." He also told me that
he "absolutely" found Volkman to be a trustworthy narrator of what
happened in Ohio and was generally convinced of Volkman's account of
being railroaded.

It included one of Volkman's bridge-playing pals from Chicago, who
was a retired CEO and graduate of Yale (undergrad), Harvard (law school),
and Stanford (business school), who told me that what Volkman was doing
in Ohio sounded like Doctors Without Borders, the Nobel Peace Prize–
winning organization dedicated to bringing medical care to conflict zones.
He said that Volkman struck him as a "very sincere well-meaning guy that
was only trying to do good for the world . . . and [who] has paid a terrible,
terrible price for what he did."

This list of Volkman defenders also included his daughter, Jane, who,
though she sometimes wrestled with her father's tale, spent years as a vocal
advocate on his behalf. In her words, Paul Volkman was "a gentle man,
who has never committed a violent act in his life," and who "was acting at
all times according to proven medical principles that he believed in."

After these first few days of listening to Volkman, I was aware of what
made him so convincing.

For all his tale's outlandishness and paranoid flourishes, Volkman was clearly an intelligent man. He seemed to have a perfect recall for facts, statistics, names, and details. He appeared to be widely read and fluent in an eclectic mix of subjects, from history to law to politics. And when it came to medicine, he drew from what appeared to be immense expertise.

He also wielded this expertise like a weapon, to attack people who in his view fell short of his standards of intelligence. One of the primary DEA agents who had worked on his case was a "total moron." The lawyer who had represented him in the feeding-tube lawsuit was a "dumbass." David Procter was "pathetically stupid."

And even when he wasn't on the attack, Volkman didn't pad his speech with the disclaimers and doubts that people often use. When he quoted stats or facts, he didn't say, "I think it might be . . ." or "It was around . . ." He rarely admitted uncertainty or confusion or minimized his story by saying, "Of course, this is just *my experience* . . ." When Volkman told his story, he spoke as if every decision he had made was the perfectly normal, expected, and rational course of action. He projected total confidence.

And so, when I did have doubts about his story, I would then have doubts about those doubts. Who was I to question this man, who was so much more qualified and experienced than I? Who was I to argue with a man with an MD and a PhD?

From these initial interviews, I walked away with the awareness that Paul Volkman — in his intelligence, his experience, his expertise, and the way he carried himself — came across as one of the most likely to be trusted people you could find.

And there was yet another factor in his favor. To fact-check his claims, the people in his Chicago life would have had to travel four hundred miles to an Ohio town that they had little reason to visit otherwise. If they didn't go to Portsmouth and Chillicothe, they were almost entirely reliant on him to tell them what had happened there.

I suspect that some people might have also sympathized with Volkman because of the ordeal he had experienced beginning in May 2007.

It started when he was arrested at home following his indictment. And after his bail was denied, he spent about two weeks in the Metropolitan Correctional Center in Chicago, where he said he had no visitors and was allowed no phone calls.

Eventually, he said, he was flown to a federal transfer center in Oklahoma, while manacled, in a "broken-down, rust-bucket 737 that looks like it's going to fall apart in the middle of the air." From Oklahoma, he was flown to Lexington, where he was placed in a small truck with other prisoners and driven to the Grant County Detention Center, about forty miles south of Cincinnati, which he described as dirty, overcrowded, and kept at uncomfortably cold temperatures.

After a few days at the GCDC, he started coughing and having chest pain, which he believed to be pneumonia. He managed to convince the on-site nurse of his situation, and he was taken to a nearby emergency room, where the diagnosis was confirmed. After this, he was returned to the prison but placed in solitary confinement as a quarantine measure for "ten to fourteen days."

While this was happening, back in Chicago his wife was diagnosed with a brain tumor and soon underwent surgery. Volkman told me that he disagreed with the decision to operate on Nancy, since her prognosis was already so dire. He told me that, because of the surgery, her quality of life was "devastatingly diminished," and he described the decision to operate as "really, really inappropriate care."

Due to the Volkman family's suddenly dire financial situation, after Nancy's surgery she was moved to a much smaller apartment on the other side of the city. And so in July, when Volkman finally secured his post-arrest release, he told me that he was "walking into a place I had never been before and seeing my wife in a completely devastated condition."

The tribulations continued.

As a condition of his release, Volkman was assigned to a pretrial services officer (PTSO) and placed under a number of stringent conditions. He had to surrender his passport and was subjected to regular drug testing. He was fitted with an electronic ankle monitor and prohibited from travel outside of the Northern District of Illinois without explicit permission. And he was permitted to leave home only for a narrow list of reasons, including court appearances, religious services, and medical appointments for him or his wife — all of which required preapproval from his pretrial officer.

Given the intense demands of his wife's care at the time, which included numerous appointments per week, it was almost inevitable that his legal situation would conflict with her medical needs. And less than a month after his release, it did.

One morning, his wife had a fever — which, Volkman noted as he told the story, was particularly dangerous for a cancer patient on a regimen of steroids — and she was advised by her doctors to come to the hospital and, later, to remain there. Volkman told me that, in response to this development, he left a message to update the PTSO and stayed at the hospital with his wife, whom he described as "disoriented and terrified and depressed."

A phone argument with the PTSO ensued about whether he was violating the conditions of his release by staying at the hospital. And this, in turn, led to a house call from the PTSO the following morning, after Volkman and his wife had returned home. A tense conversation led to the PTSO's determination that Volkman was in violation of his bond, which led to the issuance of a new arrest warrant. Within days, armed law enforcement returned to take him away again — this time, to a different county jail in Kentucky. In Chicago, due to her deteriorating mental state, his wife was admitted to a psychiatric hospital.

Volkman was eventually released. And over the next nine months, Nancy's condition worsened. Then, in June 2008, about a year after his indictment, she died. At this point, he made the call to my dad that had, eventually, led to this odd scene: me, with a digital voice recorder in hand, sitting in a Starbucks in Chicago on Christmas Day, and listening to a much older man describe some of the worst days of his life.

It would take me years, and quite a bit of reporting, before I felt that I fully understood Paul Volkman.

But some things were clear to me from these first few meetings. One was his intense and unremitting bitterness.

To be clear, it wasn't surprising that a man who believed himself wrongfully accused of horrific crimes was upset about it. But Volkman seemed consumed by a seething fury. And he became animated when expressing his loathing and contempt for various people.

As he told his story, he described the pretrial officer who had helped to send him back to prison as a "shithead." The Sixth Circuit US Court of Appeals, which was based in Cincinnati and which had denied his appeal of the DEA's revocation of his DEA registration, was a "bunch of fucking . . . stupid and bigoted and biased rednecks." An expert witness who had testified against him at his DEA registration hearing was "a disgusting human being" and "the face of evil." A former US attorney in Ohio was "a complete Bible-thumping Bush-ie asshole." The Portsmouth, Ohio, police department consisted of "a bunch of corrupt hacks."

If he had a favorite descriptor, it seemed to be "schmuck." This was how he described one of the neurologists who cared for his late wife, Nancy, when she had cancer. It was also how he described Supreme Court Chief Justice John Roberts ("chief schmuck"), the former lab director who refused to sign off on his brilliant post-med-school research ("a stupid schmuck"), and one of his former defense attorneys in Ohio ("a spineless, wheedling, weaseling schmuck . . . a real piece of shit").

Was it possible that such a cynical, profane, and angry man would have been working in Ohio out of compassion and concern for pain patients?

This was one of the many things that Volkman asked his audience to believe.

After he had walked me through the details of his case, Volkman described what he thought would happen next.

His trial was scheduled to begin in about six months, in June 2010. But he was confident that it wouldn't take place then. He believed that he would succeed in getting his recently appointed lawyer thrown off his case due to inadequate representation. And because of the case's complexity and the amount of time a new lawyer would need to become sufficiently acquainted with it, he thought this would push back the trial date by "easily a year." This would set up the next stage of his plan.

Volkman told me that, at some point in the ensuing months, he planned to request a meeting with Carter Stewart, the US attorney for the Southern District of Ohio and the top official of the office that was handling the prosecution of his case. And during this meeting, he planned to point out that marijuana was rapidly becoming legalized in states across the country, which was accompanied by changing attitudes about drugs in general. He would remind Stewart that President Obama had publicly stated a disinterest in using federal resources to contradict state law. As Volkman told it, he would in essence, argue, "This is a really bad case to present and push forward." He believed that if Stewart truly understood the details of the case, Stewart was likely to drop it.

For someone so who viewed himself as worldly wise, the plan struck me as astonishingly naive. But Volkman described it without a trace of irony. And he said that even if this plan didn't pan out, he was still confident about avoiding prison. If his case proceeded to a trial, and he had access to "adequate" representation, he believed he had a "99.9 percent chance I would win."

His ability to dismiss or beat the charges he faced was, in his eyes, so likely that he was already planning what he would do afterward.

He explained that the first step after exoneration would be to hire top-rate lawyers to sue the government, which he felt could yield "several hundred million dollars" in damages. After winning his case and forcing his tormentors to pay, he said he planned to leave the "disgusting and completely bankrupt" United States behind. He hadn't yet made up his mind about where exactly he would go. Israel was an appealing possibility, and so was Norway.

Whatever destination he chose, he was sure of one thing: "The day after my case is over I'm going to be on a plane."

Toward the end of one of our days of conversation, Volkman described the role I could play in this scenario.

"It would actually help me to have as much publicity as possible," he said. Otherwise, he said, he could be swept under a rug and the government could step on him any way they wanted.

He continued.

"Of course, I would need to read it and make sure there's nothing in there that I don't want to be disseminated at this time," he said.

This wasn't how journalism worked, nor was it how I viewed my role in the project. I had never suggested that we would be collaborators on a story, and I had no intention of giving him a preview of what I eventually published.

But I didn't say any of this. I was in no rush to puncture whatever illusions he had about why I had traveled all the way to Chicago.

And soon enough, he had changed the subject to his plans to win his criminal case and "spend the rest of my days suing the government for what they've done."

A STATE OF EMERGENCY

The closure of Paul Volkman's Chillicothe clinic in 2006 had not brought an end to the pain clinic industry in southern Ohio. In fact, the opposite had occurred.

At the time of my first visit in May 2010, Scioto County, a rural county with a population of seventy-six thousand, was home to at least eight non-hospital-affiliated pain clinics. They had names like Southern Ohio Complete Pain Management, Ohio Pain Relief Center, Greater Medical Advance, Health Maintenance Partners, Tri-State Primary Care, and Lucasville Medical Specialist.

One of these clinics was in Tri-State Healthcare's old building on Findlay Street, in Portsmouth. Another was about ten miles east of Portsmouth, in the town of Wheelersburg. It was run by a local doctor named Margaret Temponeras, who had started her career in family medicine. The clinic accepted only cash for payments, and patients traveled long distances, sometimes more than a hundred miles, to see the doctor. Those patients frequently walked away with large prescriptions for opioids, sedatives, and muscle relaxers. And as with Tri-State, when local pharmacies stopped filling her scripts, Temponeras responded by opening an on-site dispensary, where employees served customers from behind thick glass. In 2009, her clinic ordered more than 650,000 oxycodone and hydrocodone pills.

Scioto County was awash in pills. Between 2000 and 2008, more than 115 people died from apparent overdoses in the county, which was an average of about 1 death per month. In 2006, unintentional overdoses surpassed motor vehicles as the county's leading cause of death. By the time of my arrival in 2010, the county's death rate from prescription drug poisoning was now more than double the state average and rising.

And it wasn't just overdoses.

In recent years, the area had seen an alarming spike in homicides linked to the prescription drug trade.

In 2008, three people were found shot in a mobile home in Franklin Furnace, a small town about fifteen miles east of Portsmouth. Police arrived after a six-year-old boy, who was covered in blood, ran to a neighbor's house to report what happened. At the ensuing trial, one attorney stated that the victims "were up to their necks in the OxyContin trafficking in this county."

In 2009, in Lucasville (ten miles north of Portsmouth), the owner of a local pain clinic was found stabbed to death in a truck that had been lit on fire. The man convicted of the murder was a patient at the clinic and, according to court filings, had "taken pain medication for most of his adult life, and . . . has admitted to being addicted to Oxycontin." At trial, one witness testified that the killer's motive was "the pills and the cash."

In 2010, a man and a woman were shot inside a home in Lucasville. In this case, too, a young child witnessed the incident. Three suspects, including the male victim's son and his girlfriend, were ultimately charged with the crime. Trial testimony indicated that the incident began as an attempted robbery of pills.

And there were other effects from the region's inundation with pills.

The region's booming black market for pills was seen as a driving force behind an overall rise in crime. "In a period of ten years, we've more than doubled the number of adult felony cases in the county," the Scioto County prosecutor told me when I visited his office. In a separate interview with a reporter at the *Portsmouth Daily Times,* I was told that the vast majority of the area's crime "centers back to one thing, and that is the need to purchase drugs."

Meanwhile, the county's rates of hepatitis C, which tend to correlate closely with intravenous drug use, had surged to the highest in Ohio. Local hospitals were also seeing an alarming rise in the number of babies who were born physically addicted to opiates due to the mother's drug use during pregnancy.

One local health official told me that when major employers came to town seeking job applicants, they had to interview five people to find one who could pass a drug test. "We know that the town is economically depressed; that's obvious," she said. "But that part will never get fixed unless the addiction part and all of the easy access gets taken care of."

By early 2010, the prescription drug abuse crisis had gotten so bad that the Scioto County health commissioner, Dr. Aaron Adams, declared a formal state of emergency. A few months later, during one of my first visits, I watched a presentation delivered by Lisa Roberts, who worked for the City of Portsmouth's health department. When discussing Adams's recent emergency declaration, she said, "I think it's the first time, probably ever, in the history of the world that a public health emergency has been declared by a doctor, as a result of something that other doctors are doing."

As it turned out, my first trips to Portsmouth in May and July 2010 took place as the community was swinging into action. Just a few months before I arrived, a former Scioto County coroner had declared his candidacy for the Ohio House of Representatives. Dr. Terry Johnson had, in his official capacity, signed death certificates for at least two of Volkman's patients.* And in his campaign communications, he talked about how the wave of prescription-related overdose deaths had motivated him to seek office. Once the campaign was under way, he had paid for a billboard in town that read PROVEN LEADERSHIP FIGHTING RX DRUG ABUSE FOR OVER A DECADE. In his stump speeches, he spoke about plans that he had for legislation to clamp down on the local pill mill problem.

Meanwhile, in February 2010, local citizens had created a Facebook group called Fix the Scioto County Problem of Drug Abuse, Misuse, and Overdose, which quickly gained thousands of followers. Some people shared news articles about drug issues in the region and across the country. Others shared updates about drug-related crimes.

Amid it all was a steady flow of messages of grief.

"I lost my little brother to a drug overdose," one post read. "I would love to help take back our community."

Another, which accompanied a photo, read, "This is my nephew, Ryan, who we lost to an OxyContin overdose on June 29, 2009 [from] medicine that he obtained here in Scioto County . . . He was such a gentle, sweet soul."

A third read, "These so called doctors are getting rich at the expense of the lives of our children."

The Facebook group was an organizing space for a series of protests aimed at local pain clinics. The idea seems to have started in May 2010, when a gathering for the National Day of Prayer in a park in the center of town had turned into a march to the nearby pain clinic on Findlay Street. Once they arrived, participants held signs and sang "Amazing Grace" on the sidewalk outside.

A few months later, local citizens expanded the protest with a campaign they dubbed the Pill Mill Farewell Tour. With the help of nearby businesses that allowed use of their parking lots, participants set up mini-protests near various local clinics. Participants carried signs that read STOP THE PILL MILLS; PILL MILLS KILL!; PAIN DOCTOR OR LEGALIZED DRUG DEALER? Cars honked as they drove past.

At one protest, two girls with blond hair held signs above their heads. One sign read YOU KILLED MY MOMMY, with a symbol of a heart broken in two.

---

* At Volkman's trial in 2011, Johnson was among many coroners who testified.

———

When it came to Portsmouth's prescription drug problem, nobody seemed to know more than Lisa Roberts.

Roberts was a petite woman with shoulder-length brown hair who had grown up in Scioto County and graduated from Shawnee State University with a degree in nursing. For more than twenty years, she had worked for the City of Portsmouth as a public health nurse. At the time of my arrival, she was working in the Portsmouth Health Department's Office of Injury Prevention. Her job involved collecting data on how and why the city's citizens were dying.

Due to her proximity to the opioid crisis, Roberts had become a kind of de facto spokeswoman for the town's fight against addiction and overdose. And I soon came to appreciate the many traits and skills that suited her for the role. She had grown up in the region and clearly cared about its future. On top of this, she was well versed in the technical aspects of addiction and medications thanks to her experience as a nurse. She also was down-to-earth and approachable, while able to forcefully express the anger she felt when watching her home county swarmed by unscrupulous doctors. When I first arrived, she had recently told a newspaper reporter that the local pain clinics "make an insane amount of cash, and . . . basically throw their ethics out the window."

As part of her work on the local overdose problem, Roberts had become a historian and statistician of the crisis. And she was invaluable for helping me understand the role that Paul Volkman had played in contributing to it. Soon after we met, she emailed me an essay she had written for a grant application seeking funds to address the situation. The essay began, "Once known for its thriving steel mills, Scioto County has now come to be known for its thriving 'Pill Mills.'"

In the essay, she explained how David Procter and John Lilly had helped make Scioto County one of the first places in the country affected by the opioid epidemic. "Scioto County, with its high disability, poverty, and addiction rates, had become 'fertile ground' for future enterprising Pill Mills," she wrote. This was when Paul Volkman had arrived on the scene.

In Roberts's telling, there was little difference between Volkman and the region's previous crooked doctors. He and Denise Huffman were simply "carry[ing] on the profitable tradition." And when they were taken down, other doctors swooped in to take their place.

Roberts's essay explained that local pain clinics thrived by exploiting regulatory blind spots. There was no state agency that monitored pain clinics with on-site dispensaries. And by accepting only cash, the clinics also eluded oversight from insurance companies and the state's workers' compensation system.

The results of this lack of oversight had been catastrophic. "These establishments are a major contributor to Scioto County's extremely high overdose death rate, as they create a community-setting that is conducive to prescription drug overdose," she wrote. "They have induced an unprecedented level of narcotic addiction within the community, as well as an unprecedented number of overdose deaths."

During my trips to Portsmouth, I was both a tourist and a journalist.

I had driven ten hours from New York to learn about the drug problem and Volkman's role in it. But I was also intent on simply getting to know the place where most of his alleged crimes had occurred.

And so, over the course of my visits, I walked around town, reading plaques and taking photos. I ate dinner at the most celebrated local BBQ joint, the Scioto Ribber. I flipped through old newspaper clippings in the local history room at the public library. I walked through the campus of Shawnee State University and the galleries of the Southern Ohio Museum. And I also visited the city's most distinct architectural feature: a tall, thick, concrete floodwall that was built in the aftermath of Portsmouth's catastrophic flood of 1937. In the 1990s and early 2000s, the wall was painted with dazzling, colorful murals that depict and celebrate the city's history, with panels dedicated to the region's indigenous Native American tribes, the town's early history, the shoe and steel industries, and notable hometown heroes like Roy Rogers, whose face needed to be repainted multiple times before locals were satisfied with the likeness.

During this sightseeing, I found Portsmouth to be a charming place, with natural beauty and a rich history. But the city had clearly seen better days. The sidewalks around town were eerily empty and quiet. Nearly half of the storefronts on Chillicothe Street were shuttered or gutted. Some had notes of explanation taped to their windows: BJ'S BURGERS OUT OF BUSINESS; KIDZ BIZ IS CLOSED INVENTORY BEING SOLD ON AMAZON.COM.

Between my first and second trips to Portsmouth, a memorial for local overdose victims appeared in one of those storefronts, in the window of a long-empty former department store. Amid brightly colored paper butterflies and hummingbirds were photos of young people — boys in high school football uniforms, girls wearing prom dresses — along with their names and dates of birth and death. One was thirty-four years old. Another was twenty-nine. Another was twenty-two. Another was twenty. Another was eighteen.

A sign in the window read DRUG RELATED DEATHS.

I still had Volkman's story of his innocence echoing in my ears during these visits. And as I explored the town, I asked people what they thought about some of the things he'd said.

When I spoke with Ed Hughes, the CEO of one of the area's largest drug and alcohol rehab centers, I asked if he felt there was a real need for these pain clinics, as Volkman had claimed. His answer was adamant: "No, no, no." He explained that true, conscientious pain management was a complex process that required doctors to be trained in identifying and addressing addiction. None of that happened at the local pain clinics, he said. He described the clinics, and the underground economy they helped to fuel, as a "huge criminal enterprise."

Lisa Roberts told me that, contrary to Volkman's claim that Scioto County was medically underserved, the region had a strong physician-to-patient ratio. And in her experience, local doctors were perfectly willing to treat their patients' pain, and capable of it. "Your regular doctor can treat your pain plus your sinus infection and your rash and everything else," she said. The pain clinics were here just to make cash, she said. And they made a lot of it.

When I met Aaron Adams, the health commissioner who had declared a state of emergency, I asked what he thought about Volkman's argument that southern Ohio was a region that had more per-capita chronic pain issues than elsewhere. He disagreed. Scioto County was "no different . . . than anyplace else," he said.

During an interview with Wayne Wheeler, a local physician and former deputy coroner who had testified against Volkman at his pre-indictment DEA registration hearing in Columbus, he expressed concern about pain doctors who didn't accept insurance and weren't on staff at local hospitals.

At one point in that conversation, I mentioned Volkman's claim that he was the victim of an out-of-control War on Drugs.

"Somehow I don't believe that putting three or four hundred oxycodones in the hands of a drug addict who's going to sell part of them [is] being a victim," Wheeler said. "That's being a contributor. That's being an enabler."

———

During these visits, I also spent time scoping out the locations of Volkman's former clinics.

I drove past 1200 Gay Street, Tri-State's first Portsmouth address, which was located near a Kroger supermarket, a State Farm Insurance office, and a handful of fast-food restaurants, including Subway, Domino's, and Arby's. Next door was Hallmark Health Care Inc., a medical supply show-room with oxygen tanks and wheelchairs visible through the windows.

Not far from there was the building on Findlay Street, which had a wall of tinted windows facing the street and a semicircular blue awning marked 1219 over the main entrance. Next to the building was a gravel lot ringed by a fence with barbed wire strung across the top. Black tires were stacked on metal racks and clustered in piles on the ground. Nearby, a metal ware-house was labeled MITCHELL BROTHERS TIRE.

On another day, I visited Center Street.

Center Street, I learned, was in a neighborhood off the city's central grid, where the streets swerved and changed names and ended abruptly. Driving slowly, squinting to read street signs, I eventually found it: a 150-yard strip of red brick lined with modest houses with A-shaped roofs. Some of the homes on the street looked abandoned. Traffic was minimal.

I spoke with some people on the street and, like others around town, they were extremely skeptical of Volkman's legitimacy. One said, "What kind of a doctor would open up an office on this street? . . . It's not even a commercial street."

My longest conversation was with a woman who had been Volkman's next-door neighbor. Sammie Ishmael's house had a row of neatly trimmed bushes planted in front of the porch. A white flowerpot sat next to the front steps with a small American flag sticking out. We sat on the porch on a hot, humid day.

"You should experience a pain clinic next door to you," she said while dipping back and forth on a rocking chair. "That's an experience."

As she spoke, I got the sense that this episode, which had taken place almost five years prior, stuck out in her memory.

The trouble all began with his briefcase, Ishmael explained. She worked an overnight shift at a facility for adults with developmental disabilities on the adjacent street. And when returning home one morning, she noticed a briefcase on the front step of the house next door. She took the case inside and called the landlord's office, and someone there said that they would call the man who rented the house. Eventually that doctor, Paul Volkman, came by to pick up the briefcase, though he never thanked her.

She shook her head and said, "I thought, 'My God, you'd think he'd be a little bit more appreciative!'"

Things remained quiet for the time being. Dr. Volkman went to work on weekdays, kept to himself in the evenings, and disappeared on weekends to Chicago. Then one morning in the late summer of 2005, Ishmael came home to find a group of men standing on the porch next door. She asked if they were waiting on the doctor, and they confirmed that they were. They said that this was the new pain clinic.

This idea struck her as outlandish. "I was like, 'What are they talking about? There's a pain clinic *next door*?'" she said.

Life became unpleasant after that. The first trickle of patients quickly turned into a flood of cars, some with license plates from Indiana, Kentucky, West Virginia, and Michigan. Ishmael's husband, who has a prosthetic leg and walks with crutches, could no longer park in front of the house. He had to start driving up the street, looking for parking spots.

On days when the clinic was open, crowds of people spilled out of the house and onto the front porch and backyard. To control the crowds, Volkman hired a security guard, who wore a gun holstered to his belt while he patrolled the premises. For Ishmael, it was an unsettling development.

After a few weeks of this, she said that she was furious. She was losing sleep. In the weeks that Volkman was working there, she said she called someone to complain every day. Some days, it was the mayor's office. On other days, it was the police. Another day, it was her preacher. "I was gonna lose it," she told me. "There [was] a man out here walking around with a *gun!*"

When the police finally did come, they hung yellow crime-scene tape across her front yard to the porch next door. There were officers in the backyard of 1310 Center Street checking the ID cards of patients who were present. Others carried boxes of files out of the house. At some point, a TV news crew showed up.

Ishmael was overwhelmed with a mixture of happiness, relief, and fatigue. Her friends warned her that, with all the fuss she made about the clinic, someone might come and shoot her out of retribution.

She didn't care, she said. She finally had peace.

ADAM AND ELIZABETH

Adam Volkman was born in the summer of 1975, about a year after his father graduated from medical school. In Adam's telling, Paul was the quieter of his two parents. For much of his childhood, Adam said he could rely on his dad to drive him to practices and games for his soccer and hockey teams. And if someone got injured during a hockey game, he remembered how his dad would toddle out onto the ice to tend to him.

Paul was the family's main financial provider, and Adam grew up believing that his dad was a good and conscientious doctor. But he was also aware that his dad lacked certain softer skills. Despite his dad's obvious intelligence, his emotional awareness was low or nonexistent, Adam said. He seemed unable to connect with people on a personal level.

Adam told me that for most of his childhood, he saw his dad as a supporting actor to his mom, who was louder and livelier. Adam described his mother as fun, charismatic, and sociable, with a sense of humor. She was a great cook, and people liked to be around her. When his parents were together, he said that his father "couldn't get a word in edgewise." At various times in our conversations, he described his father's role in his upbringing as that of a "prop." Visible but inanimate.

Above all else, Adam said that his mom had an eye for *appearances*. With the help of a personal decorator, she was the one who outfitted the houses and apartments where the family lived. She was the one who bought clothes for Paul to wear and gave him instructions about how to wear them. And she was the one who had so many clothes of her own that she created a "look book," which, Adam explained to me, was a photo album that contained photographs of her wearing various combinations of her clothes, as a reference to help her choose a day's outfit. "Appearances — she had those down," Adam told me.

Adam told me about one moment, after Paul's indictment and Nancy's cancer diagnosis, that he found particularly revealing. It was a chaotic time, and, in the rush to accommodate his mother's severely downgraded financial situation, Adam and his wife, Elizabeth,* were helping Nancy move out of the Lake Shore Drive apartment to the much cheaper place across town. During this process, Adam was wearing a white T-shirt while moving boxes out of the apartment. Despite everything else going on in

---

* Not her real name. Adam and Elizabeth spoke to me under the condition that I change their names and leave out other identifying information. I agreed to these conditions.

her life, Nancy was embarrassed by his appearance and asked him to put on a nicer shirt.

He remembered thinking, "Are you kidding me?"

For college, Adam attended a small liberal arts school in the Midwest.* While there, he fell in love with a student named Liz. They moved to Chicago after graduation and got married a few years later. He and Liz had recently welcomed their first child when, in short succession, Adam's father was indicted and his mother was diagnosed with a brain tumor.

Adam was drawn into the vortex of his father's case in various ways.

First there was the fact that his mother and sister were too shaken by the recent events to take the necessary action to move Adam's parents out of the Lake Shore Drive apartment while Paul was in jail. As a result, the task fell to Adam and Liz.

And in late July 2007, a few weeks after his mother's brain surgery, Adam also traveled to Cincinnati to testify in a hearing about their father's ongoing incarceration. Paul and his attorney were fighting prosecutors' claim that Paul was a flight risk by arguing that, in fact, Paul desperately wanted to go home to Chicago to care for his ailing wife. Adam and Jane each testified as witnesses in support. In Adam's case, it involved explaining, under oath, that he had never heard his dad mention plans to flee and also that, having reviewed his parents' finances, he knew of no offshore accounts in the Bahamas or anywhere else.

Adam was in his midthirties when I first reached out to him in 2010. He and Liz lived with their two young children in a midwestern city. Adam told me that he was aware that what had happened with his dad was a "fascinating story." And the fact that a journalist had knocked on his door was, to him, "another amazing twist in the tale." So, in August 2010, after my first trips to Portsmouth and a second series of interviews with Paul in Chicago, I made my way to their town.

Adam doesn't have much in common with his dad, personality-wise. During our first conversations — which took place on two subsequent nights on the couple's screened-in porch — I sensed little, if any, of his dad's bravado, cynicism, or contempt. He was not an angry guy. Nor was he prone to attack other people's intelligence or credibility.

---

* By coincidence, Adam's college town was the location of one of his father's many locum tenens stints. Adam recalled meeting up with his dad when Paul was working there.

He struck me as thoughtful and down-to-earth and someone who, by his own admission, had gone through a fair amount of therapy. Both he and Liz seemed like people who were intentionally constructing a life that differed from that of Adam's parents.

Paul's pain-management years had taken place at a time when Adam's relationship with his parents was already quite strained. So we didn't spend much time talking about Paul's case. We focused instead on family dynamics. Shortly after we sat down for our first interview, Liz said, "There were a lot of issues in this family before May 21, 2007," the day of Paul's arrest.

In Adam's telling, his father was an egotistical and stubborn man who was supremely confident when it came to his own ideas and dismissive of the views of others. "To disagree with him is very difficult," Adam said. He described him as "brilliant" in some areas of life but strikingly ignorant in others, most notably in relationships.

Meanwhile, Adam said that his mother's bright and vivacious surface hid a lot of fear and insecurity. She and Paul bickered constantly, often including threats of divorce. He described their household as a "war zone" and said, "I always thought she married the wrong guy for a variety of reasons."

But there were apparently things that made the marriage work. Paul had a very high opinion of himself, and Nancy apparently spoke highly of herself, as well. Adam told me that one of his mother's favorite sayings was "It's lonely at the top," which she apparently meant as a comment on their family's place in the world.

Adam and Liz both felt that his parents also had a symbiotic relationship when it came to finances, since Paul was able to pay for a lifestyle that Nancy couldn't afford on her own. Liz described Nancy as "the best-dressed public [school] librarian Chicago ever saw."

Together, Paul and Nancy were a volatile duo.

Although Liz and Adam hadn't started dating until they were seniors in college, their school was small enough that, during their freshman year, Liz remembered hearing about a student whose parents had threatened not to continue paying their son's tuition if he didn't get straight As in his first term. It struck her as "awful." That student turned out to be Adam.

This transactional approach remained evident after Adam and Liz got together. When the couple was planning their wedding, Paul and Nancy threatened not to attend the wedding if the couple didn't take his and Nancy's wishes about the event more into account. Later, Adam's parents committed to pay for a portion of his graduate-school tuition and then rescinded the offer at the last minute. "There was a lot of conditional love with my parents," Adam told me.

Over time, Adam said he became more and more frustrated with his parents, and their relationship would go into "deep freezes" where they wouldn't speak for months. Then, after Adam and Liz had their first child in 2006, things reached a breaking point.

When they brought the child home, Paul — the child's grandfather and the former pediatrician — mentioned what he thought were alarming signs about the baby's health. This put Adam and Liz in an uncomfortable position. On one hand, their relationship with Paul was already strained, and his commentary was unwelcome and unsettling. On the other hand, neither of them was a doctor, and he was. What if there really was something wrong?

They decided to tell Paul that they didn't like how he was handling the situation, and, going forward, they would appreciate it if he kept his opinions to himself. But they also consulted with their child's doctors, and none believed that there was any kind of problem.

Afterward, Paul remained skeptical and described the doctors as idiots. At this point, Adam told his father that he needed to stop. He said that he and Liz needed Paul to be a grandfather, not a doctor. Then, about a week later, Paul made another comment about the child's health.

Liz later told me that Paul's behavior involving her newborn fit a "horrible" pattern. She said that it seemed like he had some kind of savior complex. "I think he needs to feel like a hero . . . and he has to create emergency horrible scenarios that he has to fix for the people in his life, whether they're patients or whether they're family," she said.

Those incidents, plus many others in which Paul came across as, in Liz's words, "hurtful and argumentative and aggressive and reckless and insulting," prompted Adam and Liz to draw a firm boundary. They told me that they reached a point where they felt Paul was negatively affecting their parenting quality, and he was no longer welcome in their home.

In fact, they said the tension between them and Adam's parents had partly inspired them to move hours away from Chicago, an act that Liz described, at one point, as having "fled" from her in-laws.

By the time I met the couple in the summer of 2010, Paul was not involved in their lives. "He's dangerous to our family," Liz said.

———

During these conversations, I learned that Paul's indictment had happened after Adam had mostly cut his father out of his life. And this explained his emotional detachment about the case. "I don't know if he's really innocent or not," he said at one point. But he did know that his dad was a "broken family man" who had made some "very stupid decisions." And he said that because Paul was "such a jerk as a person," he had no plans to attend his father's trial.

At one point in our conversations, which stretched across two evenings, Liz told me a story that seemed to sum up her feelings about Paul. It involved an encounter that took place on the day of Nancy's shiva when, at one point, Paul approached Liz with a proposal. Paul told her that, after giving the matter a lot of thought, he felt that Adam and Liz ought to fire their nanny and allow him to take over as their kids' stay-at-home grandfather.

At this point Liz didn't like or particularly trust Paul. And she said that Paul's suggestion struck her not just as surprising but "delusional." When she heard it, she felt like she was going to throw up. "I was terrified that he thought that was a viable option," she said.

She said that if Paul managed to beat the charges he faced, she would probably seek a restraining order against him.

THE PHARMACIST

Harold Eugene Fletcher, the Columbus-based pharmacist, was federally indicted on September 23, 2010.

The bulk of the 227 charges involved the improper possession or distribution of controlled substances, including oxycodone, hydrocodone, diazepam, and alprazolam. Another two dozen counts outlined cash deposits totaling more than $245,000 to Columbus banks over the four-month period when Volkman sent his patients to Columbus to fill scripts. Authorities alleged that those cash deposits, which ranged from $7,900 to $9,990, were intentionally structured to evade federal reporting laws for cash deposits of more than $10,000. This pattern of structured deposits was itself a crime. On page two of the indictment, Paul Volkman was described as Fletcher's "physician co-conspirator."

By the time that Fletcher received a second indictment in December, which added two charges of filing false tax returns, Fletcher had, like

Volkman, been issued a DEA Order to Show Cause, which suspended his registration to dispense controlled substances. And like Volkman, he had chosen to fight that order in an administrative hearing, which took place across five days in November 2009 and March 2010.

The government's case in that hearing included testimony from the former Volkman patient who said she was so high during some of her visits to Fletcher's pharmacy that her stumbling gait and slurred speech would have been hard to miss, and that she was "probably drooling" at the time.

Another former Volkman patient testified about how her sister-in-law had "sponsored" her visits to Volkman by paying her visit fee and then splitting the pills she later obtained at Fletcher's pharmacy. This patient testified that she was addicted to opiates during her time as a Volkman patient.

After the hearing, the administrative judge issued an opinion recommending that Fletcher's registration be revoked. The judge wrote that Fletcher had "ignored numerous 'red flags' when dispensing controlled substances to Dr. Volkman's patients," including the long distances Volkman's patients drove to the pharmacy, the large amounts of controlled substances in their prescriptions, and the lack of individualization across customers.

According to the judge, Fletcher was experienced enough to know which questions he should have asked customers to ensure the legitimacy of his operation. But he chose not to. "In six months he filled over 4,900 prescriptions without seeming to consistently engage in such conversations with Dr. Volkman's patients," the judge wrote.

Fletcher filed an appeal to that decision, which sent it to the DEA's deputy administrator for review. The administrator upheld the judge's decision, and, in doing so, called Fletcher's record of dispensing controlled substances "abysmal."

Fletcher had been initially defiant in the face of the DEA scrutiny.

In an interview with a Cleveland-based newspaper in early 2010, Fletcher — who, for unclear reasons, was not quoted directly and instead had his comments summarized — reportedly "wanted to know if it was because his pharmacy is located in a minority neighborhood; and most certainly, he wanted to know why his pharmacy was singled out for this kind of treatment."

In the same article, the pharmacist's lawyer, Bradley Barbin, said that Fletcher's pharmacy had only filled prescriptions for "real people with real medications and real doctors." The attorney added that Fletcher's pharmacy had been in the community for twelve years and that the pharmacist had sponsored the local Little League.

Later in the year, Fletcher and his lawyer raised the stakes by filing a seventeen-page federal lawsuit against five DEA agents and officials, accusing them of a multipronged effort to illegitimately run the pharmacist out of business. The complaint stated that the agency had "arbitrarily, capriciously and unconstitutionally selected" Fletcher for prosecution and alleged a series of dirty tricks that DEA agents supposedly employed as part of a baseless campaign against him.

The lawsuit claimed that in January 2008, one of Fletcher's pharmaceutical wholesalers abruptly, and without explanation, refused to continue supplying him; the next month, a second company informed him that he "had been put on a blacklist by DEA." It also claimed that the DEA had played a part in a series of unflattering print and TV news stories intended to taint the local jury pool, which the complaint said reflected a "standardized method by DEA." The lawsuit further said that the DEA had conducted an unannounced inspection of Fletcher's pharmacy at a time when agents knew that his lawyer was out of state and was thus "unable to protect [the] Plaintiff's constitutional rights." It added that DEA investigators had made a series of false and misleading statements about his pharmacy during interviews, in affidavits, and in his immediate suspension order from November 2009. The lawsuit claimed that these errors were not corrected, despite repeatedly being brought to the attention of investigators.

The complaint was built on the presumption that Fletcher was a law-abiding, legitimate pharmacist. And it included two explanations for why Fletcher's pharmacy attracted customers from such long distances. One reason was low prices. The complaint mentioned a "citywide low price pharmacy competition in Columbus" that Fletcher had won in the early 2000s, and mentioned customers who told investigators that Fletcher had once promised to beat prices at Walgreens, Walmart, and any other chain pharmacy. The second reason for the pharmacy's success, the filing said, was that DEA agents had engaged in a pattern of intimidation against southern Ohio pharmacies, warning them not to fill scripts for certain doctors and advising them in a manner "not authorized by statute, regulation or administrative rule" that they weren't permitted to fill scripts for customers outside of a thirty-five-to-fifty-mile radius. This, too, had sent patients with legitimate prescriptions north toward Columbus, according to the complaint.

In the lawsuit, Fletcher asserted that these alleged DEA actions — the blacklisting among suppliers, the media smears, the false information submitted in the process leading to the suspension of his DEA registration — had violated his Fourth, Fifth, Sixth, Thirteenth, and Fourteenth Amendment rights. The complaint ended with a demand for a legal order acknowledging the breach of those rights, plus an award of compensatory damages, punitive damages, and attorney's fees.

But then, in early 2011, in the days before his criminal trial was scheduled to start, Fletcher changed his mind. Facing more than two hundred charges, he pleaded guilty to three: one count of illegal dispensing of oxycodone (a prescription for 480 thirty-milligram pills that he filled for a Volkman patient in February 2006), one count of illegally structuring bank deposits to avoid legally mandated reporting requirements, and one count of filing a false tax return. As part of the plea deal, he agreed to a permanent ban from the field of pharmacy. That month, Fletcher, through his lawyer, also announced that he would drop his lawsuit against the DEA.

Fletcher's change of plea followed guilty pleas from Alice and Denise Huffman in late 2010. And so, with Volkman's trial date approaching in March, the three people with whom he was most closely affiliated in southern Ohio were now convicted felons. Only Volkman continued to maintain that, during his time in pain clinics in southern Ohio, he was a conscientious, law-abiding professional working in the best interests of his patients.

JANE

Paul and Nancy's second child, Jane, was born in May 1978. And while her brother, Adam, described a tumultuous relationship with their parents, Jane told me that her role in the household was "rather obedient and dutiful." She spoke of her parents in much warmer terms than Adam. She told me that her mother was a "wonderful" and "very caring" person who had "a beautiful, loving spirit." She said that, when she was growing up, her father was "always a sweetheart with me."

But there were other ways in which her story echoed Adam's. She described her parents' marriage as a "failed relationship," and she acknowledged that arguments between them were common. "Conflict resolution and forgiveness were not modeled in the home," she said. She felt that both of her parents came from backgrounds where emotions were suppressed rather than communicated or processed in a healthy way.

She believed that her parents were also alike in the way they both received affirmation through their professional lives. Everyone that I spoke to, including Adam and Liz, believed that Nancy excelled at her job. Jane told me that she was inspired by how much her mother enjoyed helping kids learn to love to read. "She was very devoted to her job and was beloved by her students," she said.

Jane also echoed Adam and Liz's assessment of the ways that Paul and Nancy came to rely on each other. She said that Paul felt gratified and affirmed by financially providing for Nancy, and Nancy, in turn, "liked to buy stuff to decorate the house, or fancy skin care stuff." At one point, Jane observed, "It was almost like the only fun my mom could have involved working and spending." The money for this came almost entirely from her husband's career.

Eventually, as an adult, Jane told me that she was forced to confront the way that she had absorbed some of her parents' values. "I became obsessed with work [and] achieving yet could not process my own feelings well or communicate well," she said. "I became like them in that respect."

Jane was a strong student in high school and, for college, attended the University of North Carolina at Chapel Hill. After graduating, she returned home to Illinois to attend law school. And this was when a series of crises rocked her family.

First came the DEA's shutdown of her father's office, which Jane said deeply affected her. Afterward, she felt constantly anxious and couldn't sleep. "My mental health started crumbling along with my mom's," she said.

When her father was indicted the following year, Jane was an outspoken defender. In comments to the *Chicago Tribune*, she said that her dad had been trying to relieve the suffering of his patients in Ohio, called him "completely innocent," and added, "He was vigilant in his drug testing and was in touch with leading researchers to devise even more accurate methods [to detect drug abusers]." In a separate interview with the Associated Press, she said, "We're going to fight this."

Jane's testimony at Paul's July 2007 bail hearing in Cincinnati provided a glimpse of her mother's health while Paul's criminal case was unfolding. From the witness stand that day, Jane described how during the month before Paul's indictment, Nancy began experiencing pain and dizziness. When Nancy went to the hospital, tests showed swelling and fluid inside her skull, which doctors initially thought was some kind of brain virus.

When antibiotics didn't work, Nancy returned for more appointments and tests. One MRI showed that the mass in her brain had changed shape, which prompted the diagnosis of an aggressive tumor located in her right temporal lobe. Shortly thereafter — and after her husband had been hauled away in handcuffs — Nancy underwent brain surgery. As Jane described it, the doctors "lifted a flap of her skull and took out as much as they could, [as] very carefully as they could."

Paul's custody hearing took place just a few months after that surgery, when Nancy — who remained in Chicago — prepared to begin radiation and chemotherapy. As Jane described from the witness stand, sometimes tearfully, her mom was in terrible shape. Nancy was bedridden and in so much pain that she sometimes curled into the fetal position. She continued to suffer from spells of dizziness and confusion, as well as a diminished memory. She was able to take a shower, but only if there was someone in the bathroom to make sure that she didn't fall. She was terrified and lonely.

Jane testified that her mother needed her husband, "to help to be less scared and take care of her." Plus, she said, the family had "no money" to pay for other caretakers.

While Adam had described being relatively unaffected by his father's case, Jane was a different story.

She had completed law school but missed a bar-exam review course due to helping care for her mother while her dad was in jail after his initial arrest. By this time, she had neither the interest nor the mental energy to pursue law as a career. She once described this period in her life as "free falling psychologically." Instead of seeking law jobs, she started teaching fourth grade in a Chicago public school while taking night courses toward a teaching certification. Meanwhile, she said, she was "trying to pretend like everything was okay."

In the fall of 2009, two and a half years after her father's indictment and a year after her mother's death, Jane said she tumbled into a deep depression. At this time, she was living with her boyfriend, Steve, whom she had met when he was working as a doorman at her parents' building on Lake Shore Drive.

She said that after Steve began reading the Bible regularly, she noticed "beautiful changes coming over him"; he was gentler and more humble. They started watching sermons by the Texas-based pastor Joel Osteen together, and Jane found herself moved by one of the hymns.

Later, in a narrative she published about her spiritual journey, she described hoping that Jesus would send the Holy Spirit into her heart. And then, as she wrote: "In God's perfect timing at age 31, I met Yeshua Messiah!"

When I first reached out to Jane in August 2010, she was thirty-two years old. She was recently married and had also recently converted to Messianic Judaism, a small religious group known by various names (Hebrew Christianity, Jewish Christians, Jews for Jesus) in which adherents identify as Jewish and observe Jewish holidays while also reading the New Testament and viewing Jesus, whom many call Yeshua, as God.

From our first Facebook exchanges in August 2010, Jane expressed trepidation about speaking with me. In one message, she explained that she was "still too vulnerable from the emotional toll this has all taken on me."

But she was also curious. And when she asked me about the questions I had for her, I sent her some. Slowly, we began to talk. We exchanged a few Facebook messages over the next few months, though she continued to express reservations. In one note she wrote, "My heart tells me to leave it all behind as much as possible. It is such a sad story."

But then, in January 2011, with her father's trial just a few months away, something shifted. Jane told me that she had wanted to remain close with her father "no matter what," especially after Nancy's death. But she said that Paul's actions made that difficult. She described his behavior as "hurtful and manipulative." She believed that her religious conversion had something to do with the friction between them. But the main cause of the conflict was money — specifically, as Jane put it, "my unwillingness immediately to do exactly as he has demanded with the money my mother left to me."

Paul, with his assets seized, was mostly reliant on others to help fund his post-indictment, pretrial life. This apparently involved leaning heavily on his daughter, to whom Nancy had left money when she passed away. Jane told me that she had made it clear to her father that she wanted to help him and had given him what she felt was a "generous" sum. But she would not agree to send him as much money as he demanded. In response, he had sent her what she described as "unbelievably sharp-tongued emails" and, at one point, called her a "Nazi." She hadn't budged, and this had led to their rift. As she explained it, "As soon as I refused to fork over tons of cash to him, our relationship was over."

By the time that we began exchanging frequent messages via Facebook in early 2011, Jane said that nothing she said to her dad seemed to elicit any kind of warmth. She had sent him cards expressing her love, but his replies were short and dismissive. "His only concern is money, which seems to have been his motivation during his years in Ohio," she told me.

As we corresponded over the next month, Jane was strikingly critical of her father. She described him as a "loner" who "did not form any friendships of which I am aware." She said that he rarely had kind words to say about anyone, adding that he was fiercely stubborn and wouldn't take direction from others. "He always thinks he knows best," she said.

When I asked her if she believed her dad was an honest person, she said that he told the truth only sometimes. After his initial arrest, for example, he had asked her to fill out paperwork that would allow him to access some of Nancy's retirement funds to help pay for a lawyer. When Jane advised him to use a public defender instead, he told her that he had met with one who was intent on pleading guilty against his wishes. Jane knew from her legal training that this would be a violation of professional ethics and was upset to hear about it. "Later he admitted that this was a lie," she said.

Overall, she said, he was glad to obscure the truth "if he would have something to gain or if it would make his life easier." Though, she noted, his lies never seemed to actually make his life easier.

When it came to her father's legal case, Jane's thoughts were mixed. She had not traveled to Ohio to visit the clinics, nor had she had met Alice, Denise, or any of the clinics' patients. What she knew came from conversations with her father or from selected court documents and news reports.

She felt that her father's motivations were not nearly as pure as he claimed they were. "He explained the work to us as a great source of cash," she told me. And she believed that her father's greed — that was the word she used — had "blinded him to the reckless nature of his actions and even helped him to overlook the grave risks to human life that he had a part in propagating."

When I asked her about her dad's insistence that he had merely tried to earn a "decent living" throughout his career, she pushed back. "I did not perceive his career as a struggle to make a decent living," she said. She said there were so many aspects of her upbringing that made the Volkmans "richer than so many": clothes, vacations, expensive dinners at restaurants, the Lake Shore Drive apartment, the ability to pay for her and Adam's college tuition. "To me a decent living means paying the bills plus an infrequent luxury dinner or special gift," she said. Her father wanted more than a "decent" living; "he wanted a rich man's living," she said.

In these conversations, Jane recalled how Paul would say dehumanizing things about people struggling with addiction. And she said that, whatever rationale or analysis he used to justify what he was doing in Ohio, "he misses the human piece" of the situation. For example, she felt that he didn't appreciate how upset families might be at a doctor who gave large amounts of dangerous pills to their loved one.

She told me that both she and her mother had expressed concerns to Paul about the safety of his practice in Ohio, but he had been defensive. He had pointed out the differences between him and other doctors in the area who had gotten into trouble (which he had done during my interviews as well) and reminded them of the drug tests he used to ensure patient compliance. But she said that even Paul admitted that the tests were imprecise, and therefore limited in their value.

She was perhaps strongest in her belief that Paul could have, and certainly *should* have, stopped practicing when the DEA first raided his office. Even if his intentions were pure, even if his practice was thorough and conscientious, and even if his prescriptions were justified, she thought that he should have left it all behind for his family's sake. At the time, her mother was still employed as a librarian in a Chicago public school. Jane said that the couple could have lived comfortably on her salary and been richer than "at least 50% of Americans."

Overall, she felt that her father's fierce defensiveness was revealing. She believed that somewhere deep within him, under layers of psychological armor, was a knowledge of his own guilt. "I believe that he fights this conviction of his heart with all of his strength," she said.

And yet despite these criticisms of her father, Jane had reservations about the legal basis of the case against him. At one point, she said, "If a doctor instructs patients about the proper way to take medicine, and then the patient takes it improperly and suffers harm, is that the doctor's fault?" She was wary of a process that pinned all the legal responsibility on him.

But these concerns were not strong enough for her to agree with her dad's decision to fight the charges. She believed that the guilty pleas of Denise and Alice alone would be "pretty damaging" to Paul's case. And on a practical level, she knew that a guilty plea would result in a shorter prison term compared with one that followed a jury's guilty verdict. As Paul's trial drew nearer, she had encouraged him to take such a plea.

Based on what she knew of the case, she also felt — in sharp contrast with her father — that Paul *was* partly responsible for the deaths of those patients. She said that she felt "just terrible" when she thought about patients who had died, and she understood why their family members would be angry. "I wish with all of my heart that he had never entered the business of pain medicine," she said.

Toward the end of January 2011, Jane told me that she was going to take a break from our correspondence. She said that she had been trying to talk with Paul for several days and that he'd been "pretty angry and mean" in response. She needed to regain some of her strength before reaching out to him again or continuing our conversation.

But during an exchange earlier that month, she had shared something noteworthy. She had said that, recently, when she was struggling with some residual pain from a broken bone, she had noticed that something unexpected had brought her relief.

"Interestingly enough," she said, "my pain has diminished incredibly since I've made a break in my relationship from my Dad."

— PART FOUR —
"A TRULY DANGEROUS MAN"

THE JUDGE

The Potter Stewart US Courthouse in downtown Cincinnati is a nine-story, art deco, gray-stone building shaped like a shoebox. The building, completed in 1939, once served as a post office, and nowadays, when visitors walk down the wide corridors of the first floor, they pass walls lined with out-of-use teller windows.

By March 2011, when the Volkman trial began, the federal agencies that once operated field offices in the building had also relocated. This made it a strikingly quiet place, with the occasional sound of heels clicking down empty hallways and people talking in hushed tones. Were it not for the metal detectors that greet visitors who enter the building, it would feel like a library.

Volkman's trial began in a large courtroom on the building's first floor to accommodate the pool of prospective jurors. But shortly after the jury was sworn in, the proceedings moved upstairs to a smaller, windowless courtroom with a burgundy carpet and pew-like benches. Oil paintings hung from the walls, including one portrait of a black-robed woman with bright blond hair holding a book in her hand.

This was Judge Sandra Beckwith, who would preside over Volkman's trial.

Beckwith grew up in Cincinnati and initially thought she would follow her grandfather, Reed Shank, into the field of medicine. Shank was a prominent surgeon who served on the staffs of multiple hospitals in the Cincinnati area and worked as team physician for the Reds and Bengals. When he died abruptly from a heart attack, at age sixty, the news made the front page of the *Cincinnati Enquirer*. The article described him as one of the city's "most colorful and prominent figures in medical, scholastic and sports circles."

Beckwith took premed courses during her first three years of college at the University of Cincinnati but instead decided to study law. She remained at the University of Cincinnati for law school, where she was one of just three women in her class. After graduating with honors, she began her legal career working with her father, an attorney, in a private practice in the small town of Harrison, Ohio, outside of Cincinnati. Within a decade she embarked on a remarkable campaign of "firsts" in elected or appointed office. In 1977, she became the first woman elected to municipal court in Hamilton County.

In 1987, she was the first woman elected to the Hamilton County Court of Common Pleas' Division of Domestic Relations. In 1989, she was the first woman appointed to the Hamilton County Board of Commissioners. And in 1992, after she was appointed to the federal bench by President George H. W. Bush and confirmed by the US Senate, she became the first female district court judge for the Southern District of Ohio.

When I interviewed her years after the Volkman trial, she told me that the federal district court fields criminal cases, civil cases, and patent cases, among other kinds. If it involves federal law, she said, "There's very little that is not within the purview of a federal district court."

In the years between her appointment and the Volkman trial, Beckwith presided over criminal cases involving crack-dealing gang members; fraudsters; sex offenders; corrupt cops, firefighters, and federal employees; a former NBA referee convicted of filing false tax forms; and a man who kidnapped a twenty-year-old woman from a Cincinnati-area motel, bound her hands with duct tape, and drove her to a cabin in northern Wisconsin. Her civil docket had included a lawsuit from a whistleblowing General Electric engineer who had raised concerns about the safety of jet engines being manufactured for the Defense Department; a dispute over whether a twelve-foot inflatable rat, erected in protest outside a local a car dealership by picketing machinists, was protected by the First Amendment; and a lawsuit against a coroner who had kept decedents' brains and other organs without proper notification or permission from families.

Beckwith's most publicized case prior to the Volkman trial involved her alma mater, the University of Cincinnati. It arrived on her desk in 1994.

The case concerned government-funded research that had been performed by UC-affiliated scientists between 1960 and 1971. The US Department of Defense, which funded the study, had hoped to gain a better understanding of how radiation affected the human body. To achieve that, the study's leading researcher, Dr. Eugene Saenger, exposed subjects to intense doses of radiation. Afterward, researchers examined subjects' urine, blood, and cognitive functioning.

There were eighty-eight subjects who participated in the studies, ranging in age from nine to eighty-four, and they were recruited mainly through Cincinnati General Hospital, where they were existing patients. Sixty percent of the subjects were Black, and most were poor. The overwhelming majority were terminally ill with cancer at the time of enrollment, and yet they were still leading relatively high-functioning lives.

Subjects of Saenger's study were kept in the dark about the nature of their treatment, the expected symptoms, and, for years of the study, even the fact that they were part of an experiment. In 1965, the patients signed forms indicating they were participating in some kind of research study. But only in the last months of the study were subjects told that the Pentagon was involved.

The results of the study were horrifying. While all the subjects were sick beforehand, the treatment almost certainly accelerated their deaths and made them more painful. As a law review article about the study from 1995 recounted, "Ten [subjects] died within forty days, the median patient died within four-and-one-half months, and the average patient survived six months." The *New York Times* would later report that "the Cincinnati study exposed patients to the highest levels of whole-body radiation and, some experts say, probably caused the most deaths of all the known Government-sponsored radiation experiments since World War II."

For decades, Saenger claimed to be proud of the experiment and said that he undertook these treatments in the interest of sick patients, with providing information to the Pentagon as a secondary concern. "We gave them this treatment to see whether we could improve their condition," he said.

Although the research prompted some concern and media coverage in the early 1970s, it did not reach the courts for decades. This changed in 1994, when the *Cincinnati Enquirer* published a series of articles about the experiments. A number of subjects' family members subsequently filed lawsuits against the university and individual researchers, and those cases were consolidated into a single class-action case before Beckwith.

A bitter legal battle ensued. Saenger, through his attorneys, sought the dismissal of the case, while a lawyer for the plaintiffs said at one point that the experiments were "no different" from war crimes committed by Nazi doctors on inmates at concentration camps. In January 1995, Beckwith was faced with a crucial decision of whether to allow the lawsuit to proceed on grounds that subjects' constitutional rights had been violated or whether, as the university's attorneys claimed, the study's government funding shielded it from litigation. She ruled for the plaintiffs, and the case proceeded. Eventually, in 1999, a settlement was reached between the university and subjects' families, which included a payment of more than $3.5 million to be distributed among the relatives and an order that the university erect a plaque acknowledging those affected by the experiments.

In June 2000, when family members of subjects gathered for the first time at the plaque, Beckwith received a standing ovation. In an interview with the *Cincinnati Enquirer*, the son of a victim said that the judge had shown "courage, moxie and guts" in the way she handled the case. Beckwith said, "It really hurts you to think that your alma mater may have been involved in something so reprehensible." In her remarks at the event, she called the experiments "a terrible breach of trust" and the lawsuit "a call of conscience for the entire country and the government."

By the time that the Volkman trial was scheduled to begin in her courtroom, in March 2011, Beckwith was an experienced and widely respected judge. In 1995, she was inducted to the Ohio Women's Hall of Fame. In a 2000 profile in the magazine of the Federal Bar Association, the former chief judge of the Southern District of Ohio called her an "outstanding judge in every category judges are measured."

Just days before the Volkman trial was scheduled to begin, the Cincinnati USA Regional Chamber had honored her as one of the year's "Great Living Cincinnatians." In a short documentary film that accompanied the award, a judicial colleague remarked that, though her manner as a judge was generally "very nice and feminine and gentle," Beckwith had a way of delivering forceful rulings without departing from that soft-spoken style.

"We called her the Velvet Hammer," he said.

THE PROSECUTION'S CASE, PART I: THE CLINICS

If jurors were expecting theatrics from Timothy Oakley, the lead attorney from the government's two-man prosecution team, they would have been disappointed. Oakley, a veteran prosecutor who wore boxy suits on the days of the trial I attended, delivered his opening statement in a quiet, casual manner. This was not a fire-and-brimstone sermon; it was a speech delivered with a low-key sense of resignation.

The story Oakley introduced was about a cash-only clinic "whose main goal was to prescribe pain pills." It was a chaotic place, where "huge" amounts of pills were prescribed, medical files went missing, guns and billy clubs were kept on hand to maintain order, bookkeeping was an "absolute disaster," and family members of addicted patients pleaded for their loved ones' treatments to stop. Oakley said that once the prosecution finished presenting its case, "you will be asked to find that Paul Holland Volkman,

MD, PhD, acted with Denise and Alice to provide these medications without a lawful purpose, and that that resulted in some of these folks' death."

For the next four weeks, the prosecution called witnesses who, piece by
piece, told the story that Oakley had outlined. And this meant describing
the beginning, through Denise Huffman.

On the stand, Denise told the story of when and why she opened
Tri-State Healthcare. She explained that she had wanted "to help people"
and that, for a long time, she had wanted to be a nurse. Though she admitted that she didn't have a lot of relevant professional experience, she said
that she did have firsthand experience with her husband's health tribulations, as well as a long history of her own health issues. And this was why,
in late 2001, in South Shore, Kentucky, she opened "a pain management
facility for chronic pain patients."

Under direct examination from the prosecutor, Denise admitted that
"basically everybody" who came to Tri-State received narcotic pain medication. She also acknowledged that after seeing just a handful of patients,
the clinic decided to accept only cash.

She went on to answer questions about the clinic's first few employees,
the locum tenens staffing agencies it used to hire doctors, and details about
the clinic's move to Portsmouth in 2003. She was then asked to identify the
doctor whom she hired at the clinic's new location across the river. "He's
seated right over here with the blue shirt and the neck tie and the suit on,"
she said.

Denise testified that Volkman's starting salary was $5,000 per week,
which she later raised to $5,500. During Denise's testimony Oakley
submitted Volkman's 1099 forms from Tri-State Health into evidence, and
Huffman read them aloud. In 2003, for work from April through December,
the doctor was paid $200,000. In 2004, he received $280,500. In 2005, for
work from January to September (when he left), he made $186,000.

During her testimony, Denise also confirmed that she herself had
become a patient of Volkman after he was hired. And as Oakley continued
with this line of questioning, she acknowledged that her husband, John,
was also a patient at the clinic, as were her daughter, Alice, and her son-in-
law, Chad.

Denise's testimony provided a factual foundation for the witnesses and
evidence that followed. But perhaps just as important, it allowed jurors to
see and hear from the founder of the clinic where Volkman had spent the
bulk of his time in southern Ohio.

At times during her testimony, Denise explained that her memory was spotty. And three times Oakley cut her off, mid-answer, to tell her that she had begun to ramble or "wander a little bit."

One juror later told me that nothing about Denise's testimony conveyed intelligence or legitimacy. "If I walked into a clinic and she owned it, I would leave," he said. "When you [saw] her, you knew that there was something going on."

Another juror later told me that, more than anything else about the trial, it was Volkman and Denise's partnership that stuck with her. She remained incredulous about Denise's total lack of medical training and how she had successfully recruited Volkman. This blew her mind, she said. "What could they have possibly said to him . . . to get him to come from Chicago?"

To add detail to the story of the clinic's early days, prosecutors called a number of pharmacists to the stand. They came from as close to Tri-State as West Portsmouth (three miles away) and as far as Kenova, West Virginia (forty miles), and Grayson, Kentucky (forty-three miles). Some worked for corporate chains, like Rite Aid or Walmart. Others, like Stephen Staker from Staker's Pharmacy and Kevin Gahm from Gahm's Pharmacy, represented family-owned businesses. Many had decades of experience. And all were there to explain why they had stopped filling Paul Volkman's prescriptions.

One by one, they recounted their reasons for their suspicion and concern. There was the fact that Volkman's customers seemed to arrive in groups of four or five at a time — "kind of a wave," as one described it. There were the striking similarities between the prescriptions written for various patients. There was the fact that the patients had traveled conspicuously long distances and tended to pay in cash.

Most concerning, however, were the quantities of the medications the doctor prescribed. One pharmacist recalled watching a Volkman patient who was eight or nine months pregnant walk into his store. He couldn't remember precisely what the script called for, but he remembered how he felt: It "just seemed wrong to me," he said. He handed the slip back and soon decided not to fill any more of the doctor's scripts.

At the end of another pharmacist's testimony, the prosecutor asked, "In your 42 years of experience as a pharmacist, had you ever seen scripts like the ones Dr. Volkman had issued?"

Yes, he said. "And I will tell you right now, the first thing I do is call the regional DEA office and say, 'Get somebody down here.'"

Having established how and why Volkman was shunned by local pharmacies, the prosecution next told the story of Tri-State's on-site dispensary.

This tale was partly covered during Denise's testimony, when she recalled her disagreements with Volkman about the wisdom of the idea. She said that Volkman had suggested the idea and argued that an on-site pharmacy would be convenient for patients, while she had said that she couldn't afford to hire a pharmacist. She was also wary of the additional time and paperwork involved. To this, Volkman apparently responded that the clinic wouldn't need a pharmacist; he had a PhD in pharmacology, and he would "take care of everything." Volkman won the argument, and they proceeded with the application to the state pharmacy board.

As part of this application process, the state board of pharmacy sent a compliance agent to inspect the clinic and to explain to the staff what their new responsibilities would be. That agent, Kevin Kinneer, testified about the stringent rules for a dispensary of the kind Tri-State sought to establish. If the clinic proceeded with its plans, the dispensary's registered physician — in this case, Volkman — would be "responsible for . . . every tablet that comes into their possession, and to make sure that when they furnish it to an individual patient, that they personally are the one who is furnishing that drug," he said.

In addition to this high level of scrutiny, on-site dispensaries also needed to keep meticulous records that tracked the coming and going of all dangerous substances. This amount of work usually convinced doctors to pass on establishing an on-site dispensary "because it takes so much time away from their patients," Kinneer testified.

But Volkman and Alice Huffman, who would oversee the logistics of the dispensary, claimed to be up for the challenge. And Kinneer said that after they signed papers affirming their commitment to following the laws, Tri-State got a green light to begin dispensing pills.

The on-site dispensary was, like the pain clinic it served, a cash-only operation. This meant that a Tri-State patient's bill for the medications that Volkman was prescribing could easily top $1,000. During Alice Huffman's testimony, Oakley used price sheets from the dispensary to show the components that went into such a price tag. He also noted, through his questioning, that the clinic served many married couples who both went to the clinic, which meant that the household costs for a single visit to Tri-State's pharmacy might top $2,000 in cash.

But the dispensary's high prices didn't necessarily translate to the quality of the pharmacy operation. As testimony showed, nobody was hired by the clinic to pick up the extra work, and many of those responsibilities fell to Alice Huffman, who acknowledged during her testimony that she, too, had "no medical training at all." At other times during the prosecution's case, former patients testified that the number of pills they received from the dispensary was less than what they had been prescribed. Alice admitted that the pharmacy's operations were "quite unorganized."

Given both the danger and the street value of the medications stored at the dispensary, it would be reasonable for the clinic to have strict protocols about who had access behind the dispensary counter. But during Denise's testimony, she rang off a long list of the people who moved freely through the back end of the dispensary. That list included Alice; Alice's husband, Chad; Denise's husband, John; Denise's two nieces, Tera and Liz, who worked at the clinic; and Tera's husband, Daniel. State rules required that Schedule II controlled substances like oxycodone be kept in a locked safe. But when asked about this, Alice testified that "pretty much everybody in the office" had the safe's combination.

Kevin Kinneer testified that, when he returned to the clinic a few months after the dispensary was cleared to open, compliance with the rules he had previously explained was abysmal. He found unmarked vials of medication and logbooks that were months out of date.* He also found that Volkman was not personally overseeing the dispensing of the medication, as he was required and had previously agreed to do.

Alice's testimony provided more detail on Volkman's approach to the dispensary. She testified that at one point he asked her to go to an office-supply store to purchase a signature stamp that she could use to "sign" prescriptions on his behalf, and told her he intended to initial those prescriptions when they were filled. But Alice said that he only initialed "some" of the prescriptions that were filled and that he never performed the counting and confirming of pills that was required by state law. Overall, when describing the dispensary, she said Volkman "wasn't in there a lot." Though she did note that, once the dispensary was

---

* A DEA-affiliated witness would testify that, at the time of the June 2005 raid, more than one million pills from the dispensary "could not be accounted for."

up and running, the amounts of medications he prescribed noticeably increased.

Other testimony revealed just how busy this dysfunctional cash-only pharmacy was. On the third day of the trial, a DEA diversion investigator described how, at some point during the agency's investigation, his office had received a request from the Cincinnati field office to perform an analysis on Volkman's controlled-substance ordering activities. The investigator testified that for the year 2004 — the first full year after the dispensary was opened — Volkman was the top practitioner-purchaser of oxycodone in the entire United States, and, during this time, Volkman himself was ordering 30 percent of all hydrocodone ordered by doctors in Ohio.

At the time, Volkman wasn't just outpacing other physicians; he was also out-ordering entire pharmacies for oxycodone and hydrocodone. For the year 2005, Volkman's ordering of oxycodone was "four to five times higher" than the national average for individual pharmacy locations, including chain pharmacies such as Rite Aid and CVS, the witness testified.

At one point, the prosecutor asked whether, in the investigator's review of such data, it was typical to see a practitioner rank so high in both oxycodone and hydrocodone purchases. It was not, the witness replied. Physicians will tend to favor one medication, and, in turn, their ordering numbers for the other are often "significantly lower."

"And if those who purchased both and were ranked in the top 100, where does Dr. Volkman rank nationwide?" the prosecutor asked.

"Dr. Volkman ranks No. 1," he replied.

Sometimes during criminal trials, jurors are taken to the scene of a crime. The Volkman jurors never made such a trip, but prosecutors still attempted to re-create the look, sound, and feel of Tri-State and Volkman's later clinics in the Cincinnati courtroom.

At different points in the trial, they showed photos of the exterior of the clinics. Jurors were also shown photos taken inside the clinics. One showed a notice tacked to a wall inside Tri-State that read ATTENTION: ALL PATIENTS WILL BE DRUG SCREENED AT RANDOM. IF YOU TEST POSITIVE FOR ANY "ILLEGAL STREET DRUGS" YOU WILL BE "DISMISSED." Another, from inside the dispensary, showed a large wooden club that was propped against an emergency exit near the cash register.

Prosecutors also called former patients who described visiting the clinic. One recalled occasionally seeing patients who were "kind of messed up" from medication in the waiting room. Another described patients looking "dopey" and "like when you can tell somebody's took Xanaxes."

There were also videos played. One was the video taken by a DEA employee during the June 2005 raid of the Findlay Street clinic, which took jurors on a slow, silent tour of the building. Another was the hidden-camera video taken by a DEA-cooperating patient from January 2004 that offered a glimpse of an average day inside the clinic's waiting room. During her testimony the patient who took the video was asked by the prosecutor whether it looked many of the people at the clinic were in severe pain. "Not all of them, no," she said.

Other witnesses described the clinics that Volkman ran after he split from the Huffmans. One former patient described the Center Street house-turned-clinic as "very, very busy" and compared the amount of foot traffic to a grocery store. Delbert Evans, Volkman's former security guard, testified in jail stripes and explained that he was serving ten years at the Chillicothe Correctional Institution for drug trafficking and conspiracy. He recalled that WHEN Volkman hired him, the Center Street clinic had "a lot of chaos." He described the scene as "patients running everywhere, money hanging out of nurses' pockets . . . people on the porch going anywhere they want to go." Evans estimated that there were at least fifty or sixty people there at a given time.

Numerous witnesses also described the Chillicothe clinic. One former patient described arriving to the clinic at seven in the morning, two hours before Volkman arrived, so he could "beat the line of people." He said that there would be thirty to fifty people when the clinic opened and that patients continued to arrive as the day progressed. Another patient testified about driving to Chillicothe and then deciding not to follow through with her appointment. She said that when she stepped inside the building, she got a "weird feeling" and "didn't like the looks of the people that were around me." With a "queasy" feeling in her stomach, she threw her paperwork in the trash and left.

The Chillicothe clinic was the focus of one of the prosecution's expert witnesses: a pain expert and assistant professor of anesthesiology at Ohio State University named Steven Severyn. Severyn had been called to discuss more than five thousand prescriptions that Volkman had written for more than 550 patients after his split from Denise. All of those scripts had been filled between early September 2005 and early February 2006 at Harold Fletcher's East Main Street Pharmacy in Columbus.

Severyn's testimony offered a statistical analysis of Volkman's prescriptions. The large number of scripts he had reviewed had allowed him to spot trends in the doctor's approach, and those trends were not subtle. In the period he examined, he found that Volkman prescribed a narcotic to his patients in 98 percent of the patient visits he reviewed. Of all the patient encounters he examined, oxycodone was prescribed 89 percent of the time; hydrocodone, 81 percent of the time; benzodiazepines, 85 percent of the time; and the muscle relaxer Soma, 61 percent of the time.

And it wasn't just the individual prescriptions that stood out to Severyn; it was also the combinations of medications that Volkman prescribed. "It was very unusual . . . that 85 percent of the time that the physician and the patient had an encounter, prescriptions were written for two narcotics, not just one," he said. He added that it would have been "much more logical" for one of these opioids to be a delayed-release preparation, but Volkman had instead prescribed two immediate-release pills. Asked why the doctor might have made this choice, he said, "I am not able to provide for you a rationale why two forms of an immediate-release oxycodone would be prescribed at the same time."

Volkman's combinations of prescribed medications made his treatment riskier, Severyn said. He was struck by the frequency with which patients received the same combination of four medications: two opioids, a muscle relaxer, and a sedative (benzodiazepine). This was the case in 45 percent of Volkman's patient encounters, he said.

Severyn's review had left him with a clear conclusion about Volkman's pain-management practice: It was "not consistent with the legitimate practice of the field of pain medicine," he said.

Week after week, testimony from prosecution witnesses continued.

The prosecution called employees who had worked at one of Volkman's clinics. One, who was also a patient of Volkman at the time, said that she was so heavily drugged that she occasionally nodded off while talking to patients. Another, who worked at the Chillicothe clinic, reported that the security guard was known to accept bribes from patients who wanted to be moved up in the line to see the doctor.

Prosecutors also called more than a dozen former patients, some of whom described their past legal issues from abusing or selling pills. One witness appeared in clothing indicating she was currently incarcerated.

Another former patient explained that she had been convicted of selling pills on two separate occasions, and both times those charges stemmed from sales to her son, who had been working with law enforcement as a confidential informant. When the prosecutor asked for more detail, she explained that all her kids had become addicted to pills at some point, and so had her husband (who was also a Volkman patient). She would sell pills to her kids to get money to pay for her visits to the doctor or the pharmacy. "I guess my son had got into some kind of trouble for writing checks or something and so he agreed to wear a wire on me twice," she said.

"Is the pill problem down there that bad?" the prosecutor asked, in response.

Yes it was, she said. "Really bad."

A recurring theme from former patients was a wariness about taking their medications as Volkman advised. "If I took them like I was supposed to, I probably would have died," one said. Another patient said that she would be dead or a "walking zombie" if she had taken all the medications Volkman prescribed to her. A third former patient gave a similar answer. She said, "If I would have took all those 34 pills in one day, I believe it would have killed me."

THE DEVIL IN SCIOTO COUNTY

One week prior to the start of Volkman's trial, Governor John Kasich made a trip to Portsmouth to announce new measures meant to combat the opiate crisis, including a new task force led by a former state attorney general and an appropriation of $100,000 in state funds for a Portsmouth-area rehab facility. During the visit, Kasich said that failure was not an option, and he promised to do his part to "drive the devil out of Scioto County."

Then, on March 8 — the fifth day of the Volkman trial — Kasich returned to the subject during his "State of the State" speech at the Ohio capitol in Columbus. Prescription drug abuse was a "scourge" that demanded "unanimous bipartisan support," he said. And he was pleased to see legislation being written to crack down on pill mills. He acknowledged that the people of Scioto County may have previously felt hopeless. But now, he announced, the cavalry was arriving. "This legislature will not let you stand alone," he declared, as the room broke into applause.

One day after Kasich's speech, the Ohio State Medical Board adopted a resolution about the prescription drug crisis in the state that specifically mentioned the problems in Scioto County. The resolution included some of the statistics that the governor had recently shared: 9.7 million doses of prescription painkillers had been dispensed in Scioto County the previous year; overdose deaths from oxycodone toxicity had quadrupled in the previous three years; the majority of those overdose victims had been between twenty-five and thirty-five years of age.

Pill mills "are sometimes disguised as independent pain management centers," the resolution explained. But these illegitimate clinics were recognizable by a "constellation of certain criteria and conduct," which included accepting only cash, a lack of coordination with other doctors, the presence of security guards, patients who traveled long distances, and treatment methods of an "extremely limited scope" that mainly focused on prescription drugs.

With this resolution, the board was formally designating such activities as an "immediate and serious harm to the public," which it planned to treat as a high-priority issue. In closing, the board mentioned actions it planned to take in response, including holding expedited hearings for alleged pill mill cases and distributing a book published by the Federation of State Medical Boards called *Responsible Opioid Prescribing: A Physician's Guide.*

While discussion of Scioto County's pill problem grew louder in Columbus, the fight against pain clinics pressed forward in Portsmouth. On March 28 — Day 15 of the Volkman trial — the Portsmouth City Council passed an ordinance regarding pain clinics within city limits.

The bill included an array of new rules for the operation of such facilities. To open for business, clinics would now have to submit an application to the Portsmouth Health Department that included proof that its physicians carried malpractice insurance and that the clinic was registered with the Ohio Pharmacy Board's Ohio Automated Rx Reporting System (OARRS). Clinic operators would also have to submit an affidavit showing their affiliation with a hospital or accredited college or university within one hundred miles of the city. Without such an affiliation they could not open or operate. If approved, a clinic would also have to pay a $1,000 fee to obtain a license to operate, as well as an annual permit fee of $1,000.

Approved clinics would also be subject to random and unannounced inspections by the Portsmouth City Health Department.

Notably, the ordinance did not allow existing clinics to be grandfathered in, which made it likely that most or all existing clinics would shut down. During a TV news story on the ordinance, the city solicitor said that he recognized there were "legitimate" and "ethical" reasons for having facilities that treat pain. What they were focused on, he said, was "stop[ping] what's commonly referred to as the 'pill mills.'"

On the day after the measure passed the city council, members of the local prescription-drug-focused Facebook group were jubilant. In one post, Lisa Roberts wrote, "No longer will Portsmouth be synonymous with Pill Mills. No longer will we be the big black-eye of Ohio!"

After its passage, the law was challenged in court by two pain clinics. A lawyer for those clinics argued that the ordinance violated the state constitution and that the job of regulating businesses fell to the state medical and pharmacy boards, not the city.

Before the dispute could be settled in court, a judge in Portsmouth held a hearing on the question of whether the clinics would remain open. On the day of the hearing, the gallery of the courtroom was packed with dozens of spectators, many wearing turquoise T-shirts emblazoned with the logo of a local support group for mothers who had lost children to overdose. While the hearing took place, some spectators wiped away tears. A camera filmed the scene for the night's evening news.

The judge denied the clinic owners' request for an injunction, which meant that the clinics would be closed until the issue was fully settled. When the hearing ended, the crowd cheered. Afterward, Lisa Roberts spoke to a reporter for the *Portsmouth Daily Times* and called it a major win for the community. The judge's ruling had prompted "an outpouring of joy," she said.

While this activity was taking place in southern Ohio, media outlets continued to raise alarms about the severity of the region's pill problem.

In December, four months before Volkman's trial, the Associated Press had published an article about Scioto County that opened with two alarming facts:

> Nearly one in 10 babies were born addicted to drugs last year in southern Ohio's Scioto County. Admissions for prescription pain-killer overdoses were five times the national average.

The article drew a direct line between the flood of prescription drugs and area pill mills, which it defined as "clinics or doctors that dole out prescription medications like OxyContin with little discretion." In the piece, Lisa Roberts said, "I would describe it as if a pharmaceutical atomic bomb went off."

The following month brought an article about Portsmouth in *Men's Health* magazine. The trend of drug deaths in this "economically struggling industrial city . . . on the banks of the Ohio River" was overwhelming, the reporter wrote. This article, too, pointed to the striking number of pain clinics in the rural county. And the author was particularly interested in the phenomenon of on-site dispensaries. "These in-house pharmacies create a troublesome conflict of interest for even the most ethical of doctors," she wrote. "The more prescriptions they write, the more money they and their clinics make."

She added, "All of this is legal in Ohio."

Then, on April 19 — two days before closing arguments in the Volkman trial — the Scioto County overdose crisis hit its biggest stage of all: the front page in the *New York Times*. The article was titled "Ohio County Losing Its Young to Painkillers' Grip." In the piece, Portsmouth police chief Horner said that he was seeing third and fourth generations of families struggling with prescription drug abuse. Other interviewees searched for words to convey the severity of the problem. "It's like being in the middle of a tornado," Ed Hughes said. Terry Johnson, the coroner-turned-state-representative, called the problem "the darkest most malevolent thing you've ever seen."

While the crisis raged, the *Times* article noted that there had been some progress in the fight against it. At one point, the piece mentioned that a "doctor from the area, Paul Volkman, is on trial in federal court in Cincinnati and accused of illegally disbursing prescription painkillers."

THE PROSECUTION'S CASE, PART II: THE DEATHS

Prosecutors called dozens of witnesses to describe what took place inside Volkman's pain clinics. But these people — pharmacists, law enforcement officers, former employees, former patients — made up only about half of the government's case. The other half focused on patients who died.

Jurors would eventually face a two-tiered decision when they discussed the patients mentioned in the indictment.

First, they would be asked to answer the question: Had Paul Volkman illegally dealt drugs to this person? This meant being convinced beyond a reasonable doubt that Volkman had prescribed pills — in the language of the Controlled Substances Act — "outside the scope of medical practice or . . . not for a legitimate medical purpose in the usual course of a professional practice."

And if the answer to this first question was yes, jurors would then be asked whether they believed that the patient in question had died *as a direct result* of this illegal prescribing.

To answer these questions, prosecutors assembled a procession of specialists who had played a role in analyzing these patients' deaths. All told, the jury heard from more than twenty toxicologists, coroners, and pathologists. And they also heard from five family members of deceased patients who described their loved ones' lives and final days.

Testimony from the family members of Volkman's deceased patients continued a theme from the testimony of former patients. While many of Volkman's patients did have painful ailments that had prompted them to seek treatment, this pain was eventually eclipsed by drug use.

Jeffrey Reed's widow, Cheryl Posey, acknowledged that her husband had sustained injuries during a construction-site accident in the mid-1990s. And she described how Jeff had tried, and failed, to return to work afterward. This was the reason he started going to pain clinics and taking pain pills, she said.

But at some point, his legitimate treatment had shifted into something destructive. In his desperation for cash to pay for his doctor's visits and pills, his wife said that he would pawn "everything he could get ahold of," including guitars, VCRs, and his daughter's television. She described moments when Jeff was so drugged that he would nod off while eating and his periods of despondency and sickness when his pills ran out.

"Was he abusing those medications?" the prosecutor asked at one point.

"It didn't start out that way, but it ended up that way," she said.

During Melissa Ratcliff's testimony, she described the back problems that her husband, Ernest, had struggled with since a football injury in high school. But Ernest was also a drug user, she said. And she had no doubt that he was addicted to his pain medication.

She explained that Ernest would snort pills, sell pills, and buy pills from friends, acquaintances, and "anyone that had them." He would take a month's worth of pills in just a few days. When the prosecutor asked her why Ernest had gone to see Volkman, she said, "Because he knew that it was a pain management clinic and that he could go there and get large quantities of pills."

The family members of deceased patients also offered a glimpse at the raw emotion that Volkman's clinics elicited. One day during the trial, Diana Colley took the stand to tell the story of her visit to the Center Street house-turned-clinic and how she threatened to shoot Volkman if he continued to prescribe pills to her son.

Steven Hieneman's mother, Paula, described a similar white-hot rage that she felt due to the fear that her son's life was endangered by his visits to Tri-State. She testified about calling the clinic multiple times and instructing Denise not to let Volkman continue writing prescriptions for Steven.

But beyond revealing the emotional impact of Volkman's actions, this testimony also served a more direct purpose. In many cases, it was loved ones who had first found the patient after their death and who could therefore describe the scene and circumstances. Melissa Ratcliff told the story of her husband Ernest's final hours and how she found his lifeless body in bed. Cheryl Reed recounted finding her husband, Jeff, sitting, cross-legged, on the floor of their bathroom, with his head hunched over. Stoney Carver described waking from a nap to find his wife, Mary, "sitting on the couch with her head laying on the coffee table in front of her in a sleep position."

Carver was not just testifying as the spouse of a deceased patient; he was also a former Volkman patient himself. And this combination of factors led to one of the trial's most haunting moments. After he had finished narrating the scene of his wife's overdose death, he recalled how he had nevertheless returned to the pain clinic for another doctor's visit. He said that there was little acknowledgment of his wife's death. People at the clinic acted "like it really never even happened," he said.

When the prosecutor asked him why he had decided to go back, Carver replied, "I was hooked on drugs."

While family members of Volkman patients helped to describe the circumstances of these deaths, the subject of *why* those deaths occurred was mostly left to the specialists.

They were an experienced group. One forensic pathologist testified that he had conducted autopsies in hundreds of cases where the cause of death was determined to be an overdose. A drug chemist at the Kentucky State Medical Examiner's Office said that of the four thousand or so cases per year in which her office performed toxicological analysis, about half were overdoses. A deputy coroner from eastern Kentucky testified that he had been to the scene of "many, many overdoses," sometimes as many as one or two per day. Another witness described overdoses as an "epidemic" in the state of Kentucky and said that he had seen "an overwhelming number."

Over the course of the trial, these witnesses offered jurors a 101-level course in how an overdose death occurs. One forensic pathologist who had conducted autopsies for two of Volkman's patients explained that, while opiates can decrease a person's pain, they also slow down their breathing. The technical term for this is *respiratory depression*. When a person is experiencing an overdose, he explained, "their respiratory rate goes down and down and down" until they eventually lose consciousness. At some point, they may stop breathing altogether.

Other witnesses described how, during this process of slowed-down breathing, the body tries to compensate for the drop in oxygen. One physical response to that process is the expansion of blood vessels in the lungs to allow more oxygen-carrying blood to flow through. As these blood vessels expand, they become leaky and fluid seeps out. Thus, one sign of an overdose during a postmortem exam is lungs that are heavier than normal due to the fluid they contain. Another indicator is the presence of stomach contents in the lungs, the result of the person vomiting and then being unable to cough or swallow to protect their airway.

During the prosecution's case, numerous witnesses testified about the heightened risk for an overdose among patients taking more than one medication that depresses the central nervous system. In such a situation, these multiple medications would, at the very least, have an additive effect. As one witness explained, "So if I take alcohol with another [central nervous system] depressant or two CNS depressants in tablet form together, they're going to work together to make my central nervous system more depressed than if I just took one of them alone."

But beyond additive effects, witnesses explained that opiates can have a synergistic, or "super-additive," effect on other medications. This means that the cumulative effect of the medications is more than just the sum of each medication's individual effect in isolation. As one witness put it: "It is almost as if one plus one equals three."

———

Years after his trial had ended, Volkman would write that "none" of his deceased patients "had toxicology results which were consistent with drug overdose deaths."

But this was, like many things he said about his case, demonstrably untrue.

In fact, quite a few prosecution witnesses testified that, based on the autopsies or toxicological analyses they had performed, they believed overdose to be the cause of the patient's death.

A former employee from the Kentucky State Medical Lab who performed a toxicological analysis for Dwight Parsons testified that Parsons had an oxycodone level that was "consistent with a lethal level."

Another forensic pathologist testified that the toxicological analysis for Danny Coffee showed "phenomenally high levels" of both oxycodone and hydrocodone and that, when considered with other drugs found in his bloodstream, "with reasonable certainty I can tell you that he died of drug intoxication."

Another forensic pathologist who conducted the autopsy for Charles Jordan testified that he found an "extremely high level" of oxycodone in his blood, which, even if divided in half, "would be sufficient in my opinion, in and of itself, to account for his death, even if he were physiologically tolerant of that particular narcotic."

When describing the combination of substances found in Steven Hieneman's bloodstream, a pathologist from the Kentucky State Medical Examiner told the jury, "This could kill a normal person just in combination."

A drug chemist at the Kentucky State Police forensic lab who performed a toxicological analysis on Ernest Ratcliff said that, among the various medications identified in Ernest's bloodstream — the diazepam, nordiazepam, hydrocodone, and methadone — his oxycodone levels alone were at a "very high level" that "you see associated with the deaths a lot."

The chief deputy coroner for the Montgomery County coroner's office, who had conducted an autopsy on Scottie Lin James, said that her oxycodone levels alone were "high enough to cause death by itself." He testified he believed her cause of death to be "a result of multiple drugs."

Volkman's claim that "none" of his deceased patients died from overdose also entirely ignores the testimony of the government's main cause-of-death expert.

At the time of his testimony, Dr. Michael Policastro was a Cincinnati-based physician who specialized in both emergency medicine and medical toxicology. He was also an assistant professor in the department of emergency medicine at Wright State University, in Dayton. Early in his testimony, Policastro defined *medical toxicology* as the "diagnosis and management of drug and poison overdoses." He also mentioned that, during his fellowship at the University of Cincinnati, he had taken calls in the drug and poison center at a local children's hospital.

In preparation for his testimony, Policastro spent more than 170 hours reviewing records from deceased patients provided to him by the DEA. Those records included notes from doctors who previously treated the patients, notes from their visits to Volkman, diagnostic tests (X-rays, CT scans), prescription histories, plus autopsy reports and toxicological analyses.

In his analysis of those records — specifically, of the twelve deceased patients who were the focus of his testimony — Policastro noted that Volkman's prescriptions showed little evidence of individualized medical care. Each of those twelve patients had received prescriptions for a combination of opioids and sedatives, and three-quarters of them had been given scripts for two opioids and two sedatives. Half of the patients in that group had been prescribed the same exact combination of medications: oxycodone, hydrocodone, benzodiazepine (Xanax), and Soma.

Policastro mentioned two other trends from his review. Three-quarters of the deceased twelve patients were under the age of forty, which was an age range less associated with heart attack death and more associated with drug overdose. He also observed that eight patients had died within two days of visiting Volkman, and eleven had died within five days of their last visit to the doctor. Nearly all of the patients had also received an increase of their prescribed medication on their last visit.

When offering an opinion on individual patients' cause of death, Policastro acknowledged that some patients' records showed signs of underlying heart disease. But in case after case — for Aaron Gillispie, Charles Jordan, Daniel Coffee, Mary Catherine Carver, James Estep, Kristi Jo Ross, Dwight Parsons, Steve Hieneman, Scottie Lin James, Ernest Ratcliff, and Mark Reeder — he attributed the primary cause of death to a toxicity of drugs.

THE DEFENSE'S CASE

By the time his trial began, Volkman had cycled through several attorneys. There was a Cincinnati-based lawyer who had advised him during his time in pain management, following the DEA raid of the Tri-State clinic on Findlay Street.*

There was Kevin Byers, the Columbus-based attorney who had represented him during his pre-indictment asset-forfeiture case and DEA registration hearing.

There was Dennis Lieberman, a Dayton-based criminal defense attorney (who had previously represented the convicted Portsmouth pain doctor John Lilly) who represented him in the post-indictment detention hearing at which his two kids had testified.

At some point after his indictment, Volkman ran out of money and was paired with a court-appointed defense attorney from Cincinnati named William Gallagher. Within months, Gallagher sought to withdraw, writing in a court filing, "The relationship between counsel and client has deteriorated to the point counsel believes it would not be in the best interest of either for counsel to remain." He officially left in December 2009.

After Gallagher came Wende Cross, an experienced Cincinnati-based defense attorney who, earlier in her career, had spent nearly a decade as a prosecutor in two local US attorneys' offices, in the Eastern District of Kentucky and the Southern District of Ohio.

Cross and Volkman also had a rocky start.

A month after her appointment, she filed a motion to withdraw from the case. During a March 2010 hearing about Volkman's frequent lawyer-switching, she explained that "Dr. Volkman and I have not had one pleasant communication between us since I came on this case." She said she officially decided to withdraw after a particularly "hostile" phone call during which he personally insulted her. Volkman, during the same hearing, said, "From the beginning, Ms. Cross took exception to any kind of direction that I attempted to give her with regard to what type of preparations should be immediately undertaken."

Prosecutors objected to the idea of yet another lawyer, arguing that Volkman ought not be able to prompt further delays in the trial schedule. The judge — who, for this hearing, was not Beckwith, but a temporary fill-in, Susan Dlott — agreed. She described Cross as one of most qualified attorneys in Cincinnati and told Volkman, "You have the right to counsel, but you don't have the right to infinite counsel."

Dlott then changed the terms of Volkman's pretrial release to demand

---

* When I reached out to her via email, her response was brief: "I acknowledge that I am familiar with Paul Volkman but do not wish to share any other information related to him at this time."

that he cooperate with his attorney. She told him that he couldn't curse at Cross or raise his voice or be antagonistic. If he broke these conditions, his bond would be revoked, and he would await his trial from jail. Before the hearing ended, she ordered Volkman to apologize.

And Volkman — in what is perhaps the only time I saw, heard, or read about him apologizing — said, "Mrs. Cross, I'm sorry for offending you."

"I accept," Cross replied.

This court-enforced reconciliation seemed to improve their working relationship. And in short order, due to the size and scope of the case, a second publicly appointed attorney joined the team. Her name was Candace Crouse. A West Virginia native, graduate of Ohio State's law school, and a former clerk for a federal judge in West Virginia, she had worked in various Cincinnati-area firms as a criminal defense lawyer since 2002.

It was this two-woman defense team, Cross and Crouse, who represented Volkman during his trial.

"This case is about an experienced and caring doctor who treated people that he believed were legitimately in pain and who were not receiving adequate pain care anywhere else."

So began Candace Crouse's opening statement on behalf of Paul Volkman on morning of March 3, 2011.

While the prosecution's opening statement had barely acknowledged Volkman's pre-Ohio life, Crouse proceeded to spend significant time on it. "Before I tell you what we believe the evidence is going to show in this case, I want to introduce you to Dr. Volkman," she said. At one point, she walked behind her client and placed a hand on his back, as if to show that he was an approachable man, and not the monster the prosecution would portray him to be. Volkman offered a meek smile.

Crouse described Volkman's upbringing in Washington and the fact that he was a high school valedictorian. He was, she said, a "self-proclaimed nerd" who later received an MD and PhD from the University of Chicago. She described how he went into private practice in pediatrics and family medicine in the early 1980s and how, later, he began seeking locum tenens work, which she described as "basically . . . temping for doctors."

She presented this pivot in Volkman's career as a response to an external need rather than his own personal motivations. Small towns and rural areas are often short on doctors, she explained, and Volkman was helping to fill this gap. This was what brought Volkman to Portsmouth in the mid-1990s, years before he worked at Tri-State. "He went down to the Southern Ohio Medical Center and worked in the emergency room as an emergency doctor, and that's how he got to know Portsmouth and the surrounding area," she said. During her narrative of Volkman's career, she noted that he was board-certified in pediatrics, emergency medicine, and, later, pain management.

Crouse made no mention of the malpractice lawsuits that had prompted a career crisis for Volkman. Instead, she moved quickly from his locum tenens career to his work in a southern Ohio pain-management clinic as if this were a natural, logical progression. She said that Volkman's Tri-State salary of $5,000 per week might sound like a lot of money — but jurors would hear from witnesses who would testify that "that is not an outrageous salary for a doctor, especially for a doctor who's practiced for over 35 years." Her description of Tri-State's origins was conspicuously vague. "This pain clinic was already established and already being run by Denise Huffman," she said. "It had been open for about two years and it had other doctors who had been working there."

Instead, she focused on pain. She told the jury that they would hear testimony that seventy-six million Americans suffer from chronic pain and that, due to uneasiness among doctors about treating patients with narcotics, millions of them suffer needlessly. This was why pain-management clinics existed, she explained: to give pain patients the medications they need. And this, she said, was what Paul Volkman was doing in southern Ohio: addressing a public health gap, alleviating needless suffering, and prescribing vital, yet stigmatized medications. She said Volkman preferred to prescribe opioids because they were the "best medicine available for pain."

As she discussed Volkman's tenure in pain management, she emphasized that he never treated patients who didn't provide medical records, spent "considerable" time with patients, and responded to each patient's unique needs with individualized courses of treatment. This sometimes included referring patients to the Cleveland Clinic for "various things," she said. She also highlighted the measures he had adopted to prevent diversion and abuse, including pill counts and urine tests.

As she wound down, Crouse told the jury that the prosecution's case would last for several weeks. She also acknowledged that they would hear testimony about twelve patients who had died. "But please keep an open mind until you get to hear our side of things," she said.

Crouse closed by drawing a distinction between a criminal case and a malpractice dispute. This trial was not about whether the jury agreed with every decision Volkman made but about whether he was trying, in good faith, to treat his patients.

"We're confident that the evidence is going to show that Dr. Volkman was acting as a doctor," she said.

The defense's case was much smaller in scale than the prosecution's. Volkman's lawyers called just ten witnesses, compared with seventy from prosecutors. His lawyers submitted a relatively small number of exhibits next to the hundreds submitted by the government.

Perhaps this was due to a lack of resources — after all, Volkman's lawyers were local attorneys who, for this case, were serving as public defenders. Then again, there was no disagreement from the defense that Volkman had worked for Denise Huffman, or that their clinic had an on-site dispensary and armed guards and accepted only cash, or that the doctor had prescribed the medications in the amounts that prosecutors had described. There was also no dispute that Volkman had worked out of his house on Center Street or that several of his patients had died during the time in which they were in his care.

At its core, the case was not a dispute over facts but about what those facts *meant*. And the bar for success was lower for the defense. Paul Volkman was innocent until proven guilty. And to succeed, his lawyers didn't need slam-dunk proof of his legitimacy. For him to walk free, they would just need to sow enough reasonable doubt for jurors to vote "not guilty" on each of the charges.

Because of the length of the prosecution's case, much of the work of defending Volkman took place through cross-examining government witnesses.

During the testimony of various pharmacists, for instance, Candace Crouse asked questions to confirm that several had never actually called Volkman to discuss his prescriptions before they decided to stop filling them. In another instance, Crouse focused on what a pharmacist had described as Volkman's patients' suspicious lack of visible pain. "Is it your experience that people who are chronic pain patients who are taking meds as prescribed are going to look like they're in pain?" she asked. Later, she said, "Is that not the point of pain medication: To stop people's pain?"

During the testimony of a DEA agent who had played a leading role in the

Volkman investigation, Wende Cross got him to confirm that the DEA had attempted to send in an officer posing as a pain patient and that the officer had been turned away because he did not have the proper medical records.

During the testimony of another DEA employee — the one who walked jurors through a slideshow comparing Volkman's prescribing with that of other physicians — Cross's questions aimed to defuse jurors' shock at the high numbers of hydrocodone pills Volkman had ordered in a six-month window. Her questioning showed that if that number was divided by six, to show the average being ordered per month, it dropped significantly. Then, if this number was divided by five hundred patients, it equaled around seventy-five pills, per patient, per month. And when the number seventy-five was divided by the thirty days in a month, it fell even further. "So when we see a graph like this and you break it down . . . what we're really talking about is two and a half pills per patient per day," she said.

During her cross-examination of Jeffrey Reed's widow, Cheryl, Cross asked if Jeff had died with methadone — a medication that Volkman had never prescribed — in his system. He had, she confirmed.

During the testimony of Ernest Ratcliff's widow, Melissa, Candace Crouse asked, "Your husband had been living with pain for quite a few years?" and "And the pain got so bad that he actually had to stop working?" The answer to both questions was yes.

During the testimony of Alice Huffman, Wende produced an email Alice had written during Volkman's tenure at Tri-State. It was an email discussing a Portsmouth-area physician who had treated Alice while she was pregnant with twins. During her cross-examination, Wende asked Alice to read aloud from the document.

"Doctor Volkman is my choice of physician," she had written. The letter went on to describe how, after Alice had received poor care from this physician at Southern Ohio Medical Center in Portsmouth, she consulted Volkman, who had referred her to a doctor in Cincinnati who had advised bed rest and daily monitoring of both babies by ultrasound and also placed Alice in the of a "team of specialized high risk OB/GYNs." When discussing Volkman, Alice had written, "I might not have my nine-month-old twins today if it had not been for him."

One memorable example of the defense's cross-examining took place on the trial's eleventh day, during the testimony of a former Portsmouth police narcotics officer named Todd Bryant. In Bryant's direct examination, the prosecutor had submitted a photo taken during the Center Street raid that showed an open safe containing an unorganized pile of cash. "To me it's almost like a drug dealer with the way the money is just wadded up and thrown in the box," the officer said.

During cross-examination, Wende Cross returned to that comment and asked Bryant whether the mere fact of cash in a safe was an indicator of drug dealing. From here, she asked, "Since you're testifying as to the habits of drug dealers, do drug dealers typically ask for photo ID's and make copies of it for their client, their customers?"

He responded, "Drug dealers on the street? No."

The back-and-forth continued:

> Cross: And is it your experience that drug dealers are typically concerned with their customer's health when they're dealing drugs to them?
>
> Bryant: No, drug dealers don't care about nobody's health.
>
> Cross: And is it your experience that drug dealers give receipts to customers when they give them cash for their drugs?
>
> Bryant: Never got a receipt before.
>
> Cross: Do drug dealers, in your experience, give their customers drug tests to make sure that they're taking the drugs they're giving them?
>
> Bryant: No.
>
> Cross: Or that they take — they give them drug tests to make sure they don't have any other drugs in their system?
>
> Bryant: No.

After his trial, Volkman would viciously criticize his attorneys, stating that he felt his lawyers had been "working hand in glove with the judge and the prosecution" to create the appearance of a fair trial. But such a view is hard to square with exchanges like the one between Cross and Bryant, as well as numerous people I spoke to — including the judge, the prosecutor, and multiple jurors — who believed that his attorneys had done as effective a job as possible under the circumstances.

The prosecution in *US v. Volkman* rested after seventeen days of testimony, spanning five calendar weeks. On April 12, 2011, the defense called its first witness: a yoga instructor named Charlene Ballard.

At the time when Volkman arrived at Tri-State, Ballard was employed full-time at a hospital in Huntington, West Virginia, about an hour's drive from Portsmouth. From the stand, she described being contacted by Volkman, who explained that he had used yoga himself, and it had helped with a back problem. He thought it would be useful for his Tri-State patients.

Starting in July 2003, Ballard began commuting to Portsmouth to teach free yoga classes for Tri-State patients. During the months that followed, she taught four classes per week that served an average of twelve to eighteen patients per class. Initially the classes were held in a space at Shawnee State University. But when the clinic moved to Findlay Street, classes took place in a room upstairs.

Ballard explained that the ninety-minute classes covered traditional yoga poses that were, in some cases, modified to accommodate the lack of mobility among patients with chronic back, neck, and shoulder issues. Her classes would end with breathing exercises meant to encourage deep relaxation.

The classes were a success, and Ballard testified that patients frequently told her how much better they felt afterward. "I can't speak for every patient that came to every class," she said, "but overall I felt that the people were responding favorably."

But after less than a year, she had to stop due to the distance of the commute. And under cross-examination from prosecutors, she explained that she had not taught all of Volkman's patients, she had never worked at the Center Street or Chillicothe clinics, and when she left the clinic, the staff never asked for the name of a potential replacement.

Volkman has estimated that he saw somewhere between five hundred and seven hundred patients during his time in Ohio. And yet his defense team called just two to testify: a married couple, David and Tammy Powell, from South Shore, Kentucky. (The prosecution had called sixteen former patients to testify, and eighteen in total, if you include Denise and Alice Huffman.)

David Powell was a former brakeman and conductor for CSX railroad who had stopped working after thirty-five years due to disability. He had been in a motorcycle crash in the 1970s that left him with a split pelvis, and his railroad job had been physically grueling. He had suffered from neck pain, lower back pain, and migraines for "at least" a decade before going to Volkman.

Tammy suffered from poor circulation, muscle spasms, and herniated disks in both her lower back and her neck, and the reasons for these issues were numerous. She had been in a seventeen-year relationship with an abusive, alcoholic husband who beat her when he drank. And in the early 1980s, she had been in an auto accident during which she was, in a mind-boggling series of events, thrown from her car and subsequently bitten by a copperhead snake. The snakebite went untreated for five weeks until her leg swelled and her foot turned black, leaving her with scars that were still visible thirty years later. She said she began seeing Dr. Volkman after her primary care physician acknowledged that the pain pills she was receiving weren't getting the job done and advised her to see a pain specialist.

The Powells' testimony was clearly intended to reframe Volkman as a conscientious, thoughtful physician who practiced according to exacting standards. Tammy recalled how Volkman "insisted on you having medical records" before he agreed to see you. And both she and her husband described how, once patients were cleared for treatment, Volkman took his time in visits with them. David said that his visits took anywhere from fifteen to forty minutes, and Tammy testified that hers ranged from thirty minutes to an hour. Both testified that Volkman performed thorough physical examinations. Tammy said that Volkman watched her touch her toes, checked her reflexes, examined her spine, and worked on her neck. David said that Volkman had closely examined his neck and back to see exactly where his pain was. David recalled how the doctor had, at one point, sent him out for an MRI. Tammy testified that he had prescribed physical therapy.

Both Tammy and David acknowledged that Volkman had prescribed them controlled substances. And both were adamant in describing the relief they got from those pills. David said that medications he was prescribed allowed him to fully function and "helped [him] out quite a bit" at work. He added that he never became addicted to the pills and had no side effects aside from "a couple of night sweats."

Tammy told a similar story. Before seeing Volkman, she said she couldn't sit or stand for very long due to the pain and, in her job as a customer service representative for ATT, had needed to use a phone headset with a long cord so she could get up and walk around while talking to customers. She said that the meds Volkman prescribed helped her sit for longer periods of time and, in doing so, helped her better serve her customers.

Volkman struck her as a "very caring individual," which was why she continued to see him after his split with the Huffmans.

"I liked his care," she said. "I liked him as a doctor."

Four former employees also testified on Volkman's behalf.

One was Ida Renee Ames, who had started as a Tri-State patient in early 2003 while seeking relief for numerous ailments, including a shoulder injury, a past abdominal surgery, and bladder issues. "It was like chronic torture, not just chronic pain," she said, of the reasons she had first gone to the clinic. Ames also had a personal connection to the clinic: Denise Huffman was an aunt to her two youngest children.

Ames, who was a registered nurse, explained how she started working at Tri-State in the fall of 2003 when she was unable to pay the clinic's patient costs and Denise offered her a work-off-the-bills program. Her work at the clinic was mostly administrative: answering phones, tracking the medications patients received, ordering tests and referrals at Volkman's direction, and taking faxes.

Sally Scott, Ames's sister, was a registered nurse from Vanceburg, Kentucky, who had nearly twenty years of nursing experience at the time Volkman hired her. She worked for Volkman for five months, starting on Center Street.

Jennifer Tilley — Sally Scott's niece — worked at the Chillicothe clinic as a secretary from October 2005 to its close in February 2006. Her duties included answering phones, faxing, filing paperwork, and making appointments.

Elizabeth Santos-Mauntel was a veteran nurse who had worked in a variety of settings, including hospitals, nursing homes, and doctors' offices. She lived on the outskirts of Chillicothe and explained that she stopped in at Volkman's office after it opened because she saw "a lot of people there." She worked at the Chillicothe clinic for its final three months, from November 2005 to February 2006. Her duties mostly involved patient-intake interviews and paperwork.

As a group, these former employees expanded on the Powells' portrait of Volkman as a conscientious doctor who ran a high-quality medical operation. Scott testified to the fact that she was a registered nurse and that three other employees were either licensed practical nurses or certified medical technicians, which meant that everyone on Volkman's post-Tri-State staff had some medical background. According to Tilley, it was clear from looking around the waiting room that patients were in real pain. Some were visibly anxious. Quite a few had canes, braces, walkers, or wheelchairs. Others were "keeled over in the chair," she said.

Other testimony covered Volkman's strict protocols for screening potential patients. One former employee said that Volkman did not accept walk-ins. Another recalled how he insisted that patients provide past medical records in order to be seen. According to Scott, this intake process also included reminding patients that misrepresenting symptoms to obtain narcotics was a felony.

The employees also described the ways Volkman tried to ensure patients' honesty and compliance with his advice. They recalled how patients were required to track their symptoms in pain journals and show proof that they had purchased a safe for securely storing their medications. They said that patients were also subject to frequent blood tests as well as urine screens during which they were accompanied to the bathroom by a clinic employee to prevent tampering with the sample. Sally Scott testified that in the last four to six weeks of the Chillicothe clinic's operation, she had begun to conduct informal background checks on patients who seemed suspicious. This involved calling the local district court to see if the patient had any past drug or alcohol charges and, if she found something, taking the information to Dr. Volkman; according to her testimony, he would then dismiss the patient because "they were too high-risk to treat."

If the former employees' testimony was to be summed up with one word, it could be *normality*. In response to a question about whether she felt comfortable voicing concerns about patients, Tilley said that she was because she knew Volkman was willing to do "anything that a normal doctor would do to take care of the situation." During testimony about how Volkman's post-Tri-State clinics accessed patients' prior medical records, Sally Scott said that it was "like a normal doctor's office."

There was even an attempt from one of witness to pull the most glaringly abnormal portion of Volkman's southern Ohio tenure — his time on Center Street — into the realm of normalcy. During her testimony, Scott admitted that the house-turned-clinic was small and chaotic, that some of the patient-intake work took place in the kitchen, and that the cramped nature of the house and the traffic problems on the street made the situation difficult. And yet it was still, to her eyes, fundamentally legitimate. "I come from a rural county where, you know, back in the olden days . . .

physicians actually did treat patients in their house," she said. "It was that kind of an atmosphere."

After weeks of brutal testimony from prosecution witnesses, the former employees — three of whom only worked for Volkman after his years at Tri-State — gave the defense a chance to place some weight on the other side of the scale.

And from each of the witnesses came a quote that encapsulated their belief in Volkman. Santos-Mauntel testified that she believed he was "really making an effort" to dismiss drug seekers who were not in actual pain.

Tilley said that she believed his office was run "better than any doctor's office that I had seen."

Ames was effusive in her praise. She said Volkman was a well-educated man who cared deeply about his patients. He didn't stigmatize his patients for needing pain medication, she said, and he would have worked "24 hours a day for his patients." She said that he was a very good doctor and that she would have "walked on hot coals" to help him.

Scott echoed many of her former coworkers when she said that Volkman spent a longer time with his patients than any doctor she had previously seen. She believed that his concern for patients in pain was real.

During her cross-examination, however, Timothy Oakley was quick to point out that, in her job application for the hospital where she currently worked, she hadn't mentioned her past employment with Dr. Volkman. When he asked her why, she responded, "It was highly publicized the day that they shut Dr. Volkman's office . . . I felt it would be in my best interest not to put that down because of the publicity."

The majority of Paul Volkman's defense fell to three doctors.

One was Forrest Tennant, a prominent figure in the fields of pain management and addiction treatment.

Tennant's interest in these subjects arose after medical school while serving as a US Army physician during the Vietnam War. "I treated many of the addicted soldiers and I vividly recall prescribing my first dose of methadone to withdraw an army soldier addicted to opium," he once wrote. In 1975, he set up a California clinic for research on and treatment of both issues, including detox programs and methadone maintenance therapy. By the end of the decade, he had become, as he later wrote, "one of very few physicians in the United States who was researching opioid addiction and treating severe chronic pain."

This expertise led to his recruitment as an expert in two high-profile criminal cases involving opiates, pain, and addiction. The first such case followed the death of Howard Hughes, the reclusive, eccentric billionaire, who passed away, without a will, in 1976, which sparked intense curiosity and speculation about the circumstances of his death. Dr. Wilbur Thain, the physician who pronounced Hughes dead, was one of a group of highly paid aides who faced drug-related charges after Hughes's death for, allegedly, illegally providing Hughes with medications. As part of the case, Tennant was asked by the DEA to provide a report on Thain's prescriptions to Hughes.

A second case took place a few years later, when Tennant was asked to testify for the defense in the criminal case of Elvis Presley's personal physician, George C. Nichopolous, who, after the musician's sudden death at age forty-two, faced criminal charges for wrongfully prescribing medication. Tennant was the defense's key expert. Upon reviewing Presley's files, he became convinced that the singer had numerous serious medical issues, and he testified that Nichopolous's care for Presley had been "comprehensive" and "exemplary." A jury acquitted Nichopolous on all counts.

In the Volkman case, Tennant was called mainly to respond to a book that many prosecution witnesses had relied on when assessing whether the levels of substances found in Volkman's patients' bodies had factored in their deaths. That book, by a toxicologist named Randall Baselt, was called *Disposition of Toxic Drugs and Chemicals in Man*, and it was considered a kind of Bible among toxicologists and pathologists. Many of the prosecution's witnesses had confirmed that they had used its data about toxic and lethal levels to determine if Volkman's patients had overdosed. The book, known simply as Baselt, was a pillar of the prosecution's case.

Tennant felt that Baselt and other widely cited resources didn't properly account for the physical tolerance to opioids among pain patients who had been taking steady doses of the medications for a long time. And he had conducted a study to substantiate these views. The data for that study was voluntarily submitted by physicians of chronic pain patients whose ailments included lupus, fibromyalgia, migraines, osteoporosis, diabetic neuropathy, and spine degeneration and who were taking medications including codeine, fentanyl, hydrocodone, methadone, morphine, and oxycodone. The results of the study were published in the journal *Practical Pain Management*, of which Tennant was executive editor, in 2006.

Those results showed that many of the patients' opioid levels were above levels believed to be therapeutic, or even toxic, for non-opioid-tolerant patients. And because these patients continued to work and "function quite well," they had clearly become tolerant to these seemingly high dosages. Therefore, one stated conclusion of the study was: "A high opioid dosage cannot automatically be blamed for an unexpected death or accident based solely on a[n] opioid blood level taken post-accident or at autopsy."

Tennant's blood study, with its dramatically different interpretation of opioid blood levels among chronic pain patients, was tremendously important for Volkman's defense team. Whereas Baselt indicated that Volkman's prescriptions were likely to harm, or perhaps even kill, patients, Tennant's study argued that blood levels alone were insufficient to show harm. Tennant's study also suggested that, if anything, those levels might indicate a completely normal and proper course of treatment for opiate-tolerant patients.

Under direct examination on the twenty-first day of the Volkman trial, Tennant explained that tolerance was common and expected among long-term pain patients taking opioids and that such patients could take high doses of opioids (or what seemed like high doses when compared with amounts that would be toxic for opioid-naïve patients) and still lead high-functioning lives. They worked. They drove cars. They cared for their families.

Shortly thereafter, defense lawyer Wende Cross asked Tennant a question that allowed him to deliver his thesis to the jury. "Patients who have titrated their dosage up to a very high level can still function and carry very high dosage levels, which would be several times that of a dosage that would frankly kill all of us in this room, and would be much higher than what is normally seen in autopsy reports," he said.

While Tennant was called to discuss a general principle behind the defense's case — opioid tolerance — another physician was called to specifically rebuke the notion that Volkman's patients died from overdoses.

Dr. Harry Bonnell was a veteran in the field of forensic pathology. He had worked in the medical examiner's offices in three major American cities (Seattle, Cincinnati, and San Diego) and held teaching appointments at local universities in each case. At the time of his testimony, he had performed more than seven thousand autopsies and supervised thousands more by trainees. He had also published numerous articles in peer-reviewed journals. As he explained in his testimony, for about a decade he had been self-employed as a full-time expert and had testified in more than five hundred judicial proceedings across eighteen states. Most of those cases had been criminal trials, and his participation had been split fairly evenly between prosecution and defense.

Unlike many of the prosecution's death-focused witnesses, Bonnell had not personally performed any of the autopsies or toxicological analyses that he discussed from the witness stand. He was relying on the medical records, autopsy reports, toxicological results, prescription history, and other documents that were provided to him.

Bonnell explained that in four cases, the patients whose files he reviewed had not undergone autopsies, which meant that he could not offer a conclusive opinion on their death. Commenting on the case of James Estep, for whom no autopsy or toxicological analysis were performed, he said that without a postmortem physical exam, there was no telling precisely why he had died. "He could have been hit by lightning," Bonnell said. "He could have had a stroke. He could have had a brain aneurysm. He could have had pneumonia."

In three of these no-autopsy cases, Bonnell's lack of information was compounded by what he viewed as flawed methods for toxicological analysis. In the case of Kristi Ross, the analysis had been performed using fluid from her eye, not her bloodstream, a method that Bonnell said was not viewed as scientifically accurate. In two other instances, non-autopsied patients had undergone toxicological testing from an unspecified part of the body and this, too, made the analysis unreliable because, he said, "the significance would vary whether it was from the heart or peripheral from the groin area."

Bonnell's testimony about the deaths of remaining Volkman patients fit a pattern. In each case, he determined that the patient would have been tolerant to the medications Volkman had prescribed to them and thus far less likely to have been injured by those medications. And he focused on other identified substances in their systems, or medical issues that were identified in their autopsies, that he believed to be the true cause of their death.

In the case of Scottie Lin James, he testified that he believed it was the cocaine found in her bloodstream that had been the true cause of her death. And in the cases of seven deceased Volkman patients, he believed that the evidence pointed to heart disease, not overdose, as the cause of death. He noted that Bryan Brigner's autopsy had found his right coronary artery to be 75 percent blocked, his left anterior descending coronary artery 50 percent blocked, and that the heart itself was "severely enlarged" at 485 grams. He testified that Mark Reeder was morbidly obese, at 456 pounds; that his heart was "massively enlarged," at 590 grams; and that his left anterior descending coronary artery was 65 percent blocked. He said that Steve Hieneman's autopsy showed a 60 percent obstruction of both the left main and the left anterior descending arteries, and 70 percent obstruction of the right coronary artery. Mary Carver, meanwhile, had a 50 percent blockage of her left anterior descending coronary artery. "Based upon her drug levels and her cardiac findings, I would have signed her out as a cardiac death, not as an overdose," he said.

Overall, based on his review of the patient files provided to him, Bonnell testified that he found no case where the patient appeared to have died because of an overdose from medications Volkman prescribed.

The defense's third and longest-testifying witness was Dr. Hal Blatman, a local pain-management specialist. Blatman, who had been treating pain patients for more than two decades, would provide the defense's answer to the overall question of Volkman's legitimacy.

This had been discussed in great depth by the prosecution's last witness, a pain-management expert named L. Douglas Kennedy, who had reviewed records from Volkman's practice to determine whether a legitimate doctor-patient relationship had existed. Kennedy's testimony, which stretched across multiple days, was punctuated by expressions of alarm and disbelief. Discussing one patient's prescribed medication, he said, "I've never seen a regimen like this, period." In another case, he said that he struggled to understand why Volkman had asked for 540 pills of oxycodone for a patient who would be working away from home for three months. Refills for three-month supplies of opioids weren't legal, Kennedy said. Of another patient's drug regimen he said, "If they did get them filled and took them, they would end up in the emergency room or dead. Or severely ill." Discussing another, he said, "I mean, this isn't medicine."

Before Volkman's trial, Blatman had testified in a variety of cases, including malpractice cases, lawsuits involving car accidents, and hearings before the Ohio State Medical Board. But this was his first time in federal court.

At the start of his testimony, he explained that, at his clinic, he saw patients with various kinds of non-cancer pain, "from an ankle sprain, to osteoarthritis of a knee, to chronic low back pain, to low back pain after surgery where surgery hasn't worked, to migraine headaches." His treatment approach was multidisciplinary, involving diet and nutrition, psychological counseling, chiropractic care, massage, trigger point injections, and "of course, medication."

To set the stage for his remarks about specific Volkman patients, defense lawyers elicited two answers that were generally helpful to their case. The first was that, in Blatman's words, chronic pain was a "huge and under-treated issue" in this country. There were forty million people in pain in the country, he said.* He also explained that there were a lot of doctors who specialized in treating pain, but "nowhere near" the number needed to meet the overall need. Blatman identified many reasons for this under-treatment of pain. Some were based on the nature of pain itself: It was hard to recognize and diagnose, and it didn't always show up on physical exams or medical tests. But he also said that doctors feared "scrutiny of regulatory agencies, which would be the state medical boards and the DEA," based on their prescribing of certain medications.

Blatman also spent time on the witness stand discussing the field of pain management itself. While the prosecution's experts had attempted to portray the specialty as well established in its customs and practices, Blatman described disagreements about basic clinical questions. He testified that there was "no general agreement" among pain physicians about what constituted an appropriate physical examination, and that doctors' approaches varied widely. He said that some doctors only saw patients once a year, while others saw them every six months or three months, or on a monthly basis. He also testified that, as long as a doctor understood the patient's history and spent enough time with them to develop a plan of treatment and communicate, a visit "can vary anywhere between five minutes and an hour." There was, similarly, no standard number of patients for a doctor to see in a given day. He had been in offices that saw ten patients a day and other offices that saw seventy-five.

While the prosecution's experts had reviewed Volkman's prescriptions records with an unforgiving eye, Blatman's review seemed grounded in a deep and abiding sympathy. At one point, he said that he believed that the

---

* This number — forty million — was significantly lower than the seventy-six million Candace Crouse had mentioned in her opening statement. The disparity was never addressed by Volkman's defense witnesses or his attorney's closing arguments.

doctor's prescribing had been "for the most part . . . safe and effective" and "did a wonderful job at relieving these people's pain."

Blatman said that he didn't find Volkman's practice of prescribing two short-acting opioids medically unreasonable. It was a legitimate choice, he said, for multiple reasons: "effective pain relief, return to function, and lower cost."

Whereas a lack of documentation for some patients had struck the prosecution's expert as suspicious, for Blatman, it seemed like an honest mistake. He acknowledged that he had not been able to form an opinion on whether Volkman had a legitimate doctor-patient relationship with Danny Coffee because Coffee's files had been lost. But when Candace Crouse asked whether he assumed that such a record had never existed, he replied that he did not. "Medical records get lost [or] get misplaced," he said. And for other patients, he believed that Volkman was "fairly meticulous" in his record keeping. "I would figure that . . . if he prescribed anything for Daniel Coffee, he had a medical record," he said.

And so it went. In many places where the prosecution had raised red flags, the defense called Blatman to lower that flag and raise a green one in its place.

Blatman's belief in Volkman's legitimacy carried over to his review of specific patients. When discussing Volkman's treatment of Mary Carver, for example, Crouse asked, "With regard to the prescribing of controlled substances, was that doctor-patient relationship adequate for prescribing the controlled substances on the initial and then the subsequent visits?"

"Yes," he replied.

"And what is your opinion regarding whether Dr. Volkman prescribed controlled substances to Ms. Carver for a legitimate medical purpose?" she asked.

"That he did prescribe for a legitimate medical purpose," he answered.

He offered similar approval for Volkman's treatment of other patients including Bryan Brigner, James Estep, Aaron Gillispie, Steven Hieneman, Scottie Lin James, Charles Jordan, Dwight Parsons, Kristi Ross, Jeffrey Reed, and Mark Reeder.

At the end of this questioning about individual patients, Crouse asked about his overall view of the patient files he had reviewed.

"Based upon your review of all twenty-seven files, why do you believe that Dr. Volkman formed a doctor-patient relationship with his patients?" she said.

Blatman replied that it was his job, when reading through the charts, to try to figure out what the doctor did and whether he had established a legitimate relationship with those patients. Based on the "thorough details" in the charts that he was provided, he believed that Volkman had.

Crouse continued. "And why do you say that Dr. Volkman prescribed controlled substances for a legitimate medical purpose?" she asked.

"The objective of controlled substances is to reduce and relieve pain, to reduce and relieve suffering," he replied. "That is a medical purpose for prescribing pain medicine and Dr. Volkman did that."

Oakley's cross-examination of Blatman included some of the most tense and confrontational exchanges of the entire trial.

One strategy that Oakley employed was creating space between Blatman's own practice of pain management and the doctor whom he so staunchly defended.

At one point, the prosecutor asked if Blatman made psychological help readily available for his patients. He did, the doctor acknowledged.

And do local pharmacies fill his prescriptions? Blatman answered, "Yes."

Oakley continued.

Had Blatman ever hired an armed guard for protection of his clinic? He had not.

Had he ever had a mother come into his practice and threaten to kill him if he gave her son, who was an addict, more drugs? He had not received death threats.

When he opened his office, were there people who had been waiting there for hours to get in? There were not.

At one point, when Blatman continued to defend Volkman's prescribing practices under aggressive questioning, Oakley said, "Well, these people were dying, though, weren't they?"

Blatman responded: "There were a few deaths."

The exchange continued:

> **Oakley:** Just a couple?
> **Blatman:** A few.
> **Oakley:** Twelve?
> **Blatman:** Twelve.
> **Oakley:** Is that okay, during his experimentation, figuring this out? . . . Is that a legitimate experimentation to see how these pills work as people die around you?

> **Blatman:** You know, every choice a patient makes and every prescription a doctor makes is an experiment, whether it's a cholesterol drug or diabetes drug. Our patients are all in some ways lab rats of that sort.

This was clearly a major slip-up on Blatman's part. As useful as his testimony may have been for the defense, it's hard to imagine any scenario where they would have wanted him to describe patients as "lab rats."

And at another point during cross-examination, the discussion of one particular patient reflected some of the issues at the heart of the case.

In his review of Scottie Lin James's case, Blatman had looked at her medical chart, plus records of her office visits from both 2003 (at Tri-State) and 2005 (on Center Street). And just as he had sympathized with Volkman in his review of other patients, during his direct examination, Blatman testified that Volkman seemed to have had a legitimate doctor-patient relationship with James. He also believed that the medications Volkman had prescribed her were for a legitimate medical purpose.

Oakley returned to this point in his cross-examination, and the conversation turned into a debate about the responsibility for determining whether a patient is being truthful with a doctor. Under questioning from Oakley, Blatman described James as a "master manipulator," a "drug addict," and "a liar." He portrayed Volkman as essentially powerless against such a patient.

"Scottie James has probably been manipulating people since she was a child," he said.

At another point, he added, "This guy" — meaning Volkman — "doesn't have a chance."

Oakley pushed back, asking Blatman to tell him who was the professional in this situation: Dr. Paul Volkman or his patient?

"I would suggest that Scottie James is just as much a professional with what she does as Dr. Volkman is with what he does," Blatman replied.

CLOSING ARGUMENTS

Because the government faced the burden of proving Volkman's guilt, prosecutors had two chances to offer closing arguments. First up was prosecutor Adam Wright.

Wright was a graduate of Harvard Law School who had worked in large firms for five years before joining the Ohio US attorney's office in 2009. As the junior member of the government's two-man prosecution team, he had shared the duties of examining and cross-examining trial witnesses with Tim Oakley. Now, on the morning of April 21, 2011, they would each deliver a closing statement.

Wright spent an hour laying out the case for Volkman's guilt. Toward the beginning of his remarks, he said, "This is a case about the defendant taking responsibility for his decision to give drugs to anyone who walked in the door with enough cash to see the doctor, no matter if they were addicts, no matter if they were dealers, no matter if they had health conditions, no matter if there wasn't anything wrong with them." Shortly afterward, he added: "No matter what the patient, no matter what the situation, the answer was always the same: Pills, pills, and more pills."

At one point in his remarks, Wright cast doubt on the defense's argument that most of Volkman's patients had died from heart attacks, not overdoses. "It's news when someone dies under the age of 40 because of a heart attack," he said. "Nine out of twelve did here."

Wende Cross, the senior attorney on Volkman's defense team, began her closing statement with a definition of a reasonable doubt. A reasonable doubt is a doubt based on common sense, she said. It's the kind of doubt that would make a reasonable person hesitate to act in the most important of his or her affairs, such as deciding where to live, whether to take a particular job, or whether to proceed with a medical operation for their child. The standard of "beyond a reasonable doubt" is critical, she said. "That's the standard you have to apply when deciding this case."

She then attempted to plant seeds for such doubts at various points in the government's case. She cast doubt on the idea that a high number of prescribed pills or a clinic's decision to accept only cash was, by itself, a sign of a doctor's illegitimacy. She encouraged jurors to dismiss pharmacists' testimony because those pharmacists weren't examining or treating any of these patients, and therefore were in no place to judge a prescription's legitimacy. She reminded the jury that many of the former patients called by the prosecution had described legitimate pain issues when they went to see Volkman. She reminded them that Volkman, as a salaried employee of Tri-State, made the same amount of money "whether there were two patients or 2,000 patients." She attempted to dismiss testimony that had discussed whether Volkman's patients had looked like they were in pain. "Throughout this trial we have learned that pain is . . . very subjective and you cannot tell by simply looking at someone," she said.

She went on to argue that, in fact, Paul Volkman had established a legitimate doctor-patient relationship with the people he saw at his clinics. This was clear from the fact that he interviewed patients about their symptoms, conducted regular follow-up visits, suggested yoga and physical therapy, referred patients to other doctors, and prescribed medications for non-pain-related issues such as blood pressure, circulation, and asthma. And when it came to the deaths of patients, she reminded jurors that many of the deceased patients had health conditions such as heart disease and morbid obesity and that, in multiple cases, no autopsy or toxicology report existed, so the cause of death couldn't be determined with certainty.

Mainly, she wanted jurors to remember that if they were uncertain about any aspect of the case, it meant they had doubts, which meant, because of the threshold for conviction she had stated at the beginning of her remarks, they must choose "not guilty" for that charge. And at one point, she argued that the question of her client's legitimacy was an all-or-nothing proposition. "Ladies and gentlemen, Dr. Volkman was either a doctor or he wasn't," she said. "He wasn't a doctor on this day, at this time, and then two hours later he wasn't a doctor, and then two hours [later] he was." That didn't make any sense, she said.

In her retelling of the story, the evidence was clear. "Dr. Volkman was an experienced and caring doctor who treated people who he believed were legitimately in chronic pain and couldn't get adequate pain relief anywhere else," she said.

She closed by stating that there was "no question there is a prescription drug epidemic in this country." But she said that there was also an epidemic of chronic pain that affected more than thirty million people. Because of an uneven focus on the first epidemic, she said, "pain doctors like Dr. Volkman who . . . try to help people end up being called common drug dealers."

This was not a medical malpractice case, she said; it was a criminal matter. And as a criminal matter, the standard of proof needed for a conviction was the highest that our system requires.

"Is there plenty of reason to doubt?" she asked. Yes there was.

"So say so by returning a verdict of not guilty on all counts," she said.

———

Last to speak was lead prosecutor Tim Oakley, who delivered the prosecution's rebuttal. And at one point Oakley pounced on a word that Cross had used in her statement to describe Volkman's tenure on Center Street. She had acknowledged that those weeks had been "chaotic" but stressed that the house was just a temporary situation.

"Somehow 'chaos' excuses the fact there was absolutely no legitimate purpose for those medications prescribed by Dr. Volkman," Oakley said. "How does 'chaos' allow for death?"

He then gave a recap of some of the most damning testimony jurors had heard. He reminded them that within three months of Volkman's arrival, pharmacies in a hundred-mile radius of the clinic refused to fill his scripts, prompting Tri-State to open its on-site dispensary. He reminded jurors of the intake forms Volkman's patients signed in which they promised not to sue him. He reminded them of the fact that, after Volkman was threatened by the mother of a patient at Center Street, he didn't notify the police; instead, he hired an armed security guard. Oakley rapidly ticked off various health issues — obesity, high blood pressure, breathing issues, and clear signs of heart disease — that Volkman mostly ignored during his patient visits. "He didn't even do a cholesterol check," Oakley said. "He just let these people die."

Oakley was dismissive of the clinic's measures that purported to prevent abuse and diversion. The blood tests that supposedly tested patients' levels of medication "had no medical scientific credibility at all," he said. And the safes that Volkman advised his patients to buy, as a supposed measure against theft, were also a sham. "Can anybody please explain to me how that stops me from using my pills that are in my safe that I have the combination to?" he said.

The motive behind all of this was clear: money. *This* is what the case was about, not pain, he said. As Oakley told it, Volkman had been hired at Tri-State for a simple task: to write prescriptions for pills. For two and a half years he did this, and he made almost $700,000 in the process. After that, when he set out on his own, he hit the "jackpot," the prosecutor said. Every week, when Volkman flew back to Chicago, he "left town with his money, leaving behind in his wake the addictions . . . and the families mourning their dead," he said.

Toward the end of his remarks, Oakley asked jurors to envision a scenario in which a doctor had just told them that they, or a loved one, were gravely ill. In such a scenario, he asked, would they feel comfortable going to Paul Volkman for a second opinion?

INSIDE THE JURY ROOM

In one of our early interviews, Volkman had described the jury he expected for his criminal trial. He said they were likely to be a "bunch of chronically unemployed, ignorant, bigoted, biased, morons that have no understanding of medicine to start with and probably no sympathy for pain patients either."

The jury that he got was, in fact, a mix of working professionals, including an elementary school teacher, a bank executive, an engineer, a financial officer at a cemetery, a truck driver, a high school athletic trainer, a manager at an Olive Garden, and an employee at a Walmart. The ages ranged from midtwenties to late sixties. Women made up a slight majority. One juror was Black, while the rest were white.

I wound up speaking with four of those jurors, one of whom told me that the group had worked "faithfully and diligently" to find the truth. "They're all good people with integrity and seriousness," this juror told me. "I'm so proud of them."

The four jurors I spoke to recalled different aspects of the case that made a strong impression.

One juror remained stunned that Volkman had gone into business with two women who had no medical background. "I still can't wrap my head around the fact that someone would open a pain clinic that has zero medical experience," she told me. "How does that even happen?"

Others remembered the sheer number of pills that Volkman prescribed and dispensed. "The amount of medication just still, to this day, blows my mind," one told me. A third juror described testimony from a DEA agent about how Volkman's purchasing and prescribing compared with other doctors, regionally and nationally, as "totally mind blowing." And as soon as it was finished, she said, she was "all the way" convinced of Volkman's guilt.

Another juror was struck by the unyielding *consistency* of Volkman's activity. He said jurors were willing to give Volkman the benefit of the doubt for one or two patient deaths. But Volkman had not stopped after just one or two deaths. Jurors kept hearing about the same outcome over and over and over. "He never changed," the juror said.

To him, this was a story about "a doctor who knew better but didn't give a damn." And when I asked him if anyone in the jury room had sympathized with Volkman, he responded, "How can you sympathize with a man who has no sympathy?"

———

In terms of its sheer scale, the jury's task was formidable. They had heard from eighty witnesses and seen hundreds of exhibits, and they were asked for verdicts on twenty-one separate counts of illegal activity.

They approached the job through a division of labor. Each juror was assigned to the file of a different patient to whom Volkman was charged with dealing drugs. They would then study that file closely, comb through the details about that person from evidence and testimony, and write their findings on a large sheet of paper, which would be posted to the wall of the room. Each juror would then present their findings to the group, and the jury would discuss that portion of the case.

It was a slow process. Days went by, and the amount of paper on the room's walls multiplied. After the information about a particular deceased patient was presented and discussed, the group took a vote on whether Volkman was guilty or not. If there was unanimous agreement, they moved on to the next count. If not, they kept debating, or moved on with a promise to return to the subject later. "It continued that way until all 12 deaths were gone over, discussed, picked at, and eventually agreed upon," one juror told me.

The discussions were not always peaceful. One juror explained that deliberations marked the first time that jurors finally got to hear what their peers were thinking after weeks of being prohibited from discussing the case. "And some people's perspective was offensive to others," they explained. Another juror said that deliberations were sometimes "very intense" and "heated."

When they spoke with me, numerous jurors described assigning responsibility for patient deaths as the jury's hardest task. Where did the responsibility fall between the doctor and the patient?

In my interviews, I heard about one juror who didn't think Volkman had caused any of the deaths. In his view, drug-addicted patients were themselves to blame when they obtained pills and overdosed. At other points during deliberation, jurors discussed the fact that some of Volkman's patients had been addicted to drugs before they saw the doctor.

But then other members of the jury would push back. As one juror told me: "There [were] times when we could have walked out of there . . . but it was a couple people saying, 'I will *not* let him off for killing that person.'"

———

Outside the deliberation room, one incident bears mentioning.

On Wednesday, April 22, the day after jury deliberations began, Volkman sent a Facebook message to a former Chillicothe clinic employee who had testified for the prosecution.

"How much jail time were you facing for selling pills?" he wrote. "What deal did you make with the DEA to come into court and lie on Dr. Volkman? . . . How do you look at yourself in the mirror?"

At the end of the note, he wrote, "You are truly disgusting."

That message was eventually handed over to Volkman's pretrial services officer, who then presented it to the judge, along with a request that Volkman's bond be modified. The new condition they sought was for Volkman to "avoid all contact, directly or indirectly, with any persons who are or who may become a victim or potential witness in the subject investigation or prosecution."

Beckwith approved the request.

Eventually, over seven days, jurors arrived at a consensus on all counts Volkman faced. And the four jurors I interviewed agreed about certain underlying aspects of the experience.

They all agreed that Volkman had gotten a fair trial and that the jury had taken its responsibilities seriously. One juror told me that she was struck by the weight of the decision she was making. It was a decision she knew she would carry with her for a long time after the trial ended. "You're determining someone's fate, and the rest of their life," she said.

Another juror told me that she was proud of the way the jury had given each count the scrutiny it deserved and thoroughly discussed it with one another. This commitment was partly fueled by a shared desire not to be deadlocked and render the previous months irrelevant via a mistrial.

Another told me, "What made it extraordinary was that here we were, twelve strangers with all our backgrounds and differences, charged to work as one. Somehow or another, we did that."

None of the jurors I interviewed expressed regret or reservations about the verdicts. One described a feeling he had of "satisfaction [that] the right thing was done." Another told me that she wanted my readers to know "how very dedicated we all were to finding the truth."

She added, "I believe justice was served."

VERDICT

A few minutes before 5:00 P.M. on Monday, May 9, 2011, the Volkman jurors filed into the courtroom.

"Ladies and gentlemen, I understand that you have reached verdicts in this matter, correct?" the judge asked.

The jury foreman confirmed that they had.

The judge instructed him to hand the verdict forms to her clerk, who would read them aloud. Soon, the clerk began to read: "In *The United States of America versus Paul H. Volkman*, Case Number CR-1-07-60, Defendant No. 3 . . ."

The first count of the indictment was by far the longest, running twelve pages in the original document. This was the count that described the alleged conspiracy between Paul Volkman and the Huffmans to distribute drugs. For jurors, it was their first chance to answer the question at the heart of the trial: Was Paul Volkman a drug dealer?

The clerk read their answer. "We, the jury, in respect of the charge of conspiracy to distribute controlled substances as set forth in Count 1 of the Indictment, do find the Defendant Paul H. Volkman: Guilty."

From there, the clerk read verdicts for nineteen additional counts. If an observer had been following along with the indictment as reference — as I later did — they would see that the jury found Volkman guilty of operating drug houses at each of the two Tri-State clinic locations and also at his home on Center Street and the final clinic in Chillicothe.

The jury also found him guilty of illegally dealing drugs to patient after patient: Charles Jordan, Danny Coffee, Jeffrey Reed, Mary Catherine Carver, James Estep, Kristi Ross, Steven Hieneman, Scottie Lin James, Bryan Brigner, Ernest Ratcliff, Mark Reeder. And in four instances, the jury exercised its option to not just find the doctor guilty of drug dealing but to also find him guilty of *directly causing a patient's death* via that drug dealing. Those four patients were Kristi Ross, Steve Hieneman, Bryan Brigner, and Ernest Ratcliff.

Volkman was acquitted of dealing drugs in Count 4, the first drug-dealing count that connected to a specific patient's death: Aaron Gillispie. He was also acquitted of one count of gun possession, although he was convicted of another.

All told, the jury found him guilty for eighteen of twenty counts.

Before the proceedings ended, Judge Beckwith delivered brief remarks. "I hope none of you will ever need a jury to decide anything in your lives," she said. "But if you do, I hope it will be one as dedicated and hardworking as you all have been." She added that, at long last, she was lifting her oft-repeated instructions to jurors not to discuss the case with anyone under any circumstances. They were now free to discuss their experience as jurors with whomever they wished.

"Thank you so much," she said. "You are discharged."

In Portsmouth, the reactions online were ecstatic. Comments on social media read: "Praise the lord!!!!!" "Thank goodness this murderer is gone!" "Thank God he has been convicted. Angels are smiling."

On Facebook's Fix the Scioto County Problem of Drug Abuse, Misuse, and Overdose page, Dr. Aaron Adams, the county health commissioner who had declared a state of emergency in Scioto County in 2010, wrote, "Perhaps others will learn from Dr. Volkman's dishonored oath to 'do no harm,' arrogance and personal entitlement to exploit our region by way of his home in Chicago!"

Lisa Roberts said, "I hope they send a few million dollars of those confiscated asset seizures our way, since we were left destroyed and to handle disaster clean-up from this operation."

Two days after the verdict, Volkman's conviction was the top story on the front page of the *Chillicothe Gazette*, under the headline "'Pill Mill' Doctor Convicted in 4 Deaths." Other articles on the verdict ran in papers as far away as Fort Collins, Colorado; Jackson, Mississippi; Fresno, California; and Bradenton, Florida.

A summary of the case even made it into the *New York Times*, in a section containing news briefs from around the country. On page A16 of the May 11 edition, the story ran under the headline "Ohio: Doctor Found Guilty on Drug Counts."

The article read, in its entirety:

> A doctor who the federal authorities said was one of the largest national dispensers of Oxycodone, a powerful prescription painkiller, was convicted on Tuesday of illegal distribution. As a result of the verdict, in federal court in Cincinnati, Dr. Paul H. Volkman of Chicago could face life in prison for illegal distribution of a controlled substance that resulted in the death of four people in

southern Ohio, where he practiced. Such a sentence would be the first of its kind in Ohio, where the authorities are trying to strengthen laws to combat the drug scourge, one of the worst in the nation.

Meanwhile, in Volkman's adopted hometown of Chicago, the verdict received more prominent billing. During a 6:00 P.M. news broadcast for the local ABC affiliate, an anchor announced, "A doctor from Chicago has been convicted of running one of the nation's largest so-called pill mills, where he sold pain medication like candy, regardless of any medical need."

The anchor then handed the story to a reporter, who described Volkman as once having a "promising future" in the 1970s after graduating from the "prestigious" University of Chicago. Now, he said, "an incredible violation of the Hippocratic Oath has Volkman headed to federal prison."

He proceeded to recap some of the facts of the story. And at one point, he gave Volkman a new nickname: "The Pill Mill Killer."

INSIDE HIS MIND

As far as I know, Paul Volkman never underwent a psychological evaluation during his criminal case.

And over the years we spoke, he claimed to be in perfect mental health. In one letter, I asked, "Have you ever been diagnosed with a personality disorder or mental condition? Have you ever doubted your own sanity?" His response was brief: "As to my mental health, it has never been better."

At other times, he described his outlook and behavior as an appropriate response to his circumstances. "A person is not paranoid, if they really ARE out to get him," he wrote.

Once, many years into our relationship, I cut and pasted a list of signs and symptoms of narcissistic personality disorder from the website of the Mayo Clinic into an email and asked if he had ever suspected that he might have NPD or been officially diagnosed. In response, he said he was "glad" I had done some research on NPD but said that it was *me*, not him, who was exhibiting symptoms. "Self awareness does not come easily for [one] such as yourself," he wrote. "You are not even embarrassed by exhibiting such stupidity."

Thus, any discussion of Volkman's psychology must state at the outset that it is not based on a formal diagnosis from a mental health professional and also that Volkman staunchly maintains his own mental fitness.

It's also important to note that the ethical guidelines for mental health professionals are clear in advising against diagnosing people who have not undergone an in-depth, in-person examination. The experts whom I interviewed for this book mentioned these restrictions when I spoke to them, and, being familiar with this policy, I did not expect them to diagnose Volkman.

But with all of that said, Volkman's psychology is important to this story. And over the course of this project, I have used the tools of journalism to see what I could learn about the workings of his mind.

An inquiry into Volkman's psychology would naturally begin with his family. And though I didn't learn much about his parents or earlier generations, I did learn about his older brother, Alan.

This information came from Alan's only child — his son, David — who, when I first met him in 2011, was a financial adviser living with his family in the suburbs of New York City. David was born in 1970, which made him a few years older than both of Paul's kids. Though he hadn't spent much time with his cousins or uncle growing up — Paul's loathing for his brother was apparently mutual — he could tell me about his dad. We wound up speaking many times, both in person and via phone and email, and I found him to be smart, kind, and credible. And the story he told me was unforgettable.

Alan Volkman was born in June 1943, three years before Paul. His birth name was Seymour Alan Volkman, though he went by his middle name. He attended George Washington University, in Washington, DC, and participated in Reserve Officers Training Corps (ROTC) activities for the US Air Force during his time there.

After college, he apparently spent some time in the air force but didn't stay long in the military. Paul once told me that his brother was in the air force for six weeks or two months before being "brought home in a straitjacket." David also believed, based on conversations with his mother, that his father was indeed committed to a psychiatric facility in Texas during his early adulthood. But it was unclear to him whether this hospitalization was due to a genuine psychiatric condition, a feigned illness to avoid deployment to Vietnam, or some combination of the two. "Either way, he didn't go to Vietnam," David said.

Alan was married in 1966 and then divorced in 1979, at which point Alan's ex-wife, who won full custody of David, moved to Wilkes-Barre, Pennsylvania. David would briefly move back with his father before permanently returning to live with his mom. And after this point in the early 1980s, the details of Alan's life go dark, even to his own son.

When I met David, he didn't know with certainty what his father did for a living, beyond his vague awareness that he had a background in computer programming. And when it came to Alan's whereabouts, he told me, "You can never pin him down to even a state where he is." Their relationship was extremely strained.

David told me that strangers meeting his dad were likely to be impressed by him. He said that Alan was strikingly intelligent and well read, and he spoke in a professorial way that seemed based on prodigious amounts of research. David said that if you asked his dad a simple question he might give a lengthy, detailed response that would sound like it was taken from a textbook.

David said that his father had a few friends who knew him superficially. He could envision those men speaking to his dad and walking away thinking, "Wow, this guy's really got his stuff together." But those who knew his dad on a deeper level saw a different side. Once you went beyond the surface, he said, you would find "a monster."

David's in-person memories of his father were mostly limited to the first fifteen years of his life, but they had clearly left an impact. David recalled that, as a kid, his father would give him spelling tests, but when David submitted his answers, there was no attempt at coaching; his father simply pointed out which words were misspelled. His father would tell him to "figure it out" and stare at him, while commanding him to stay at the table until he got the answers right.

After David's parents divorced and his mother moved to another state with him, Alan aggressively lobbied his son over the phone to resist the new arrangement. Using what David described as considerable powers of persuasion and intellectual domination, Alan convinced his son that his mother was evil, that David had moved to the "worst shithole on the planet," and that his only hope for a decent future was moving back to Maryland to live with him. "He literally brainwashed me through the phone," David told me. "How am I, as a 12-year-old, going to compete against a grown man who is a lunatic?"

David's reunion with his father lasted less than two years. The breaking point was when David forgot to take out the trash one day, which infuriated his father, who, David said, came home from work, threw his briefcase down, gritted his teeth, put his fist in his son's face, and told him, "I'm so mad I could punch your fucking teeth down your throat." Alan was a large and imposing man, and the incident left David terrified; decades later, he said he still remembered it vividly. After this, when David went back to Pennsylvania to live with his mother, his father saw it as an unforgivable betrayal. "He's upset that he couldn't control me and that I left him," David said.

David's relationship with his father never really improved.

When David got married, he said that Alan told him that he wouldn't be attending if David's mother was in attendance. Alan apparently also told his son that, if David had kids, he wouldn't attend the baby naming or bris if his ex-wife was there; nor would he even attend David's funeral if his ex-wife went.

Later, when David and his wife had two sons, his dad showed no interest in meeting them, or speaking to them over the phone, despite his invitations. David said that his dad's version of fatherly wisdom involved encouraging him to adopt many of his own intensely private habits, like avoiding smartphones, and advising him to "stay as much off the grid as possible." When Barack Obama became the Democratic nominee for president in the 2008 election, David said that Alan sent him long and elaborate emails about the impending Marxist takeover of the United States.

Because of his paranoid approach to the world and his proficiency with computers, Alan was capable of chilling feats of surveillance. In one instance, David told me that he was driving on the upper level of New York City's George Washington Bridge when his father called him and said that he knew exactly where David's car was, down to the specific lane he was in. David couldn't explain how Alan knew this. Had he accessed traffic cameras? Had he placed some kind of tracking device on his car? "It was almost like something out of a spy movie," he said.

There were rare instances when his father would show a softer side. And David said that when Alan wanted to, he could easily act like a "warm fuzzy bear." But this was not how he acted most of the time. Generally, he was a source of significant pain and unease in his son's life. At various times in our conversations, David called his father a "devil," an "ogre," "fucking crazy," and "terrifying."

In Judaism, there is a tradition at funerals where loved ones of the deceased take turns with a shovel to toss a bit of dirt on the coffin after it's been lowered into the ground. When I first met David, he told me that he didn't want anyone else to get a turn with the shovel at his father's funeral. He wanted to shovel all the dirt himself. "That's gonna be the only way I can, in a quasi-crazy way, try to put some distance between him and his pain and his anger, and make sure that I'm burying it," he said.

He never got the chance.

In December 2022, while living in Green Bay, Wisconsin, Alan contracted COVID. (He had refused to be vaccinated and tried to advise David against it as well.) He apparently tried self-medicating with Theraflu for a period, but his condition worsened. Then he fell at home, injured himself, and had to be driven by a friend to the hospital. Upon his arrival, he was confirmed to be COVID-positive. He was placed on a ventilator on December 26, and he died on December 30.

At no point during these events was David notified of his father's illness or death. And due to snowstorms in Wisconsin, it took more than a week for Alan's body to be transported to Falls Church, Virginia, where he was buried next to his parents. There was no funeral.

David learned of his father's passing on January 15, 2023, when, on a whim, he happened to search his father's name online and found a short obituary.

Because of Alan's estrangement from Paul, David Volkman didn't know his uncle very well. He estimated that he'd seen him a dozen times at family functions. He said that all his interactions with Paul were "sane, rational, uncle-to-nephew types of relations."

He told me that he had learned about his uncle's criminal case when his father sent him a news article about it. David was flabbergasted. But he said that his father seemed to take some satisfaction in the news. It seemed to offer Alan validation in their decades-long mutual loathing. "He's a killer," David recalled his father saying.

When it came to making any public comments about the case, Alan tried to command his son not to speak with the press. David recalled the language his dad used: that he was not "authorized" to speak to the media about the case. It sounded almost like an order a military officer might issue to a lower-ranking soldier. An argument ensued, during which, at one point, Alan told David, "If you care about your family, you'll follow what I say."

David remained strongly concerned about speaking with me for this book until his dad's passing, at which point those concerns dissolved. He was then eager to share what he knew about his dad, including the fact that, after his dad's death, David had learned that Alan had once been diagnosed with Asperger's syndrome and paranoid personality disorder.

Based on what he had learned about Paul from his conversations with Adam, David was convinced that his father and Paul shared a similar obsession with control. "Control of wealth. Control of others. Control of information," he said. "[Adam] and I escaped from all of that."

At another point, he told me, "I think that the similarities between Paul and my father, from a personality standpoint, are uncanny."

The stories that David told me about his father — Paul Volkman's lone sibling — were alarming. But let's say, for the sake of argument, that Alan Volkman's life and personality have no bearing at all on Paul's. Even so, there is still a pronounced pattern of disturbing tendencies in Paul Volkman's life.

My research into Volkman's life made it clear that he had difficulty maintaining relationships. He spoke about his parents and brother in unrelentingly negative terms. And his familial relationships as an adult did not appear to have gone much better. He admitted that his marriage had been "unhappy."* And at one point in our conversations, he referred to having kids as "life's largest single mistake."

Meanwhile, both of Volkman's children told me that they knew of no close friendships their father kept. "My Dad was always such a loner," Jane said. In a separate conversation, Adam added, "I couldn't name one friend that he ever had."

He also spent most of his professional life working alone or in temporary settings. As a pediatrician, he never worked with a partner or group practice, and his career as a traveling locum tenens doctor seems to have prevented him (perhaps intentionally) from making any lasting associations.

In our conversations, he described various colleagues with contempt, whether it was a supervisor at Duke during his residency whom he

---

* Volkman, in a characteristically non-self-effacing way, pinned most of the responsibility for this on Nancy. He once wrote to me, "All of the happiness which should have gone along with [having a] family was mostly ruined by my marriage to a depressed, angry, bitter wife who hated men."

believed was performing unnecessary surgeries, the lab director back in Chicago who refused to cosign his supposedly brilliant research, or the small-town doctors whom he worked with as a traveling ER doc. In fact, judging solely by its duration of nearly two and a half years, his partnership with Denise Huffman appears to have been one of his longest-lasting working relationships.

Another theme in Volkman's life is his apparent unwillingness or inability to empathize.

Diana Colley told me that, when she went to Volkman's house-turned-clinic on Center Street and barged into his session with a patient, his response to her concerns about her son's addiction was, "That's his problem, not mine."

During one of my trips to Portsmouth, I spoke with the attorney who had represented Paula Eastley in her wrongful-death claim against Volkman in local court. He said that he had only spoken to Volkman once, briefly, over the phone. He recalled the doctor saying something to him along the lines of, "What are you doing all of this for? This guy was just a drug addict, anyway." The attorney was disgusted by those comments and hung up.

And although Volkman didn't testify at his trial, witnesses described comments that fit this pattern of coldness and detachment.

Alice Huffman testified that there were a "couple times" when she had spoken with family members of patients who called the clinic after their loved ones died and that she had relayed those messages to Volkman. She recalled how, in response, he told her that if those patients wanted to kill themselves, they could use Drano or anything else; he felt it had little to do with the pills he had prescribed. His logic, she testified, was that he hadn't forced them to abuse or overuse their medications, and if they were taking them properly, they would have been fine. "So, basically . . . he wasn't responsible for the fact that they overdosed," she said.

Later in the trial, a former employee from Chillicothe recalled how Volkman had informed her that his patient Mark Reeder had died. Volkman had just landed in Columbus and was heading toward the clinic when he called to share the news. As she recalled, he said, "The SOB is dead . . . He overdosed."

She said that she was "floored" by how Volkman delivered the news; it struck her as heartless. When she asked the doctor what she ought to do with Reeder's file, he instructed her to write "Deceased" on the front of the folder and place it at the bottom of one of the drawers of his filing cabinet. So she did.

But she described it as a turning point in her feelings about the doctor.

One trait of Volkman's that I know well is his erratic relationship with the truth. His tendency to make misleading or false comments was so pronounced that, during this project, I created a classification system to identify different kinds of less-than-credible statements.

One folder contained things that Volkman had said that I knew to be verifiably untrue, like his claim in a letter to a judge after his arrest in 2007 that he had "no history of any actions against [me] by any state medical board," which ignores the Illinois Medical Board's attempts to suspend or revoke his license as part of the Frey case.

Another category focused on instances when Volkman's description of events was at extreme odds with others, such as his description of his actions in the Frey case as "heroic" when others believed they had led directly to the child's death.

Other documents tracked his misleading use of statistics, the baseless political conspiracy theories that he embraced, and even medical claims he made that had no basis in established research, such as his statement that he believed his wife's brain tumor was the result of stress from his criminal case.*

At one point in my research, I spoke with a psychology expert who offered a framework by which I might better understand this behavior. Nancy McWilliams is an emerita professor at Rutgers University, a former president of the psychoanalysis division of the American Psychological Association, and the author and editor of numerous books on psychology and psychoanalysis. During our conversation, we spent some time discussing people with a grandiose self-image, which certainly includes Volkman.

McWilliams told me that truth is not a particularly high priority for people who want or need to preserve a grandiose sense of themselves. "The truth is a very secondary thing to them," she said.

She explained that such people learn early in life that *image* and *appearance* matter more than substance and that who they *invent* themselves to

---

* When I emailed a professor of neurosurgery at Columbia University about this, he told me, "As far as I know a brain tumor is not specifically brought on by emotional stress." Although Volkman's explanation does, conveniently for him, enhance his narrative of victimhood.

be "can be more rewarding than who they really are." The truth gets in the way of such a project.

The full truth of any human being's life is not particularly flattering, she said. But people with this tendency toward grandiosity cannot abide such failings. "So if you're trying to be perfect and superior to all the rest of humanity, you don't want to be bothered by the facts," she said.

Over the course of this project, I spoke with numerous people about Volkman's psychology. One former patient memorably described him as an "over-educated madman." But perhaps the most detailed psychological portrait came from his daughter, Jane, with whom I corresponded for more than a decade.

Jane seemed to struggle with the facts of her father's case. She said that she found the degree to which he ignored others' advice and wishes "mind-boggling." She thought that his choice to reopen his office after a DEA raid defied explanation. She said that it was a "terrible idea" that a single doctor would even be allowed to order the amounts of controlled substances he ordered while working at Tri-State Healthcare. At another point, when discussing the period after his split from the Huffmans, she said, "I just cringe at the thought of his office in a home. Obviously the whole neighborhood would hate him."

When it came to explaining how this all happened, she wouldn't point to a single reason. Instead, she said that it had taken a "special cocktail of shortcomings and bad decisions" for her father's life to turn out the way it did. And over many conversations, she identified some of the ingredients of that "cocktail."

She believed that growing up, her father's only affirmation from his "exhausted and discouraged" parents derived from academic achievement. She also said that, throughout his life, he also "suffered . . . with wanting to be all-knowing intellectually" and that he exhibited an intense and "incredibly alarming" tunnel vision when it came to others questioning his decisions. She said that he seemed either unwilling or incapable of "integrating others' emotions into his perspective on his own behavior." She believed that, as an adult, he maintained so few close relationships with others that, as a result, "relying on his own judgment was all he knew."

When it came to explaining why he began working in Ohio, she said that he was "desperate to maintain the status quo in his life." And at another point, she said that this desperation wasn't just financial but also psychological. "He needed the personal affirmation of being a doctor because without it, he did not know who he was." She also believed that there was an element in her father's relationship with Denise that appealed to him. "Denise easily played him and made him feel like a big powerful guy who was doing a great thing," she said. "In reality on the inside he felt unimportant and emasculated so he loved how he felt, I think."

At other points, Jane said that her father approached his pain management work in overly legalistic terms. He would frequently mention a Supreme Court case that he felt provided legal protection for his activities and she said, "He convinced himself that by following rules he could get his desired result." At another point, she said, "He had this delusion as if saying something made it so." She also believed that he had an "unusually limited social awareness," which may have made him an easier target for deceitful patients.

So when it came to explaining the unusual trajectory of her father's life, Jane would often mention numerous factors at once. "I think my dad was easy to deceive AND felt a desperation to maintain a profession AND was pleased with the money he was making," she wrote.

At another point, she said, "[The] bottom line for me is that my dad was desperate to maintain the status quo in his life and was afflicted with an astounding, irrational amount of pride in his own intellect while yet having very little emotional intelligence."

She added, "He ended up living in his own reality I think."

BUTLER COUNTY JAIL

After his trial, Volkman was held at the Butler County Jail, about thirty miles north of Cincinnati, in the city of Hamilton. For nine months until his sentencing hearing, he was inmate #154945.

In a letter to me from the fall of 2011, he described the place as a "human garbage dump" and said, "Every drifter, grifter, drunk, gang punk, wife beater, child rapist/abuser, child porn aficionado, drug addict, drug dealer, serial killer, alcoholic manslaughterer picked up within 50 miles in any direction lands here."

By this time, I had graduated from my program at Columbia and moved back to Rhode Island, where I had a part-time job teaching writing at the Rhode Island School of Design for the fall semester. I had also resumed contributing articles to the *Providence Phoenix*, the alt-weekly paper I had written for prior to grad school.

These months wound up being a period of intense correspondence with Volkman. Between July 2011 and January 2012, he sent me more than seventy pages of handwritten letters, and I responded with typed and printed letters of my own.

Some of Volkman's letters described everyday life at his new home. Breakfast, he explained in one note, consisted of a slice of bologna between two pieces of Wonder Bread, plus two ounces of cold Cream of Wheat. After doing yoga in the morning, he was allowed out for "rec" rime, during which he said he climbed a flight of stairs forty times and walked around the gym for an hour. He was done with his exercise by ten, after which he had a cup of coffee and got a fifteen-minute call with Clara. Lunch would be at eleven, after which he would nap for most of the afternoon and, once a week, speak to a friend from Cincinnati who came to visit. He said the jail had plenty of good books, and, since arriving, he had finished Mary Shelley's *Frankenstein* and Thomas Hardy's *Return of the Native*.

He said he missed his wife terribly. He wrote, "I miss seeing trees and the sky. I miss edible food. It is total sensory deprivation in the midst of a human sewer." At another point, he added, "There is no one here I would have had anything to do with in my far-distant, long-lost existence."

There was at least one person with whom Volkman enjoyed conversing: a corrections officer in his late twenties. Volkman said the topics they covered included the news, government corruption, the War on Drugs, and the officer's career and plans for his wife and kids. "It makes a big difference to have someone with a functioning cerebral cortex to interact with," he said.

Volkman also used these letters to update his tale of persecution with details from his trial.

He claimed that the federal government was "vicious" and "completely corrupt"; that his lawyers were ineffective; that the judge had routinely made illegal rulings and colluded with the prosecution; and that the government's witnesses had peddled "deliberate junk science, distortions, speculations, [and] outright lies." At one point, he also offered a conspiratorial explanation for why the jury may have convicted him. He claimed that, near the end of trial testimony, the Obama administration had sent the head of its Office of National Drug Control Policy to Cincinnati to deliver a speech about the evils of prescription drug abuse, which was meant, in his words, "to make sure the jury understood what was expected of them."* He said that the jury was an "angry mob" that had received the czar's message and proceeded to "punish me for everyone they had ever known or heard about who had ever had problems with drugs of any kind."

By this time, I was accustomed to Volkman's version of his story and the bitterness and cynicism with which he told it. Still, during this posttrial correspondence, there were a few aspects of Volkman's personality that came into sharper focus. One was his grandiosity.

Although Volkman was now convicted, incarcerated, and publicly disgraced, his letters from jail were filled with boasts of various kinds.

Some were about chess. In one letter, he told me that during sleepless nights before his conviction, he had played thousands of games of two-minute online chess and "was one of the best in the country in those games." In a subsequent letter, he estimated that, if he were released from prison and was able to resume competitive chess, he would rank among the top two hundred players in the world and top ten in the United States. "Hopefully, I will have a chance to prove that," he said.

He also trumpeted his legal knowledge. In one letter he said that, since his last clinic was shut down in 2006, he had spent around ten thousand hours studying the law. He described himself as "an accomplished legal scholar." Elsewhere, he said that, for a case like his, he knew "the relevant law better than any lawyer (who could not possibly devote such attention to a single case) possibly could."

---

* When I fact-checked these claims, I found a number of elements to be disputed or flatly untrue.

While Obama's "Drug Czar," Gil Kerlikowske, *did* travel to southern Ohio in 2011, he did so in July, two months after Volkman's verdict was delivered. And when I spoke to Kerlikowske via email about this trip, he didn't remember any previous trip to the region during Volkman's trial and said that it would have been "odd" for him to travel to the same place, to discuss the same topic, twice in such quick succession. I found numerous press clippings about his July trip from Ohio newspapers, while I found no coverage of an event in April, when Volkman claims it happened.

It is possible that the speech Volkman is describing took place during this *July* trip to Cincinnati, when Kerlikowske unveiled the administration's National Drug Control Strategy. But even that speech — which, again, took place two months after the Volkman trial — doesn't sound like the kind of public-furor-stoking rally Volkman alleged occurred. In his email, Kerlikowske told me that, while he didn't remember the specific speech, in his five years in the Drug Czar post almost every presentation he gave was to treatment centers, law enforcement groups, or conferences for people in recovery and not to the general public.

Kerlikowske also flatly denied the claim that he was following orders from the president to influence a local jury. He said that he had no memory of Volkman and added, "The Obama WH had a strict prohibition about political appointees being in contact with DoJ about any investigations, cases, etc."

In one of my responses to these boasts, I remarked that he seemed to have limitless confidence in his intelligence. I asked, "Have you ever met anyone smarter than you?"

He responded that "I do indeed have limitless confidence in my analytic abilities and intelligence." And he proceeded to name a few people — a few of his fellow bridge players, his analyst, a rabbi he had been friends with for decades — who, he felt, had both intelligence and life experience he admired. Overall, he said, "I have not really met anybody I could not keep up with and interact with as an equal."

Volkman's most eyebrow-raising claims from the Butler County Jail related to his medical skill. In his words, he was an elite physician who, if he was ever released, would surely be welcomed to practice in any hospital or clinic outside of the United States.

In one of my letters, I asked if at any point in his training he had recited the famous Hippocratic oath to "First, do no harm." He responded that he had never given much thought to the oath, because his standards were "miles beyond the lowest common denominator represented by 'Do no harm.'" He said that during his career he assessed problems in the context of the patient's life, occupation, finances, living circumstances, religion, and relationships. "I worked hard to get 3 or 4 levels beyond the obvious complaint to grasp the totality of the medical problem."

In the same note, Volkman described the quickness and accuracy with which he conducted this analysis. He said that when he was working as an ER physician, he could size up a patient quickly based on their appearance, a few seconds of examination, and less than a minute of conversation. "I formulated a plan of action almost instantly and was putting it into action by the time the nurse had taken the vital signs, and well before the clerk had typed up a chart," he said.

Although he no longer practiced medicine, he said that he still had those same lightning-quick assessment skills and used them every day. "The only time I have made mistakes is when subsequent events provide additional information which changes the results of analysis," he wrote. "Those mistakes are not really mistakes, but failure to predict the future, like a failure to foresee a once in 1000-year event like the 9.3 [Richter scale] Japanese earthquake."

Aside from revealing his sky-high self-esteem, Volkman's post-conviction letters were notable for their rage.

"My best days are those in which I am the most angry," one note began. In his position, he explained, fury was the fuel that kept him going, and if it subsided, he would be left with unpleasant thoughts about his "disgusting" daily existence. In another note, he wrote, "Every day I get just a bit more furious and embittered."

These letters were rife with references to Nazi Germany. At one point, he said he was facing "as monstrous an injustice as my grandparents' relatives in Poland." Of Judge Beckwith, he said, "In another era she would have efficiently and conscientiously kept the trains to Auschwitz running on schedule, full to capacity." At another point, when discussing remarks he planned to deliver at his sentencing, he explained to me that remaining silent would be "far too reminiscent of my conception of WWII, as brothers and sisters of my grandfather and dozens of their children marched meekly into the gas chambers."

Volkman attributed much of his anger to what he felt was the grievous extent to which his activities in Ohio had been mischaracterized. "To be . . . accused of selling prescriptions to make as much money as I could, not even caring about numerous deaths that I brought about by indiscriminate dispensing of dangerous drugs, quite simply crosses a line in the sand beyond which violence is possible, even hard to avoid," he said in one letter. "There is some core fortress of last resort, some basic self respect as a doctor, even as a person that you cannot allow anyone to attack without an all out response."

At one point he discussed the prosecution's presentencing report that recommended he serve four consecutive life terms in prison. The report had been authored by a probation officer who Volkman said — based on what he had heard from Clara, who had been interviewed for the report — was "a moron barely able to read and write."

"Fortunately, I was not seated across a table from the P.O. when I perused her report," he wrote to me. "I would have strangled her with my bare hands, so that I would at least have earned one of my . . . life sentences."

While Volkman was writing letters about the "monstrous . . . injustice" of his conviction, a very different reality was unfolding in the region where his crimes took place.

The weeks following Volkman's trial saw a continued surge of national attention on the pill problem in Portsmouth. In May, two of the country's most recognizable TV doctors, Drew Pinsky (a.k.a. "Dr. Drew") and

Mehmet Oz (a.k.a. "Dr. Oz"), both aired segments of their nationally tele-vised shows about the city's woes.

Dr. Drew's segment, titled "Prescription Pill Use Destroying Whole Town," featured the host in a brightly lit studio, wearing a suit and black rectangular glasses. He began his interview with Ohio attorney general Mike DeWine, who joined the show via satellite, by asking, "What is going on in Portsmouth?"

DeWine responded by saying that it wasn't just in Portsmouth; it was a statewide problem. He said that most doctors were doing a great job treating their patients. But in Ohio, he said, "a handful of doctors . . . are killing people."

Dr. Oz's segment, meanwhile, was called "A Town Addicted to Pain Killers." At the beginning of the show, he spoke in voice-over narration over video footage. "In Portsmouth, Ohio, which sits in the heart of Scioto County, a new kind of terrorist is holding residents hostage: prescription painkillers," he said.

In this county, he continued, there were more addicts per capita than almost anywhere else in America. Overdoses from opioids occurred at a rate five times the national average.

"Why is this once-idyllic rural area under siege?" he asked.

On May 20, less than two weeks after the Volkman verdict, Ohio Governor John Kasich signed a bill that placed new restrictions on pain-management clinics across the state.

Aimed squarely at the kinds of clinics that had plagued Scioto County, House Bill 93 had been unofficially dubbed the Pill Mill Bill. It stipulated that pain clinics needed to be owned and operated by physicians, limited the amount of controlled substances that a prescriber could prescribe to a patient, required the Ohio Medical Board to produce standards of conduct for doctors who owned or worked at pain clinics, and empowered the state medical and pharmacy boards to impose hefty fines for failures to meet those standards. The bill was cosponsored by state representative Terry Johnson, the former Scioto County coroner (and prosecution witness at the Volkman trial) who had run for office on an anti-prescription-drug-abuse platform.

At the bill's signing ceremony in Columbus, Kasich quoted a statis-tic about the number of pills that had been prescribed in Scioto County the previous year: 9.7 million for a population of seventy-nine thousand.

Moments later he said, "Thank goodness that we've engaged the enemy now."

To sign the bill, Kasich sat down at a desk with a sign reading FIGHT-ING RX DRUG ABUSE affixed to the front and invited members of a Scioto County–based support group for mothers who had lost loved ones to overdose to gather around him. In a statement released by his office that day, the governor issued a warning: "If you overprescribe, we're going to come get you."

Momentum in the fight against pill abuse continued to build. In July, the Ohio US attorney's office appointed a special prosecutor to assist in the fight against prescription drug trafficking in southern Ohio. In October, Scioto County was among two counties in the state to be granted the federal designation as a High Intensity Drug Trafficking Area (HIDTA), which made it eligible for additional federal support to combat its drug problem.

And in December, the last pill mill in Scioto County was raided.

Dr. Victor Georgescu came to Scioto County out of desperation.

According to an Associated Press report, the physician, who had previously lived and worked in Pennsylvania, took a job at a Scioto County pain clinic called Greater Medical Advance after being "fired from four previous jobs after suffering a stroke."

Many aspects of Georgescu's clinic were reminiscent of those where Volkman worked. The patients traveled long distances to visit the clinic and included husband-and-wife duos who reportedly received identical prescriptions. The clinic's owner, Tracy Adkins, wore a gun while working there. Over a nine-month stretch in 2009 and 2010, Georgescu wrote more than fourteen thousand prescriptions. At least one overdose death was linked with medications he had prescribed. Then, in December 2011, state authorities made their move.

Georgescu and Adkins were each indicted on multiple state-level felony counts related to drug trafficking, permitting drug abuse, and "corrupt activity." Two other employees of the clinic were also charged. The Ohio attorney general's office filed papers to have the clinic deemed a "public nuisance" and immediately closed.

On hand for the raid was Barbara Howard, whose late daughter had received a prescription from Georgescu's clinic before filling it at Harold Fletcher's East Main Pharmacy in Columbus. She told a reporter that she had been praying for this outcome, and when she heard that the raid was under way, she drove to Wheelersburg to see it for herself. She felt more at peace knowing the clinic had been closed, she said. It meant that her daughter's death hadn't been in vain.

One year before the raid of Georgescu's clinic, there had been ten pain clinics operating in Scioto County. But in the ensuing twelve months, each one had either closed or been forcibly shut down. Greater Medical Advance was the last one.

As the year drew to a close, the *Columbus Dispatch* published an editorial applauding the development. The pain clinics had "undoubtedly contributed to the wasted lives, ruined health and drug-addicted newborns that are the hallmark of prescription-drug abuse, and made Scioto County one of the nation's worst for the problem," the paper said. The state's recent crackdown had given long-suffering communities like Portsmouth "reason to hope that unethical physicians willing to trade in human misery will know better than to set up shop here."

In Portsmouth, the manager of the *Portsmouth Daily Times* also penned a column celebrating the raid. "For a community that is guilty of often celebrating its shortcomings and failures, closing the final pill mill deserves a victory lap," he wrote.

Three days later, the paper's final issue of the year featured a recap of the ten biggest stories of 2011. At the top of the list was the fall of the county's last pill mill. The photo accompanying the story showed an exuberant Lisa Roberts embracing a friend at the site of a clinic raid in April.

"We've emerged on the other side of the hurricane, now victorious," Roberts told the paper. "But we do have some disaster cleanup to do."

SENTENCED

Volkman's relationship with his court-appointed attorneys deteriorated after his trial. In letters from jail, he described his lead attorney, Cross, as an "incompetent Benedict Arnold" who had been wrong "about 100 times in a row" on matters relating to his case. He said that he believed that his defense team had not actually been working on his behalf but, rather, acting "hand in glove with the judge and the prosecution" to create the *appearance* of a fair trial. The final straw, he said, was when Cross filed a presentencing memo on his behalf without consulting him.

Whether that actually happened is an open question. (Cross did not respond to a request to be interviewed for this book.) But I can confirm that, in early February 2012, she and her cocounsel, Candace Crouse, filed a motion to withdraw as Volkman's attorneys, citing "irreconcilable differences" with their client. They wrote that Volkman had expressed "strong distrust and dissatisfaction" with their representation and that their efforts to maintain a professional relationship with him had failed.

In a hearing about the motion on the day before Volkman's sentencing, Beckwith granted the motion in part. She dismissed Cross's second-in-command, Candace Crouse, from the case entirely but instructed Cross to remain as a "stand-by" attorney for Volkman who, while no longer representing him, could still advise him on technical issues, if requested. Beckwith also agreed to strike the presentencing memorandum submitted by Cross from the record so that Volkman could submit his own.

Before the hearing ended, the judge thanked Cross and Crouse for what she felt was their exemplary work on the case, even when that work was made difficult by "personalities" involved. Then she corrected herself to say: "A personality."

And with that, Paul Volkman headed into his sentencing as his own lawyer.

The twenty-eight-page presentencing memo that Volkman submitted on his own behalf was written in pencil on lined composition paper, which gave it the appearance of a grade-school student's book report. In its pages, he offered a sweeping defense of his actions in Ohio and a rebuke of the case against him. At one point, he listed the many ways he was not like a typical drug dealer. He had no criminal record. He did not have a "flamboyant life style replete with expensive, flashy clothes, jewelry, cars, home and women." He was not an addict who used drugs himself. And he had no "network or organization of unsavory associates and accomplices" who supplied him with the drugs he sold or helped him to distribute them.

He also listed the ways that a common drug dealer wasn't like him. Drug dealers don't have an office with a secretary and nurses, he said. Nor do they make appointments, give customers receipts, obtain records of prior medical treatment, perform physical exams, refer customers to other doctors, or require customers to sign a contract affirming that they will take the medications as prescribed. "The drug dealer would <u>not</u> think of performing pill counts or urine drug screens to ensure that his customers are consuming their drugs in a safe manner and not reselling them," he wrote.

Elsewhere in the document, he stated that his patients needed the medications he prescribed for their pain, muscle spasms, and sleep difficulties and that they had "improved greatly" when placed on this regimen. He said that he carefully advised his patients to take pills only as prescribed, and, in some cases, "carefully wrote out schedules for taking the medications." He stated that he had avoided OxyContin as a response to the finances of his "impoverished patients" and instead prescribed multiple daily doses of the generic, much cheaper oxycodone to replicate the same effect.*

He also went over each of the four deaths the jury had held him responsible for, and argued his innocence, whether due to an absence of sufficient evidence (such as the lack of an autopsy), evidence of heart disease or other illnesses, or the patient's dishonesty about the medications they were taking. And he said that, given the "good faith belief" underlying his prescribing, a malpractice suit or complaint with the Ohio State Medical Board would have been more appropriate than a criminal prosecution for disputing his actions. But he said that this wouldn't have been merited, either, because he had been a good doctor.

"Therefore," he wrote, "the appropriate punishment to be delivered to an innocent man in order to satisfy the interests of justice could not be anything in excess of no further punishment beyond the ordeal to which [I have] already been subjected."

The handwritten document was, in essence, the testimony he never gave at trial. Though, as the judge would later tell him, it was not admissible as testimony. There had been a time during the trial for him to take the stand and testify under oath, and he had declined.

The sentencing hearing took place on Valentine's Day, in a crowded courtroom with an empty defense table. Wende Cross wheeled her briefcase to the front row of the gallery, where she would sit throughout the hearing, taking notes on a legal pad. I flew to Cincinnati to attend the hearing, and as I scanned the gallery, I recognized reporters, family members of Volkman's patients, and what I believed to be a few jurors.

Volkman's appearance had changed dramatically in the months since his

---

* I never heard Volkman address the glaring contradiction presented by his avoidance of OxyContin for his patients' supposed financial sake, while simultaneously refusing to accept insurance or Medicaid, thus forcing patients to pay out-of-pocket.

conviction. During the trial, he had been clean-shaven and his hair was short and combed. Now his hair had grown long and stringy and he appeared to not have shaved in months. The *Columbus Dispatch* would later write, "With his long white beard, bushy white eyebrows and graying hair, the 65-year-old Volkman could have passed for a department-store Santa Claus if he'd been in a red suit. Instead, he wore chains and orange-and-tan striped jail scrubs." As he entered the courtroom, I heard the sound of clinking chains.

A notable exchange took place just a few minutes after the hearing began. While preliminary matters were being discussed, Beckwith referred to Volkman repeatedly as "Mr. Volkman." And after a few times, Volkman paused to request that she and others refer to him as "Dr. Volkman." He reminded the judge that this issue had been raised at trial, and she had agreed to it.

This was true. The question of whether Volkman would be referred to during the trial as "Dr." or "Mr." cut to the heart of the case. And in the final days before trial, Volkman's lawyers had filed a motion requesting that the prosecution be required to refer to him as "Dr. Volkman," not "Mr. Volkman." Beckwith had ruled in the defense's favor. And for the duration of the trial, the jurors had heard him referred to with the title "Dr."

But the trial was now over. And as Beckwith explained — while, once again, addressing him as "Mr. Volkman" — it was within her discretion how any person in the case was addressed. Given the fact that Volkman was no longer licensed to practice medicine, calling him "Dr." would be an honorary title, she said.

"And as we continue this morning and as a consequence of the trial, I do not believe that you are entitled to use that honorary title," she said.

The sentencing hearing was a chance for numerous people to weigh in on the question of a proper punishment.

On behalf of the government, Assistant US Attorney Adam Wright argued for the maximum sentence. The reason, he said, was that "the jury found the defendant distributed millions of pills without any legitimate medical purpose and four people are dead as a result of it." Later, he said, "This was deliberate and sustained conduct over the course of almost three years by someone with every advantage in the world, who chose to travel from Chicago to Portsmouth week after week after week to distribute pills." Volkman, he said, had betrayed his patients, their families, and the community, in general.

Wright was followed by Paula Eastley, the mother of Steven Hieneman, who was the lone speaker on behalf of the families of Volkman's deceased patients. She said that Volkman had not helped sick people; he had made them sicker.

"Dr. Volkman flew back and forth from Chicago each week for the sole purpose of writing mind-boggling amounts of narcotics and Xanax to drug addicts in exchange for cash," she said.

She said that, through his actions, Volkman provided fuel for the underground economy, which, in turn, kept local courts busy with cases involving drugs, theft, and prostitution and flooded local coroners with the bodies of young overdose victims.

"He ruined happy families," she said.

Volkman's comments during the hearing covered what was, to me, familiar ground. He cited statistics that downplayed the risks of overdose due to opioid painkillers. He attacked various people — the judge, the prosecutors, the government's expert witnesses — for their roles in a case that he called "ridiculous," "bizarre," "nonsense," and "entirely based on junk science."

He made claims that flatly contradicted the trial record, like his assertion that he had "always welcomed input from [patients'] family members who observed problems or irregularities" with his care.

He, again, absolved himself of any role in the deaths of his patients, whom he said were profoundly unwell when they came to him. "It is the particular role of a pain doctor to ease incurable symptoms, to make the quality of life as good as possible as long as possible," he said. He believed he had been successful in the role, and said, "I have no regrets about my treatments and no apologies to make."

At one point, while directly addressing Judge Beckwith, he said, "In sentencing an innocent man to death in jail, you are revealed as the heinous criminal in this courtroom."

Over the course of the hearing, as Volkman tried to air various grievances, Beckwith steered the conversation back to the order of the day. At one point, she said, "Sir, do not interrupt me. I did not interrupt you." At another moment, when he tried to interrupt, she said, "No, I've heard from you, Mr. Volkman." At various points, she told him that his critiques of trial witnesses and the jury's verdicts ought to be presented to the court of appeals.

The hearing also marked the first time that she shared candid opinions of Volkman and his actions. At various points during the hearing, she called Volkman's conduct "appalling," "inexplicable," and, when discussing the fact that he continued his activities after patient deaths, "wholly unconscionable." She told him that he had "abused [his] special skills as a physician in providing prescriptions and drugs for individuals without adhering to the standards of medical practice that should be applied and should control the distribution of medical services."

She reminded him of the various choices he had made in southern Ohio. He had chosen to get involved with Denise Huffman and to open an on-site dispensary after local pharmacies refused to fill his prescriptions. He had ignored numerous red flags in the behavior of the people whom he claimed to be treating and had continued to prescribe to them after their family members complained.

She added that she found his presentencing memo and comments during the hearing gravely concerning. "This Defendant has absolutely no remorse. He said so this morning," she said. "He has no insight into his behaviors and he is a truly dangerous man."

Toward the end of the hearing, she informed Volkman of his sentence. He would serve twenty years in prison for each of ten drug-dealing convictions. Those sentences would be served concurrently.

Additionally, for each of Counts 10, 11, 18, and 20 — the drug-dealing convictions tied to the deaths of four patients — he would serve a life term in prison. These life terms were to be served *consecutively*.*

On the day after the sentencing, a big, bold headline ran across the top of the *Portsmouth Daily Times*'s front page: "Volkman Gets 4 Life Sentences." On Facebook, the mood in Scioto County's prescription-drug-abuse-focused Facebook group was jubilant. One commenter said that she was doing a "happy dance." Another said, "Drug dealing murderer gets only a fraction of what he deserved but I am happy with that!!"

When I spoke over the phone with Volkman's son, Adam, he seemed relieved by the news. His father was a "toxic person," he told me. And for the first time in years, his family had confirmation that he would never again be a part of their lives.

---

* When I interviewed Beckwith, via phone, in 2022, after her retirement, she shared the thinking behind this sentence. She said that, on one level, she wanted to send a warning to doctors that "atrocious behavior" like Volkman's "will not be tolerated, or permitted or overlooked."

But she said the sentence was also fueled by practical concerns. Volkman struck her as an unremorseful "total megalomaniac," and she had the impression that, if he were released from prison, he would "rustle up a medical license, somehow or another" and go back to peddling pills.

"I felt that he was pretty much irredeemable," she said.

— PART FIVE —
AFTERMATH

CRIME WAVE

Volkman's sentencing marked the start of a busy year for pill mill cases in Scioto County and eastern Kentucky.

In April, the US attorney for the Southern District of Ohio indicted the owner of three pain clinics, along with six doctors who had worked at those clinics, for the illegal distribution of prescription drugs. One of the clinics was in Columbus; the other two were in Portsmouth, including one in the former home of Tri-State Healthcare, on Findlay Street. A press release about the indictment noted that the clinics' owner, Tracy Bias, had no formal medical education and that he was believed to have "secured doctors for brief periods of time ranging from one day to several years through what are known as locum tenens, or temporary service contracts, to prescribe pain medication for customers at his clinics."

Among the indicted physicians was Dr. Mark Fantauzzi, whose pre–Scioto County career included locum tenens positions in more than sixty hospitals around the country. Fantauzzi pleaded guilty, and in documents submitted before his sentencing, his lawyers explained that his work at the Portsmouth pain clinic was due to a "a perfect storm" of factors, including an economic downturn, a crumbling marriage, and personal financial struggles. The clinic owners "were able to capitalize on Dr. Fantauzzi's misfortunes and put him in a situation where he was hard-pressed to say no," they wrote. The doctor "badly needed the job."

Prosecutors were far less sympathetic, stating in a court filing that the doctor had committed "a serious offense with dangerous repercussions" and that his case was "part of a greater pill tsunami into the Southern Ohio area." Fantauzzi was ultimately sentenced to eighteen months in prison and one year of supervised release. The remaining five doctors from that case, all of whom also pleaded guilty, received sentences ranging from three months of house arrest to eighteen months in prison. Bias, the clinic owner, was sentenced to fourteen years.

One month after those six doctors and clinic owner were indicted, another pain-clinic case went to trial in Cincinnati before Judge Sandra Beckwith. The defendants were Nancy and Lester Sadler, a husband-and-wife duo who had co-run a series of pain clinics in Ohio and Kentucky.

Like Denise Huffman, Nancy Sadler had no formal medical education or training. But for more than five years, from the mid-1990s to the early 2000s, she had worked in the offices of David Procter. When Procter came under legal fire in the early 2000s, Sadler pleaded guilty to a count of wire fraud and received a sentence of probation. Nevertheless, during her period of probation, she opened a clinic in Garrison, Kentucky, using paperwork filed under her sister's name. The clinic was initially called First Care, though it eventually moved to Piketon, Ohio (twenty-five miles north of Portsmouth), where it became 1st Care Family Practice. Later, the clinic moved again to the town of Waverly (twenty-eight miles north of Portsmouth), where it eventually became Ohio Medical and Pain Management (OMPM).

OMPM followed the blueprint of many area pain clinics. It was a cash-only operation where patients — many of whom had traveled long distances to get there — underwent cursory examinations before receiving high-dose prescriptions of opioids. In response, many local pharmacies refused to fill the clinic's scripts. Summarizing the clinic's operation, a judge from the Sixth Circuit US Court of Appeals later wrote, "A 'dope sick' drug addict could walk into Nancy's clinic, hand over some cash, get no 'real pain assessment,' tell an obvious lie, and walk (or skip) out of the clinic minutes later with a drug prescription in her pocket."

The Sadlers' clinic put its own spin on the pill mill formula, however. In some instances, intake paperwork and prescriptions were prefilled for patients; in other cases, medical charts and prescriptions were generated for "phantom patients" who never set foot in the clinic at all.

In August 2010, Sadler was indicted, with her husband, her sister, her father-in-law, a separate clinic employee, and a physician who had worked at the clinic. Three of those defendants — Nancy's sister, Lester's father, and the doctor — pleaded guilty, while Nancy, her husband, and the clinic employee chose to fight the charges at trial.

The pretrial motions in that case included at least one noteworthy document. In August 2011, prosecutors submitted a motion alleging that, even after their indictment, the Sadlers continued to run a pain clinic in Columbus that brought in more than $100,000 per month and that these proceeds were being spent on shopping (at Edible Arrangements, Babies R Us, Walmart, and Best Buy, among other places) and at various casinos. "On August 6, 2010, three days after the arraignment and the submission of her Financial Affidavit, Nancy Sadler played the slots at Hollywood Casino [in southern Indiana] with over $27,000 in funds," the document read. In response, Judge Beckwith issued an order that specifically barred the Sadlers from working at any kind of medical facility or entering "any casino or similar gambling establishment anywhere at any time."

After an eleven-day trial in May 2012, the Sadlers were convicted on numerous charges, including operating a criminal enterprise, maintaining a premises for the purpose of distributing drugs, and, in Nancy's case, wire fraud and money laundering. At her sentencing, Nancy Sadler described the "dysfunctional atmosphere" of her upbringing, which included "severe physical, mental and verbal abuse." Through tears, she said, "I'm sorry that I didn't make myself available to the orderly running of the clinic. I'm sorry that this has caused so much pain and hurt to those who were directly and indirectly involved."

Beckwith responded that Nancy had seemed unrepentant and eager to blame others before the day's sentencing proceedings. "Her childhood experiences are sad and they may be a reason for a good deal of her illegal and aberrant and antisocial behavior," she said. "That's not an excuse."

Nancy was sentenced to 17.5 years in prison, while Lester received a sentence of 12.5 years. A doctor affiliated with the clinic pleaded guilty and received a 4-year sentence.

During the same month that the Sadlers were convicted, another doctor and clinic owner were indicted for illegal activity related to pain clinics in Dayton, Lucasville (ten miles north of Portsmouth), and South Point (thirty-five miles east of Portsmouth), Ohio. The indictment told a familiar story: John Randy Callihan, the clinic owner, had no medical education or background; customers paid cash to see the doctor, Christopher Stegawski, and, in return, were prescribed large amounts of controlled substances.

The clinic owner pleaded guilty and received a five-year prison sentence. But the doctor took his case to trial in Cincinnati, and it was notable for the tempestuous relationship between the defendant and his attorney. At one point during the weeklong trial, when Stegawski's attorney declined to cross-examine a prosecution witness, the doctor spoke out in the courtroom to say "of course" they wanted to cross-examine the witness. When his attorney again said no, the doctor replied that if the lawyer wouldn't do it, he'd do it himself.

A couple days later, in a conference in front of the judge, the doctor, who had previously dismissed two public defenders, said that he was having major problems cooperating with his attorney and accused the lawyer of intentionally tanking his defense until he was paid more money.

His lawyer, who disputed the claim, told the judge his client was "grand-standing" and "trying to create a scene."

Stegawski was ultimately convicted and sentenced to thirteen years in prison.

Due to cases such as these, Portsmouth was already regarded as an epicenter of the national opioid epidemic. And in the years following Volkman's case, news coverage further solidified the reputation.

In 2017, the Canadian Broadcasting Corporation (CBC) traveled to Portsmouth for a report on what the reporter called "drug abuse beyond anything we've seen in Canada." At the time of the visit, the city's overdose numbers were still climbing. Demand for foster care was surging. Emergency calls for overdoses were commonplace. At one point in his report, the journalist stood in front of 1219 Findlay Street, the former location of Tri-State Healthcare, and said, "This building behind me was one of Portsmouth's infamous pain clinics."

The CBC story ran shortly after British newspaper *The Guardian* published a report from Portsmouth with the headline, "'The Pill Mill of America': Where Drugs Mean There Are No Good Choices, Only Less Awful Ones." Soon, the *New York Times* returned to Scioto County for a lengthy story on the fallout from the city's addiction crisis. "Call them Generation O," the article said, "the children whose families are trapped in a relentless grip of addiction, rehab and prison."

Perhaps the most widely seen story of all was a book by a former *Los Angeles Times* reporter, Sam Quinones, called *Dreamland: The True Tale of America's Opiate Epidemic*. By the time of the book's release in 2015, the opiate epidemic involved two parallel crises: the abuse of pharmaceutical opioids as well as black-market heroin. And in his book, Quinones told the stories of both.

Dreamland was both a critical and a commercial success, and, in the wake of its release, Quinones appeared at events across the country, from Maine to Mississippi to Oregon.* In time, it would be viewed as a definitive history of the American opiate epidemic.

And though the book reported from numerous places across the United States and Mexico, Portsmouth was its narrative center of gravity. A photo-

---

* I was among those who praised Quinones's achievement. In a review for the literary website *The Millions*, I called it "astonishing," "monumental," and "one of those rare books that's big and vivid and horrifying enough to shake up our collective consciousness."

graph of the city appeared on the book's cover, and at different times in the story, Quinones called Portsmouth "America's pill mill capital" and "ground zero in the pill explosion."

In a few paragraphs, he even briefly mentioned the peculiar pain-clinic partnership between a Chicago-based doctor and a local mother-daughter duo. As he wrote, "Volkman and the Huffmans were only part of the story in Scioto County."

TERRE HAUTE

Franklin Delano Roosevelt authorized the construction of a federal prison in Terre Haute, Indiana, in 1938. And in 1943, an article in the *Indianapolis Star* raved about the new institution. "In planning the Terre Haute prison, daring men chucked medieval blueprints — massive cell blocks, corporal punishment, dungeon confinement," the author wrote. "They designed, instead, a hospital for men's sick souls — scientific diagnoses and treatment of causes, light and air, intelligent sympathy and understanding."

Half a century later, in 1993, the prison at Terre Haute was designated the location for the federal death penalty to be administered, and a "Special Confinement Unit" was constructed to house death-row inmates. In 2001, news organizations from around the country descended on Terre Haute to cover the execution of the Oklahoma City bomber, Timothy McVeigh.

By the time that Volkman arrived at Terre Haute in 2012, his fellow prisoners included murderers, rapists, bank robbers, kidnappers, carjackers, child molesters, gang members, and drug dealers. Among them were Zaid Safarini, who was one of the 1986 hijackers of Pan Am Flight 73, which left twenty people dead, and Dr. Ronald Mikos, a Chicago-based podiatrist convicted in 2005 of shooting and killing a patient who planned to testify against him in a Medicare-fraud investigation.

Volkman described his new home to me as "filled by design with large, vicious, ruthless people who will never go anywhere else." It was, he said, a "frightening snake pit as foreign to all of my prior life experience as the surface of Mars." Not long after arriving, he reported that he was attacked by a fellow inmate whom he described as a "Nazi skinhead."

He said that he spent the next three and a half weeks under twenty-four-hour lockdown in a tiny, dark cell known as "the Hole," for what the prison staff told him was his own protection. There were no visits, no phone calls, no email, and no desk at which to sit and write. Aside from the four hours per week of "rec" time he was given to roam in a small, caged-in area, he told me that the experience was like being buried alive, albeit with an "illiterate 53-year-old moron who has been in jail for the past 30 years" as his cellmate.

Despite these circumstances, Volkman reported that once he was released from the Hole, life at Terre Haute was "decent." He lived in a cell measuring approximately fourteen by eight feet, with a tiny desk and double bunks. He had made friends with an "enormously street smart" former biker named Ty, who had spent most of his adult life in and out of prisons. He also found a few fellow inmates with whom he could play chess.

He reported to me that, during mornings, he was allowed to walk outside on a quarter-mile track, and in the evenings, he could watch TV until lockdown. He passed the time in between with yoga, walking up and down a set of stairs for exercise, and conversations with his public defender. Meals included French toast and a banana for breakfast, and, for one dinner he described, "watery spaghetti with some chicken gravy."

It was, he said wryly, the retirement of his dreams. "No expenses. No worries," he wrote, in one letter. "I recommend it to your father."

Volkman remained a zealous advocate of his innocence from prison, and with the help of a federal defender, he submitted an appeal of his conviction to the Sixth Circuit US Court of Appeals. The court released its response in late 2013 and, over twenty-six pages, laid out the reasons for its denial.

The judges spent the most time on Volkman's argument that the jury had not heard sufficient evidence to arrive at its guilty verdicts. The panel wrote that Volkman's notion that Tri-State was a legitimate clinic "turns a blind eye to quite a bit of evidence." In his arguments, the panel said that Volkman made himself out to be a "blissfully-ignorant doctor," and they simply did not buy it. They wrote that the establishment of Tri-State's on-site dispensary was, by itself, enough for a jury to find that he and the Huffmans "executed a plan to unlawfully distribute controlled substances with no legitimate medical purpose." The existence of this in-house pharmacy, "combined with Volkman's role in rubber-stamping the distribution of prescriptions, could have easily persuaded a jury that Volkman knew of and actively participated in the charged conspiracy."

The panel also found no reason to overturn verdicts for any of the four deaths for which the jury had deemed Volkman directly responsible.

They wrote that Kristi Ross suffered from several risk factors for over-dose — obesity, hypertension, sleep apnea — plus a pending divorce and a bitter child-custody battle that further elevated her stress. "She was already at risk of breathing difficulties, and Volkman's drug cocktail exposed her to a greater risk of death," they wrote.

They noted that Ernest Ratcliff had a history of drug addiction and drug dealing and that a toxicologist had testified that oxycodone, not the methadone that Volkman hadn't prescribed, had been the most significant factor in his death. They also pointed out that he had died from a *cumulative* effect of toxicity, not just one drug alone.

When it came to Bryan Brigner, the panel found that the drug regimen Volkman prescribed "made little sense," especially in light of his underlying heart issues.

For Steve Hieneman, they found that not only was there evidence on which to "draw a causal connection between Hieneman's prescriptions and his death," but that Volkman had prescribed him controlled substances despite red flags, including his past addiction to OxyContin and heart problems.

The panel upheld Volkman's conviction and included a bit of commentary that was perfectly understandable to people without legal expertise.

"When a doctor first enters the practice of medicine," they wrote, "he or she swears to abide by a prime directive of the profession: 'First, do no harm.' Paul Volkman breached this sacrosanct tenet when he prescribed narcotics to addicts and individuals with physical, mental, and psychological frailties."

Volkman fought this decision to the US Supreme Court, which agreed to reconsider a narrow aspect of his conviction and sentence. In October 2014, the court issued a short ruling that focused exclusively on Volkman's four death-related convictions and left the other fourteen other conviction counts untouched.

In the matter of those four convictions involving patient deaths, the court vacated Volkman's judgment and sentence in light of another case involving drug-related deaths that the Supreme Court had heard after the Sixth Circuit's first ruling on Volkman's case. In that case, *Burrage v. United States*, the court had unanimously ruled that that maximum mandatory sentence could only be triggered if prosecutors had proved the drug a defendant had illegally distributed was proved to be the *primary* cause of a patient's death and not just a contributing factor. In Volkman's case, the court wanted the lower appeals court to reconsider the doctor's sentence for those four death-related sentences in light of that subsequent ruling, which had slightly narrowed the legal basis for such a sentence.

While it was a small victory for Volkman, it was hardly the broad validation he was seeking. The Supreme Court had specifically stated, "Nothing in today's order should be understood as suggesting that petitioner is entitled to acquittal." And in 2015, the Supreme Court's question to the Sixth Circuit was answered resoundingly when the lower court, once again, upheld Volkman's conviction and sentence, even after factoring in the *Burrage* case.

Appealing his conviction was just one of the routes Volkman pursued to try to overturn the verdict against him. In 2011, shortly after his trial ended, he filed a motion for acquittal and/or a new trial, which was denied. In 2013, he filed a motion to "Dismiss Appeal & Declare Judgment Void for Fraud Against the Due Administration of Justice," which failed. In 2016, he filed a variety of motions "to disqualify each and every federal officer implicated in the arbitrary and fraudulent exercise of civil law 'judicial power' from Congress," "for bail or release on movant's recognizance," and to "void proceedings and for equitable relief." All were denied.

That same year, he also filed two motions seeking to specifically disqualify and recuse Judge Beckwith from his case, which were also denied. In her response to one of them, Beckwith stated that Volkman had not presented any evidence that would prompt a reasonable person to question her impartiality in the case. She went on to say, "Defendant continues to harangue the Court and waste precious judicial resources with frivolous motions for the undersigned to recuse." She cautioned him that "if he files one more motion, pleading, or document determined by the Court to be frivolous he will be subjected to sanctions."

But he was not done.

The arrival of the COVID-19 pandemic in 2020 provided another basis to try to argue his way out of prison. In a filing from late 2021, Volkman argued that he met the standard of "extraordinary and compelling reasons for release" because of his age (seventy-five) and a variety of medical conditions, including Type 2 diabetes, kidney disease, heart disease, liver disease, small vessel disease, hypertension, and obesity. Presenting statistics about

COVID transmission at his current prison ("over 14 inmates [deaths], and over 876 contagious during the critical period of the pandemic"), he argued that he was at risk due to both his incarceration and his health conditions, for "a negative outcome should he contract COVID-19 or any of its variants."

In a supplemental memo filed by an attorney representing Volkman, the lawyer noted that Volkman was a first-time offender with no criminal history before his current convictions, that he was an "older man," and that he was "unquestionably an educated man with a PhD and an MD from the University of Chicago, perhaps the most prestigious university in the Midwest, and one of the most respected in the nation." The lawyer said that Volkman had no intent to reenter the workforce, and no specific desire or plans to practice medicine or prescribe medication.

"Frankly, it is highly unlikely that he lives another decade whether granted compassionate release or required to serve his remaining sentence," he wrote. "But what this Court can be assured of is that he . . . will never again be practicing medicine or committing crimes."

This motion, too, was denied.

Volkman also relentlessly pleaded his case outside of the court system.

In his words, his actions and the injustice he had suffered made him comparable to some of the most famous dissidents in Western history. In a letter to friends he sent after his sentencing, he seemed to delight in the moment during his sentencing when Judge Beckwith had described him as "dangerous."

"Whether she realized it or not," he explained, "she called me 'dangerous' the way Martin Luther was 'dangerous' to the Pope, the way Thomas More was 'dangerous' to Henry VIII, the way Thomas Jefferson was 'dangerous' to George V [*sic*], the way good, principled, honest, courageous, outspoken men are always 'dangerous' to cruel, evil, corrupt, petty tyrants."

In the years that followed, he produced a torrent of written and typed words. Many of them were in letters or emails directly addressed to me, as part of our long-running correspondence. But he also sent me copies of things he wrote to other people. These writings amounted to one long telling and retelling of the story of his innocence.

At the center of his story was himself, a man he described as an "honest, conscientious physician, attentive husband, caring father and grandfather, never before convicted of any type of offense, whose apparent crime was to provide appropriate pain relief care to desperate, impoverished patients in Ohio and Kentucky."

He described his patients as people who were profoundly unwell. "Patients who suffer severe, chronic pain from various injuries and diseases are not, in general, healthy people," he stated. He said that many of his patients were suffering from "severe, chronic" pain that was a result of years of hard manual labor, other ailments (such as severe heart disease or emphysema), or the secondary health issues stemming from chronic pain itself, including hypertension, stroke, muscle cramps, insomnia, and a "vastly increased incidence of suicide."

In one email from 2021, he went much further than his defense team had argued during his trial and said, "Pain doctors are essentially hospice doctors, and to blame a hospice doctor for the death of his patients is ridiculous." At another point, he wrote that, given the poor health of the people he was seeing in Ohio, his rate of patient deaths was actually low. "During 2003 to 2006, some thirteen or fourteen of my patients out of about 500 died from their chronic conditions, actually far fewer than would have been expected from such a fragile population," he said.

The villains of Volkman's story were legion. They included the government of the United States, the Department of Justice, the DEA, the judge, the prosecutors, his own defense attorneys, and the expert witnesses who testified against him. The press was complicit as well. At one point, he referred to the well-documented scourge of overdose deaths in Appalachia as "bogus" and "public hysteria [stoked] through sensationalized, false reports in tabloid media."

In this serialized retelling of his story, Volkman was, above all else, a victim. In fact, in one essay — an open letter from 2018 that was published on a website sympathetic to convicted pain doctors — he stated explicitly, when describing his case, "I was actually the victim in that grim scenario."

He also frequently insisted that this case was much bigger than him. In one letter, he wrote, "I need help from anybody who thinks that the Constitution, The Bill of Rights, and the Rule of Law still matter." In another, he described the "demonization of the one-third of adult Americans who have legitimate need for daily, strong pain medicine, and of the pain doctors who, at great risk to themselves, try to take care of them, out of compassion and concern."

DEFENDERS

Around two weeks after Volkman's sentencing, the *Columbus Dispatch* published a letter in response to its coverage of the event. The 160-word note began with a question: "When are people going to realize that life often is unfair, and there isn't always someone to blame when things go wrong?"

The author, a woman named Pamela Filsoufi, from Columbus, continued:

> Patients came to see Dr. Paul H. Volkman. He didn't go down to the schoolyard and sell drugs to kids. Adults came to his clinic wanting relief from their pain.
>
> It's sad when someone overdoses. Their family members are justifiably upset. Most often they want someone to blame to avoid having to place blame on their dearly departed.
>
> Isn't blaming the doctor akin to blaming the automobile sales-man when a loved one dies in a car accident? As adults, we must be responsible for bad decisions that might cost us our lives.
>
> Is a grieving mother the most rational person to guide our thoughts or courts on this subject? I hope that the people support-ing the war on pain medications never need them.

Filsoufi was far from alone in voicing her sympathy for Volkman. In the years after his sentencing, I found a number of folks who were skeptical or critical of the case against him.

Sally Scott was a registered nurse who had worked for Volkman on Center Street and in Chillicothe and who testified on his behalf at trial. She told me, via Facebook message, that Volkman was a "good person" whom she cared about and respected. She seemed to believe that Volkman had been brought down by an excess of virtue. He had been too trust-ing of patients who were lying to him about their conditions in order to get medication. As she viewed it, he was, if anything, too devoted to their treatment. "He talked with each patient sometimes for hours," she said. "I believe he truly care[d] about them."

She said that despite her advice that he close his clinics for his own legal protection, he refused because he told her that "he couldn't abandon his patients." The only reason he had run a clinic out of his house on Center Street, she said, was so his patients wouldn't suffer in the time between his split from Denise and finding a new office.

In her eyes, Volkman was a purehearted and "misunderstood" man who had been "lured" to Portsmouth and preyed upon by Denise Huffman. One of Denise's motives, she guessed, was that Volkman could help her to establish an on-site dispensary. But whatever the exact reason, she believed Denise had a "hidden agenda," had "dug her claws" into Volkman, and had "exploited this poor man."

I also spoke via email to Harry Bonnell, the forensic pathologist and former chief deputy coroner of Hamilton County (where Cincinnati is located) who had testified as the cause-of-death expert in Volkman's defense. Bonnell told me that he had been providing pro bono consulting in cases of wrongful prosecution for years by the time he was contacted by Volkman's defense team, and this case struck him as "no different." He estimated that, based on his consulting fees, he would have charged around $20,000 for his review of documents and subsequent testimony. But he worked on Volkman's case for free because, as he said, "I do not charge for my labor to defend those wrongfully charged or wrongfully convicted."

Bonnell told me that, based on his review of the documents, he felt there were two reasons that Volkman was wrongfully charged with contributing to, or causing, patient deaths. One was that for many of the deaths he reviewed, it seemed that local coroners had not properly weighed non-overdose-related disease factors into their analysis. "Several [patients] had severe cardiac disease which was ignored, deferring to a drug level even though the history surrounding the death was that of a sudden cardiac death and not an opiate OD," he said.

Another error, he felt, was a misinterpretation of drug levels in the decedents' blood that ignored the likelihood that they were tolerant to opiates at the time of their death. The coroners and toxicologists who produced the records he reviewed "just knee-jerked to the blood drug levels and did not consider that the levels were in the range expected for the dosage prescribed," he said.

He felt that the motivation behind this ill-advised prosecution was a federal law enforcement system that didn't want to admit that it was losing, or had already lost, the War on Drugs. As a result, they were going after the "easiest target[s] to hit," like Volkman. He felt that the case was a miscarriage of justice and that Volkman's sentence was "overkill," the result of "attorneys and [a] judge trying to maintain a reputation."

———

Scott and Bonnell came by their skepticism of Volkman's conviction through direct ties to the case. But there were others who expressed support from a distance — or at least spoke in favor of doctors accused of similar crimes.

David Borden was the founder and longtime executive director of an organization called StoptheDrugWar.org. The group is dedicated to ending the US's long-standing drug policies and thereby halting their side effects, which, in Borden's assessment, include the overcrowding of prisons with nonviolent drug offenders, the creation of dangerous black markets in response to strict drug laws, racial profiling in drug-law enforcement, and corruption in the legal system.

Borden has also identified the undertreatment of chronic pain as one of the drug war's unintended effects, due to doctors avoiding the prescribing of opioids for fear of investigation. After the widely covered 2004 conviction of the Virginia-based pain doctor Dr. William Hurwitz, who had previously appeared on *60 Minutes* for his willingness to prescribe high doses of opioids to patients with excruciating pain, Borden called the verdict "a travesty of justice against an individual — a lynching, in effect — of an innocent doctor whose only crime is that he would not torture his patients by denying them the medicine they needed."

When I spoke with him about Volkman's case, Borden said that he hadn't done enough research to weigh in on the case's particulars. But he remained skeptical about the government's overall efforts to prosecute doctors. He had seen cases of doctor prosecutions that were "clearly unjust" and did a lot of harm to pain patients. And he was wary of law enforcement's ability to distinguish genuine criminal doctors (who did exist, he acknowledged) from ones who were well intentioned and yet made some mistakes, or doctors who were conscientiously treating pain patients who were otherwise underserved by the medical system. "Applying criminal punishments to the latter two of those three groups has a chilling effect on pain control in general, especially when we're talking about long prison terms," he said.

"We should look very carefully at accusations of this type made against doctors," he continued. "We have to keep all sides of this issue in mind, otherwise the attempts to address one side will be done in ways that do harm to the other sides that might have been avoided."

Siobhan Reynolds was, at one time, the country's most aggressive and outspoken activist on behalf of pain doctors accused of illegally distributing opioids. She had been radicalized by her attempts to access care for her husband, Sean, who suffered from debilitating pain. As she once explained, "Being with somebody in pain whom you love and being unable to help them is the most stressful, upsetting situation you could be in."

In 2003, Reynolds founded an organization called the Pain Relief Network that, in its mission statement, called chronic pain patients the "most disenfranchised and voiceless minority in America today." In the following years she produced a documentary called *The Chilling Effect — Pain Patients in the War on Drugs*. She repeatedly defended besieged pain doctors in the press, including, at one point, calling the drug war "a crime against our most vulnerable population, those in serious, chronic pain" in a letter to the *New York Times*. In 2007, during testimony at a congressional hearing on oversight of the Drug Enforcement Administration, she called the DEA an "out-of-control . . . agency that has demonstrated no respect for the rights of ill Americans, nor for the rule of law itself." And she said that, as a result of doctor prosecutions, pain patients, including veterans and children dying of cancer, "are increasingly shut out of care by doctors who were being conditioned, terrorized in fact, out of treating pain responsibly."

As part of her activism, Reynolds traveled to Texas, Georgia, South Carolina, New Mexico, California, and other states to speak out on behalf of accused doctors. During the trial of a pain doctor in Wichita, Kansas, she paid for a local billboard ad that read, DR. SCHNEIDER NEVER KILLED ANYONE.

Reynolds told me that she had spoken with Volkman in the early stages of his case. From these conversations, she seemed familiar with him and his personality. "He probably has the best résumé of any one of our docs," she said.

But she said that these conversations took place after she had decided not to get involved in cases where the defense team was unwilling to address the broader politics of pain, opiates, and law enforcement. At the time she spoke with Volkman, his lawyers weren't interested in such an angle.

When I spoke with her after his conviction, she remained generally sympathetic to him. She admitted that she found him an "unappealing person" and a bad poster child for the cause of pain doctors. And she acknowledged that a state medical board investigation could have been a legitimate place for debating his actions. But she believed that Volkman's intentions were good and didn't think he belonged in prison.

"He is a misanthrope," she said. "But . . . that's not a crime."

Perhaps the most outspoken of Volkman's sympathizers was a woman named Linda Cheek.

Cheek was a Virginia-based doctor who had been convicted of more than 150 federal counts of illegal diversion of pain medication and sentenced to thirty-three months in prison. Throughout her case, she maintained her innocence. At one point, she described herself as "a victim of illegal government persecution for doing her job and actually helping her patients heal from disease." Elsewhere she wrote that she was "an independent, female physician taking care of the expendable populations that the government wanted dead."

After her release from prison, Cheek launched a website dedicated to defending doctors accused of crimes or other misconduct related to opioid distribution. The site, called Doctors of Courage, included a database of more than nineteen hundred doctors, along with Cheek's commentary, such as a note on one page that read "these attacks have nothing to do with actual law-breaking, but simply creating MEDICAL POLITICAL PRISONERS of good, compassionate doctors by money-hungry promotion-seeking US attorneys."

While prosecutors had accused Volkman and others of writing cookie-cutter prescriptions, Cheek threw the accusation back at them, stating that the DOJ used a "cookie cutter approach" to charge and convict doctors of opioid-related crimes. She seemed to believe, on principle, that investigations and prosecutions of doctors for opioid-related crimes were inherently unjust. Included on a page on her site called "Doctors/Professionals Under Attack" were the names of more than ten convicted doctors and clinic owners from Scioto County, including John Lilly, Denise and Alice Huffman, and Nancy and Lester Sadler. It was unclear how much, if any, research had been done on these cases before the names were added to the site.

Doctors of Courage featured a blog where Cheek wrote posts expressing sympathy for various doctors. And in the years after Volkman's sentencing, she posted about his case numerous times. When Volkman applied for a petition for compassionate release from prison, she published a portion of his application with a note that read, in part, "I pray that they do give him compassionate release, and ask you to do the same." She also published an open letter from Volkman (which, having fact-checked it, I know to be riddled with distortions, inaccuracies, and untruths) in which he refused to apologize, called his case an "unconscionable miscarriage of justice," and said that he prayed that the "angry, bitter, hateful, lynch mob of [deceased patients'] relatives will ultimately realize that their government has victimized me."

In another post from 2016, Cheek used coverage of Volkman's case as the basis for her own point-by-point analysis. She said that Volkman appeared to be a high-volume prescriber of opioids because he was the "only pain management specialist in a large area," and, as long as he was "giving appropriate treatment," the number of pills he prescribed was irrelevant. She said that the long distances Volkman's patients traveled to see him was a favorable, not incriminating, aspect of the case. "In general when you run a business where people travel to see you, it is a mark of doing a good job," she wrote. She did not find his lack of malpractice insurance damning; "In fact," she wrote, "it is a reflection that he knew what he was doing, and he wasn't worried about being sued." Overall, she said, "Every case I've written about is a travesty, but this is probably the worst."

I spoke with Cheek over the phone, and during that conversation she confirmed that "of course" she had not read the transcript of Volkman trial's and did not intend to. It was "all crap" and "government lies," she said, and added, "You can't believe anything that the prosecution puts on the witness stand." But from her review of other facts about the case, she was nevertheless firmly convinced of Volkman's innocence.

When I brought up the fact that family members of Volkman's deceased patients might find the doctor's open letter she had published hurtful, she was dismissive. She felt that such relatives were blaming the doctor for the mere act of listening to their loved one and treating them "as he saw appropriate." And she said that *they* were the ones that were more responsible for these patients' deaths. "I think that the fact that they do feel responsible is why they're trying to shift blame onto Dr. Volkman," she said.

During our conversation, I asked about the fact that she was herself convicted of opioid-related crimes and had created a website dedicated to defending all such accused doctors. An observer might interpret this as one big exercise in deflection and denial, I said.

"Not true," she said. "I am just trying to right the wrongs created by our government. That's purely all I'm trying to do."

LOVED ONES

All told, I spoke with more than twenty-five people who knew Volkman's deceased patients. They were those patients' aunts, mothers, cousins, brothers, half brothers, sisters, sisters-in-law, spouses, ex-spouses, sons, and daughters. Our conversations took place in person, in some cases. In other cases, we spoke via phone, Facebook messenger, video calls, or email.

What I heard was dramatically different from what Paul Volkman said about his time in Ohio. Whereas he claimed to have been mending lives affected by pain, these people generally believed that the doctor had made their loved ones' lives worse. Whereas Paul Volkman swore that he was acting as an advocate for those who were suffering, these folks told me that the doctor had, in fact, created new and enduring sources of pain — emotional pain — that affected far more than just the patient.

Many of the stories I heard involved lives that were violently thrown off course by the abrupt loss of their loved one.

Bryan Brigner's son, who was about to turn eleven years old when his dad died, told me that, in the months following his father's death, he often cried at night when he remembered his dad's face or his laugh. He, his mom, and his brother moved around a lot after his dad's passing. For a few years, they stayed with different relatives.

Dwight Parsons's stepson, Brad, told me that, because he had been the one to discover Dwight's body after he had woken up on a nearby couch, his sleep was disrupted for years. He was scared to go to sleep because his mind was telling him, "If I wake up something horrific is gonna happen or has happened," he said.

Steven Hieneman's partner, John Kiser, described how his life had, in some ways, frozen at the moment Steven died. When I spoke with him in 2013, more than seven years after his partner's death, he had not dated anyone and had no immediate plans to. He had not watched the movie that he and Steven had been watching on the night of his death. And he had only recently moved clothes that Steven had left hanging on the back of a chair at their house. "I couldn't move 'em," he said.

More than once, I heard or read stories of family members who had struggled with substance-abuse issues after their loved one's death. In one post on Facebook, a son of Kristi Ross described how losing his mother to an overdose "sent me down a dark path." He had been on life support twice for overdoses, he wrote, and he had destroyed his marriage and lost custody of his kids due to drugs. In another post, he wrote, "Happy mother's day in heaven mom . . . If u only knew how hard it's been even tho it's been so long. For years Everyone told me to get over it. It's hard."

When I spoke with James Estep's daughter, Megan, in 2021, more than fifteen years after her father's passing, she told me that the loss of her dad was never far from her mind. Her father's death had robbed her of a parent whom she could get to know as a teenager, a young adult, and beyond. She was reminded of this whenever anyone asked her how her parents were doing. She told me that when she first met her boyfriends' parents, she had to learn how to "tiptoe" around those anxiety-inducing conversations. And on top of everything else, she said, she carried around an unsettling sense that the natural order of her family had been disrupted by her dad's death. Her great-grandparents were still alive when he died. In the years afterward, she heard people three times his age reminiscing about him. "You know how messed up that is?" she said. "Something is chronologically wrong there."

James's widow, Angie, told me that she was haunted by thoughts of how things might have gone differently. She explained that, while she wasn't able to convince James to get the addiction counseling he needed, she believed that members of his boilermakers' union might have succeeded. "I think if somebody that he respected had sat down with him and said, 'Look, we are going to have to terminate your employment here unless you go get help,' I think he would have," she said. But it never happened. And so she was left to envision alternative scenarios.

In a similar vein, Mark Reeder's sister-in-law, Kimberly, told me that her husband — Mark's brother, Matt — still wondered what he might have done differently in the hours before Mark's passing. Kim explained that, on the last day of his brother's life, Matt had been to Mark's house and seen him visibly "out of his head" on drugs. But because Matt had seen this so many times before, he hadn't done anything about it. He figured that Mark would just sleep it off, as he had before. When Mark didn't wake up, Matt blamed himself.

Kim told me that she had done her best to try to convince her husband otherwise. She had told him that Mark would have never agreed to come home with Matt that night, and that, anyway, their family had instituted a rule about Mark not visiting their house due to prior drug-related incidents. Nevertheless, she said, "Matt, to this day, thinks he could have saved Mark's life, if he would have brought him home."

Ernest Ratcliff's widow, Melissa, had been affected by his death in almost every way imaginable.

It had first affected her psychologically. She had found Ernest's body on the morning he died. At first, in the aftermath, she tried to push through the pain. She said she only took about a week and a half off before returning to her job, where she "worked and worked and worked and stayed 'til late in the night." About a year later, she said she "crashed and burned."

Later, she was diagnosed with post-traumatic stress disorder. And for a long time after his death, she avoided the town where they had been living when it happened. But she couldn't entirely escape the triggers and flashbacks. Almost anything would set her off and prompt her to start crying. She told me that it took her a "good 10 years" not to cry at the mention of Ernest's name.

Melissa believes that the psychological trauma from her husband's death is at the root of the physical ailments that followed, including thyroid issues, nerve damage in her neck and shoulder, herniated disks in her back, fibromyalgia, chronic fatigue, and plantar fasciitis. And it wasn't just Ernest's death that affected her, she said. It was also the preceding years of witnessing his addiction, which she described as "pure hell."

During one of our conversations, she told me that her current life was nothing like it had once been. She rarely goes out. She doesn't travel, doesn't go shopping, and doesn't exercise much. She stopped working because she couldn't hold down a job due to her unpredictable health issues. Some days, she'll sleep fourteen hours or more; other days, she's in excruciating pain. "I don't really live anymore," she said.

Ernest's death affected her financially, as well. Because Ernest was so young when he died, his boilermaker's pension provided only a modest monthly payment, which became her main income source when she stopped working. She recalled once asking a DEA agent if the family members of Volkman's patients would get any of the money that was seized from the doctor. She was told that they wouldn't.

This left the possibility of a lawsuit against Volkman, but she said the lawyers she spoke with after Ernest's death didn't remain interested for long. "As soon as they found out [Volkman] didn't have any malpractice insurance you never heard a word from them," she said.

Speaking with these family members, I heard a range of opinions about who deserves blame for their loved one's death.

Many of the people I interviewed blamed Volkman entirely. And even in instances when folks didn't agree to a full interview, they still said enough to make it clear whom they blamed. One spouse of a deceased patient told me, "Just to let you know up front, I hold Dr Volkmann [*sic*] responsible for my husbands death," before declining to answer any additional questions. Another deceased patient's family member who eventually chose not to speak with me said, "That bastard killed my Brother." In a third instance, the son of a deceased patient, who also didn't respond to follow-up requests, told me, "He murdered my mother by prescription."

At the same time, I also spoke with at least one family member — Jeff Swick, the half brother of Kristi Ross — who placed the responsibility mainly on his sister. Swick told me that he didn't respect Volkman, and he thought the man was "pretty much a piece of shit." But he believed that life was about choices, and he told me that his sister had made a choice to find a doctor like Volkman, and she had been fully aware what she was going to get from him. She had made the choice to take the pills she had been prescribed, he said, and she had made the choice to continue using drugs despite knowing that she was hurting herself. "She was a full-grown woman," he said. "She had every opportunity to get off 'em . . . She chose not to."

Other people I spoke with believed that the blame couldn't be placed entirely on the patient or the doctor. Dwight Parsons's stepson told me that his thoughts about his stepdad's death varied from day to day. One day he might blame Volkman; another day he might blame Dwight's friends who were using him for access to pills; still another day, he might blame Dwight himself.

"I think all [of them] hold some kind of responsibility," he said.

But while discussions of blame could sometimes get complicated, assigning *guilt* was not. In more than two dozen conversations with the loved ones of Volkman's patients who had passed away, I found no person —

literally nobody I spoke to — who believed that Paul Volkman was a legitimate physician during his time in southern Ohio.*

They came by this opinion in various ways.

Steven Hieneman's partner, John, had, as a way to confirm his suspicions, visited the clinic himself, knowing that he had no major illness or injuries. When he walked out of the clinic with "enough prescriptions that I could tranquilize an elephant," it was enough for him to make up his mind about Volkman.

Dwight Parsons's stepson, Brad, told me that he remembered his stepdad coming home from the doctor with "bags upon bags upon bags" filled with pill bottles. The word he used to describe the amount of pills Dwight got from the clinic was "astronomical." Even though he was just a teenager at the time, he still thought, "There's no way that is legitimate."

James Estep's wife, Angela, had questions about Volkman based on the fact that the clinic accepted only cash. And she had even more questions after seeing the bag full of prescription bottles that James brought home. These weren't the standard three- or four-inch bottles, she told me. "I'm talking about probably eight inches."

She was worried enough about Tri-State that one day she decided to accompany James on a visit, and what she saw didn't ease her worries. The place looked "dumpy," she would later say. There were a lot of cars parked outside the clinic, and people walking from car to car, talking with one another, like they were at some kind of social function. At one point, while she was waiting in her car, a man walked up and said, "Hey, honey. Are you going to get some pills?" Angie told him that she didn't need to be seen by the doctor. The man then offered to give her money to "sponsor" her to go in, see the doctor, obtain a prescription, and then split the pills with him afterward.

The list of reasons for distrusting the doctor goes on.

For Bryan Brigner's ex-wife, Wendy, it was about the strength of the medications that Bryan was receiving. "He wasn't dying of cancer or anything," she said. "So why put him on something that strong?"

For Melissa Ratcliff it was — among other red flags — the fact that Ernest had large and prominent scars on his arms from previous IV drug

---

* This description also extends to a civil jury in Scioto County, which, after a brief trial in 2008 in a wrongful-death lawsuit brought by Paula Eastley against Volkman and Denise Huffman, ruled in Eastley's favor and awarded her $500,000 from each of the defendants. Though, by the time I checked with Eastley's attorney in 2022, none of that money had been paid.

use by the time he went to the doctor. She felt there was no way that Volkman hadn't seen them: "You couldn't miss them."

Person after person I interviewed — siblings, children, nieces, cousins — expressed their belief that Volkman was a criminal who had chosen greed over proper medical care.

One told me, "He should have known better."

Another said, "People like Volkman cause children to grow up fatherless or motherless."

And another: "To be so uncaring of other human beings. That's the hard thing for me to understand."

And another: "This place was already going downhill and he just added to that."

And another: "Opioids destroyed most of my family and the pill pushing doctors are pure devils."

THE MAGAZINE ARTICLE

In late 2016, I was contacted by an editor at *Cincinnati* magazine who had seen my name mentioned online along with Paul Volkman's. The magazine was interested in publishing something about the case and wanted to know what I knew. After a few weeks of emails and phone calls, they agreed that I was the guy to write a story about it.

I worked on the story for a few months, conducting new interviews while compiling and distilling what I had learned up to that point. In the introductory section I wrote, "Today, more than a decade after Volkman's last clinic closed, Ohio's opiate crisis rages on, with heroin and other opioid derivatives taking center stage." I noted that, while the reasons for the epidemic were varied and complicated, there was little doubt that high-volume pill mill prescribers had played a major role in fueling it. I described the tale of Volkman and other southern Ohio pain clinics as "the prologue to a public health disaster."

In the rest of the piece, I laid out the basics of Volkman's story, including a summary of his pre-Ohio life story, plus descriptions of his tumultuous two-and-a-half-year partnership with Denise, his solo clinics, and the damage his actions had caused in the region. Given my space constraints, I could include only a fraction of what I knew.

It was important to me that the article, like this book, included Volkman's account of his life and career. So nearly eight hundred words in the piece were spent directly quoting from him or his legal filings or describing his interpretation of events. I included one of his lawyer's descriptions of him as an "accomplished, experienced, competent physician working in a rural, under-served area trying to help manage the pain of his patients." I quoted, at length, from his presentencing memo in which he ticked off the differences he saw between himself and a conventional drug dealer. I summarized his explanations for the untimely deaths of his patients. And I mentioned his overall defiance and insistence on his innocence.

The article ran in the July 2017 issue. On the magazine's website, it was given the headline "The Pill Mill That Ravaged Portsmouth."

The article marked a personal milestone. Despite the years I had spent researching the story, I had yet to publish anything based on that reporting. And it was also the first time in my relationship with Volkman that I was "showing my hand" by publicly sharing my impressions of his life and case. Knowing him and knowing what the article said, I suspected that I was lighting a slow-burning fuse.

Sure enough, he exploded.

Much of Volkman's letter in response to the article covered familiar ground. He called Judge Beckwith "corrupt" and the government's expert witnesses "whores," and he was outraged that my article had not portrayed them as such. He made a flurry of revisionist claims about his trial that I knew to be untrue. (Example: "Every one of my former patients admitted that I had taken excellent care of all of their medical issues.")

But much of the letter consisted of invective aimed squarely at me. He called the piece a "vicious, biased screed."* He said that the article showed my "absolutely amazing arrogance and stupidity." He also said — after referring to some of my recently published writing about anxiety and depression, which he had heard about via his daughter, Jane — "As an empathic physician, I do not find any glee in hearing of your mental health problems. However such issues may well be related to your vicious, hateful attacks on me."

---

* About a year after the article's publication, I was informed that the piece had won the "Best Health/Medical Story" category in a contest run by the local chapter of the Society of Professional Journalists.

Toward the end of the note he wrote, "I therefore do not expect any further communication with you, unless such displays a vastly different attitude towards me, and towards the truth."

He signed the letter, "Paul H. Volkman, M.D., PhD."

Volkman and I exchanged a few email messages after this letter, though these notes didn't yield any breakthrough in our relationship.

Before long, I received an email from CorrLinks, the service I had used to exchange emails with Volkman in federal prison. The subject line was "Inmate: VOLKMAN, PAUL H." It contained a short, auto-generated message reading, "The above-named inmate has chosen to remove your email address from his/her approved contact list and, therefore, can not receive or send messages to your email address."

Volkman and I wouldn't speak again for three years, until I contacted him after signing a book deal.

And that renewed connection, in the fall of 2021, lasted just a couple of weeks. He ended it when I refused to help him with background research for one of his legal ploys to get out of prison.

After more than a decade of conversations and correspondence, our interview was officially over.

CO-CONSPIRATORS

Harold Eugene Fletcher's sentencing took place on January 9, 2012, at a federal courthouse in Columbus. During the proceedings, Judge Algenon Marbley told the former pharmacist that he would serve two years in prison, a year of home confinement, and five years of supervised release. For the false tax returns he had filed, he would pay $275,000 in restitution plus an additional fine of $75,000. Following the home confinement, he would also complete 208 hours of community service. The judge also reminded Fletcher that two conditions of his plea deal had been "a permanent prohibition from practicing as a pharmacist and a lifetime ban from having any connection to a pharmacy."

In his remarks, Marbley called Fletcher's case "startling." He noted that Fletcher came from a stable home and was well educated. "Your personal history almost reads like a Horatio Alger tome: a hard-working man who took a detour," he said. "You could have been an icon of the American dream because you were a small businessman who did well."

Instead, his story was now an "unfortunate tale" of a man of great potential who "chose to fritter it away," Marbley said. He said that Fletcher's motivation seemed to have been "pure greed."

There were no relatives of former Volkman patients who spoke at Fletcher's sentencing hearing. However, he did hear from Barbara Howard, the mother of a thirty-four-year-old woman who had died in 2009 after Fletcher filled her prescriptions from a Scioto County pain clinic.

Howard began by saying that she lived in Scioto County, which is the "first county in history to be under a declared public health emergency due to prescription drug overdoses." She said that Fletcher had "a lot to do" with that devastation.

Howard said that her daughter, Leslie, was loved by all who knew her. "Her laughter was intoxicating," she said. She then described the events that led to Leslie's death. She had gone to a pill mill in Wheelersburg (ten miles east of Portsmouth), and afterward, none of the local pharmacies would fill that clinic's prescriptions. So the next day she drove a hundred miles to Fletcher's pharmacy in Columbus. Howard said that the pharmacy was well known in Scioto County as a business that "conspire[d] with unethical pill mill doctors and would fill anything for a price."

Leslie died within hours of the prescriptions being filled. When this happened "my world ended as I knew it," Howard said.

In closing, she instructed Fletcher not to forget her daughter's name, "because I will never, ever forget yours."

Fletcher spoke only briefly at the hearing, to thank family members and friends who had supported him during his case. He did not discuss the crimes for which he was being sentenced. And he did not apologize to anyone other than his son for "not being with him for the time which I'm going to be away."

In March 2012, three months after Fletcher was sentenced, the Ohio State Board of Pharmacy — the same regulatory agency that, during his career, had admonished him multiple times, fined him twice, placed him on probation twice, and briefly suspended his license to practice pharmacy — once again suspended his license. Then, in January 2013, the board voted unanimously to permanently revoke it.

Fletcher was released from prison in November 2013, and he appears to have returned to Columbus. As of late 2022, he was working at least

part-time as a real estate agent for rental apartments in the city. The name
H. E. Fletcher appeared online next to several listings in the Columbus
area, and when I text-messaged the phone number listed on those advertisements, he confirmed that it was the same Harold Eugene Fletcher who
once owned East Main Street Pharmacy.

He did not respond to my additional questions for this book.

Alice Huffman served her five-year prison sentence at a federal prison
camp in Alderson, West Virginia, which is about two hundred miles southeast of Portsmouth, near the border between West Virginia and Virginia.

Founded in 1927 and situated on ninety-five acres in the foothills of the
Allegheny Mountains, the complex was the nation's first federal prison for
women. Former inmates include singer Billie Holiday; Lynnette "Squeaky"
Fromme, a member of Charles Manson's "family" cult who attempted to
assassinate President Gerald Ford; and Martha Stewart, the TV personality and home decor mogul who spent five months there after her conviction for charges related to insider trading.

I exchanged a few letters with Alice in prison. The eight handwritten
pages she sent me wound up being my only direct communication from
her. When I asked her what life was like at Alderson, she said that the
campus was pretty, the food was decent, and she was allowed to mostly
do as she pleased. In one letter, she said that inmates could give one "craft
item" to family members as gifts, and she was making a blanket to give to
her son during an upcoming visit. "It's not the worst thing I could imagine
by far when you think of 'Prison,'" she wrote, "but it isn't home with my
children so I hate it every second of every day."

When I asked whether she believed she belonged in prison, her answer
was a resounding "NO!!" She felt that she was being wrongly blamed for
things that Volkman and her mother had done. She said that she didn't
own the pain clinic, didn't hire or fire anyone, and didn't make executive or medical decisions. She said in her years working at Tri-State, she
purchased office and medical supplies, handled payroll, sent out patients'
medical records in response to requests, and completed other clerical
tasks. "I didn't conspire to commit a criminal act," she wrote. "I simply
accepted a job to manage a medical clinic. I got paid a salary, $550.00 per
week (yes that's all!)."

She did think that her mother deserved to be punished, though. At the time of our correspondence in 2012, she hadn't spoken with Denise in nearly a year. "She doesn't care about people," Alice wrote.

Alice was released from prison in May 2016 and eventually moved to Ashland, Kentucky, a city of twenty thousand about thirty miles east of Portsmouth. She initially worked as a waitress but later found work as a peer-support counselor at an outpatient drug and alcohol rehabilitation center. A friend of hers whom I spoke to felt that Alice had pursued work in the field at least in part "because she felt bad for all the people's lives that were lost" due to the pain clinic.

At some point after her release from prison, Alice was diagnosed with an aggressive form of cancer. According to her friend, the pain she endured was "excruciating," and she was prescribed narcotic pain relievers.

Alice died at her home in Ashland on December 14, 2019, less than two weeks after her forty-fifth birthday. She had been free from prison for a little more than three and a half years. Her obituary read, in part, "She enjoyed more than anything being with her family whom she loved dearly, reading and traveling. She loved to give back to her community and helping others around her."

The obituary did not mention her criminal case.

Denise Huffman was scheduled for sentencing in November 2011, eight months after her testimony in the Volkman trial. But on the eve of the hearing, she filed a motion stating an intent to withdraw her guilty plea.

The motion, written by her lawyer, explained that she had been confused and intimidated when entering her plea the previous year and had done so "without sufficient time to fully digest, understand, and consider the potential consequences."

In response, Judge Beckwith denied the motion on the grounds that there was nothing in the guilty-plea proceedings to justify this request. She added that "the case had been pending for more than three years when [Denise] signed the plea agreement, so she cannot credibly claim that she did not understand the charges, especially in view of the lengthy recitation of the facts at the change of plea hearing." In addition, the judge issued an order committing Huffman, who had remained free while awaiting sentencing, to the custody of the Bureau of Prisons for psychological testing to determine if she was "suffering from a mental disease or defect rendering her mentally incompetent to the extent that she is unable to understand the nature and consequences of the proceedings against her."

After about a week in custody, Huffman, through her lawyer, filed a motion requesting immediate release. The filing argued that, while in jail, her health conditions were not being properly addressed, her "strict daily regimen" of medications had been disrupted, and she needed to be released immediately to prevent further "serious physical harm."

This request was also denied by the judge, who described it as a "misguided effort to seek release from custody before the psychological evaluation is completed." Beckwith added:

> Defendant's appearance and behavior at the November 8 [2011] hearing convinced the Court that she must be placed in a strictly controlled environment where she lacks free access to narcotics in order to properly determine if she is in fact suffering from a mental disease or defect, or is simply exhibiting signs and symptoms of an apparently long-standing dependence on narcotics and "pain killers," or some combination of these conditions.

The psychological evaluation found Denise to be competent. And the judge's denial of her attempt to withdraw her guilty plea remained.

Denise's sentencing took place in Cincinnati on the afternoon of February 14, 2012, a few hours after Volkman's. The hearing featured many of the same players from the morning's proceedings. Tim Oakley and Adam Wright represented the prosecution. Paula Eastley, the mother of Steven Hieneman, returned as the lone speaker on behalf of the families of deceased patients.

During her remarks, Eastley said that she generally applauds people who succeed in life with little or no formal education. But Denise deserved no such praise. She was "an unscrupulous woman running a physician's office with an eighth-grade education" who, Eastley said, had "received on-the-job training by a former pain clinic operator, Dr. David Procter, who is in prison now for dispensing drugs for cash."

Eastley urged the maximum possible sentence for two reasons. She thought it was important to send a message to the public that actions like Denise's wouldn't be tolerated. And she also said, "Our community does not want Denise Huffman back in it opening up another pain clinic in five years."

Oakley's comments were relatively brief. When discussing Tri-State Healthcare, he said that "the entirety of the organization was just simply to hand out pills to the people who were willing to pay for them." And Denise's role in this business was significant, he argued. She owned and operated the clinic. She hired the doctors, including Volkman. When local pharmacies refused to fill the clinic's scripts, she, along with Volkman, co-opened the dispensary. "She is as involved as anybody in this conspiracy," he said.

Oakley said that the consequences of Denise and Paul's partnership was "ongoing" more than six years after their split. Their clinics "generated countless, countless addicts [and] countless criminals, who are committing crimes to pay for narcotics," he said. In 2012, the epidemic in southern Ohio was still raging, with ever-larger numbers of people lost to addiction and overdose. Tri-State Healthcare, he said, was "one of the clinics that showed the other clinics how to start."

Huffman's comments during the hearing were brief and disorganized. She started by saying, "As you know, I'm not very well at speaking."

Then, apparently in response to what Paula Eastley had said, she said, "I'm a mother and I can understand."

The rest of her remarks, as they appear in the court record, are as follows:

> But I don't want to get into, you know — I wasn't in the clinic like I should have been. I have admitted, you know, responsibility. I was wrong.
>
> And I'm a mother. I'm a grandmother, you know. I guess I just — you know, I understand what she would feel as she does.
>
> But I can only, you know, say I'm sorry so many times. And I wouldn't go back tomorrow. I wouldn't, you know, ever go back and, you know, do anything.

After this jumbled monologue, her lawyer asked her to clarify what, exactly, she would choose not to do over again. To this, Denise offered a final statement for the court record. "It wasn't meant to be like that," she said.

During the hearing, Denise's attorney requested leniency for several reasons. He said that his client was a fifty-eight-year-old woman in poor health who had no prior criminal background. He claimed that Denise had no knowledge of the firearms in the clinic.* He maintained both the purity of Denise's intentions and her lack of influence over Paul Volkman, whom he portrayed as the bad actor at the clinic. The doctor was "his own boss," he said. "No one could tell him anything. He would belittle her. She just took a passive role with him." He also said that Denise was unaware about the exact nature of the activities at the clinic because she "did not spend enough time there."

In her comments about Denise's conduct, Beckwith was unsparing. She called Denise's criminal actions "reprehensible" and said that she had caused both physical and emotional damage to many people and their families. "She chose to involve herself in a pain clinic with full knowledge that addicted individuals were coming simply to obtain drugs to feed their addiction," she said.

At one point, she said, "I don't think it takes a medical expert to know that a small clinic in a small town like Portsmouth that dispensed in excess of one million dosage units is not fulfilling a legitimate medical need of patients or customers."

Beckwith stated that a "significant period of incarceration" was needed to reflect the severity of the offense and provide a just punishment. As the hearing wound down, she sentenced the founder and owner of Tri-State Healthcare to 152 months (twelve and two-thirds years) in federal prison.

Denise served her sentence at a federal prison in Lexington, Kentucky. Because of her general unwillingness to speak with me, I don't know much about her time there.

But public documents about her case reveal at least one aspect of her post-Tri-State life. In February 2012, two weeks after her sentencing, Denise submitted a sworn affidavit stating that she had no money. In the document, she said that neither she nor her husband was employed; she had no cash or money in any bank accounts; and she did not own any "real estate, stocks, bonds, notes, automobiles, or any other valuable property." In fact, she owed an estimated $10,000 to a nearby hospital for care she had received there.

The exact amount of money that Denise made from her stint as a pain clinic owner is disputed. At one point during her case, prosecutors had

* This strikes me as implausible. The DEA's videotaped walk-through of the Tri-State building from 2005 showed three guns in plain sight.

filed a motion seeking a forfeiture order for $3,024,198, which, they argued, represented "the proceeds . . . of her criminal activity at Tri-State Health Care & Pain Management."

An accompanying document detailed how the government had arrived at this estimate. Most of the money — $2,175,000 — was believed to have been generated from patient visit fees during Volkman's tenure at Tri-State from April 2003 to September 2005. The remaining $859,178.30 was estimated revenues from the on-site dispensary, based on price sheets and other records that were seized during the DEA's June 2005 raid. "We considered any pills that could not be accounted for to have been dispensed, sold, or otherwise distributed by Tri-State," the document noted.

But according to Denise's attorney's remarks in a 2008 trial stemming from a wrongful-death lawsuit filed by the mother of Steven Hieneman, her profits from the clinic were considerably less than that. In his closing arguments from the short trial in Scioto County, Denise's attorney referred to the pages of Tri-State bank records that had been entered into the trial record. Though the plaintiff's attorneys had submitted those pages to show the amounts of money flowing into the clinic, Denise's lawyer argued that they were, in fact, evidence of the modesty of the clinic's profits.

"There's been a lot of talk about profits," he said. "Where is that evidence, ladies and gentlemen?" He said that the records showed that, after Denise paid her bills, including payroll and orders for the dispensary, she was left with around $12,000 in profit per month. "Is that what sounds like somebody getting rich?" he asked.[*]

Whatever the amount Denise made from her foray into pain-clinic ownership, by the time she reported to prison in 2012, she was broke.

Denise was released from prison in 2020, after serving eight years. She appears to have moved back to the region where she spent most of her life. I exchanged a handful of messages with her, via Facebook, after her release, and we had previously swapped a few short notes before she went to prison. All told, over the course of my reporting, she sent me around a thousand words.

One theme of those brief conversations was her apparent sense of victimhood. In one note from 2021, she described her sentence as "unjust." In another note, she said the case had been a "real life nightmare for me

---

[*] If you multiply this sum by 28, the number of months that she and Volkman worked together, it adds up to $336,000, or a little over one-tenth of the government's $3 million estimate.

and my family." At no point did she mention any of the families whose loved ones had died after receiving pills from Tri-State.

Another theme was her eagerness to place blame on Paul Volkman. At one point she said that hiring him was "the biggest mistake I ever made in my life."

Perhaps the most prominent aspect of these brief notes was Denise's insistence that there was more to her story.

"I'm very interested if a story is written to have the <u>truth</u> written," she told me in 2012.

Later, she added, "On my part there are things that people were never made aware of that may be rather shocking. I just can't go into some things right now that can't be left out."

Sometimes, she would emphasize how unreliable Volkman's version of events was (which I don't necessarily dispute). In another case, she described how misleading the press coverage had been.

But despite her avowed interest in telling the previously unreported "<u>truth</u>," she never seemed ready to share that story. I invited her to do so, repeatedly. And eventually, as I sent more questions, she responded with four words in August 2021: "No more questions please."

This was the last time I heard from her.

ADAM AND JANE

Volkman's attack at the hands of a fellow inmate in 2012 was apparently not the only violence he experienced in prison. In 2015, he had another run-in at USP Terre Haute, which he described in detail in a letter to his son, Adam, who then passed the note along to me.

The perpetrator was, in Volkman's telling, a twenty-four-year-old "vicious sociopath" who was serving time for dealing drugs and raping a young girl at gunpoint — both crimes that, according to Volkman, the young man boasted about. As Volkman told it, the incident began after he made the "stupid" decision to lend the man $5. At some point thereafter, the man "burst" into Volkman's room, punched him in the eye (lacerating his temple in the process), knocked him to the floor, and choked him, before demanding more money.

Despite describing himself as being in "outstanding shape for a 69 [year-old]," Volkman admitted that he knew nothing about fighting and could only manage to scratch the man's face in his defense. But during the dispute a guard happened to look into Volkman's cell and brought the fight to an end. In his letter to his son, Volkman explained that he suspected that his attacker had a long-running scheme to borrow money from fellow inmates and then start fights so that he could be transferred to another prison before paying his debts. "I was his safe target this time," he said.

After the attack, both men were sent to the "Hole" — the Special Housing Unit — as a result. Once they arrived, their cells were apparently close enough that they could hear each other speak. In his letter to his son, Volkman wrote, "Last night, he said his urine is brown which likely means he is in liver failure from hep c. Hopefully he will die before he is turned loose. Like any rabid dog, he should be exterminated."

Due to these attacks, and other incidents involving being "assaulted and extorted by skinheads," in 2016, Volkman secured a transfer to a second federal prison: USP Coleman, outside of Orlando, Florida.

But the move did not bring an end to his troubles. In 2019, Volkman suffered from what his daughter described as a "surprise choking attack from a fellow prisoner." And in 2020, he was attacked by his cellmate; Volkman said he had been "severely beaten by my psychotic cellmate, breaking 3 ribs and stopping my heart for about 30 seconds." He was "almost murdered," he said.

Between these two attacks, Volkman also sustained a head injury when, according to his daughter, the leg of a chair he was sitting on buckled and he fell. In the following hours, he experienced nausea, dizziness, and rapid eye movements, which led him to believe that he was suffering from a cerebral bleed. In his daughter's telling, "he was refused medical care for some time."

By the time that these assaults and injuries befell her imprisoned father, Jane and Paul had reconciled from their previous estrangement. And in messages to me, Jane expressed regret over some of the critical things she had previously said about him. She said her feelings had changed.

The extent of those changed feelings became clearer as I read her Facebook posts and other writings defending her father. In one post from 2019, she described her father's "unjust imprisonment, serving a life sentence, after prescribing opioid relief to those he thought needed it." In another post, she wrote, "I have hope that one day the true condition of his heart — that he never intended to hurt anyone but rather only sought to alleviate suffering — will come to light and that he will be released."

In a post from 2020, she described him as "a gentle man, who has never committed a violent act in his life . . . who yet remains in prison without justification, for the 'crime' of prescribing pain relief pharmaceuticals to those who were suffering."

Jane's defense of her father escalated in 2020, when she and her husband launched a fundraising campaign to help Paul prepare a petition for compassionate release from prison based on his age and health issues. The lawyer they hoped to retain had a track record of helping doctors in similar situations, and the couple aimed to raise $5,000.

Jane and Steve's pitch on the crowdfunding website described Volkman with glowing language: a "kind man and a model prisoner," a "loving grandfather" who had "lived his entire life serving others, loving his family and saving lives." They portrayed him as a man unfairly suffering through hellish tribulations, including unprovoked beatings from fellow inmates, retaliation from angry guards, deprivation of phone calls except for a single short call per month, and confinement to a small cell in the "special housing unit" for twenty-four hours per day.

This suffering had spilled over into their own lives, the couple said. "[We] can't tell you all how gut wrenching it can be to listen to an elderly man . . . tell these stories with absolute fear in his voice, with anxiety dripping from every word that was so intense you could feel it in your soul," they wrote.

Although the plea for help was about Paul's imprisonment, there was little discussion of his case on the fundraising page.* The most direct commentary appeared in a section arguing that Paul didn't deserve to die in prison because he was "not responsible for anyone's death."

When Volkman eventually filed the motion for compassionate release (which was rejected), it included signed affidavits from both Jane and her husband stating that, in the event of Paul's release, they were willing to have him live in their home and they had the financial means to care for him.

But when I reached out to her during my final fact-checking in the summer of 2023, Jane's feelings had shifted once again. She said that discussing her father's case remained difficult because "it's so painful." But she was no longer interested in defending him.

In subsequent notes, she described her struggle with having a father in

---

* Later when I asked if she had read the trial transcript, she told me that she had not.

prison. Due to the severity of his sentence, and his tribulations in prison, she and her husband had felt sympathy for him. And, for a while, she felt that "there was goodness" in honoring him as a father by taking his phone calls and allowing him to speak with her three young kids. She felt that staying in touch with him after his conviction was a way to "salvage some relationship with him." This also involved listening to him defend himself and trying to give him the benefit of the doubt, she said. But, over time, her reserves of patience and sympathy had run out. "Recent events, where he treated even me and my family with contempt, have exhausted my openness to stay connected to him," she said.

Her thinking about the case itself had changed as well. She said that the case and its aftermath had hit her like a "tsunami," and, for years, she had been "overwhelmed and struggling and immature." Now, though, she said she had arrived at a place where she could see the facts more dispassionately, "without a stressful inward fight or flight response." She said that she had "always known that my dad did some sketchy things." But she hadn't appreciated "the extent of the nature of his personality." And, more specifically, she said he had never given her a convincing answer about why he had reopened his clinics after a raid by federal agents. She said that she did not think he was innocent. In one note, she wrote: "Today I see. A doctor who dispensed what was sought, not caring about what happened next to other people. Thought he could get away with it. Will defend himself forever."

She said that arriving at this clarity was a relief. She felt lighter. "Now I'm free of any connection to him," she said. "And that's good."

Adam and Liz had never questioned the merits of Paul's conviction.

When I spoke with them in the years after Paul's sentencing, their memories of pre-prison interactions remained fresh. Adam pointed to the "obscene negative judgments" that Paul had expressed toward him before their estrangement. And he was also troubled by the way his dad had, as he saw it, manipulated Jane into becoming an advocate for his cause. "I think the danger that he poses is more than just to patients; it's to those around him," he told me. He described Paul as a "vindictive, malicious person."

By the last time I interviewed Adam and Liz, in late 2022, they had decided to tell their kids about Paul's case for the first time, which was a conversation they had put off for years. The story that they told their daughters, and later described to me, was straightforward: Paul had overprescribed pain medication, a "lot" of people had died as a result, and his punishment was spending the rest of his life in prison. It was not a story about a wrongful conviction.

During my last conversation with them, Liz mentioned her desire to correct the record about something that Paul had written in his 2018 open letter published by the Doctors of Courage blog. In the letter, he had written that because of his criminal case, "My 43-year-old son has completely withdrawn from any communication with me."

But this was "not true at all," Liz said. She explained that there had been many issues between Paul and Adam before his criminal case, and their estrangement had nothing to do with Paul's crimes. After his sentencing, she had remained concerned about the possibility that he could get out of prison due to some kind of legal technicality. Adam said that if his dad secured a release from prison, he still had no intention of seeing or talking to him.

Over the course of my research and work on this book, I shared some documents about Paul's life and career with Adam and Liz. These included some of the malpractice complaints against him, documents from his criminal case, and his bankruptcy filing. In response, Adam said that he had a vague sense that his father had faced some lawsuits, but he knew nothing about Paul's two civil jury trials.

Liz was particularly surprised by Paul's 1998 bankruptcy filing in which, aside from two retirement accounts, he claimed possession of just a few thousand dollars' worth of clothes, furniture, and personal belongings. She was "blown away" by seeing his assets laid out in such a way, considering how she had perceived Adam's parents at the time. "They lived like they had a lot of wealth, and money was flying out the door," she said.

In one of my last conversations with Adam, I asked him if there was anything he would say to the family members of his dad's patients. Given his father's steadfast denial of any wrongdoing, I felt it was worth offering him a chance to say something.

Adam wasn't offended by the question. And he began with, "I would just say, 'I'm so sorry. I am truly, terribly sorry that this happened.'"

He said he was sorry not just for the people who died but others, too, who may have had addiction or other problems related to his dad's activity in southern Ohio. He said he felt no animosity toward these people.

He was not proud of what his father had done, and it was terrible to think about those things, he said. But he had no doubt that his father was at fault.

Of the families who lost loved ones in Ohio, he said, "They are victims."

A MAN OF PRINCIPLE

Volkman underwent at least two dramatic changes in the years after his sentencing.

The first was political.

In the years before his trial, Volkman's comments about his case had strong political overtones. In an online response to a 2007 *New York Times* article about the prosecution of another pain doctor, he was, as usual, mercilessly critical of the DEA. But in an apparent reference to the administration of then president George W. Bush, he also lashed out at "cooperating Bushie US attorneys." In one of those online comments, he wrote, "I wish I was describing Nazi Germany or Stalinist (or Putin's) Russia. Unfortunately, I am talking about the Republican States of America."

His left-leaning views remained prominent during our pretrial interviews in Chicago. He expressed admiration for two of the most liberal US senators, Bernie Sanders and Al Franken, and at one point, wished "a pox" upon the conservative Supreme Court justice Antonin Scalia. He spoke disparagingly about the "top half of a percent" of Americans controlling a vast majority of the nation's wealth. And while discussing the Department of Justice under President Barack Obama, he lamented the number of holdovers from the previous administration who were still working there. They were, he said, "the same people that have been implementing the same horrible anti-gay, anti-civil rights, agenda for the last eight years of . . . Bush."

But by 2016, his views had changed drastically. In emails from prison, he told me that he now read the *Wall Street Journal* every day and listened to hours of conservative talk radio, including the popular right-wing commentator Rush Limbaugh. His emails were peppered with insults toward Democratic politicians. Barack Obama was "a communist ideologue" who was "by far the worst POTUS in this country's sorry history." Hillary Clinton was a "a rank, money-grubbing, corrupt fascist who has never in her life accomplished anything for anyone else, and who belongs in jail." He parroted far-right conspiracy theories, like the notion that former Obama adviser Valerie Jarrett was "Iranian" (she was not) or that the mother of Huma Abedin, Hillary Clinton's longtime deputy chief of staff, was the "the editor of the Muslim Brotherhood newspaper in Beirut" (also untrue). He described the scientific-consensus-backed notion that climate change was occurring due to human activity as a "hoax" perpetrated by "Obama and his henchpersons."

A couple weeks after the 2016 presidential election, he told me that he was "very gratified that Trump won, over the communist, fascist, socialist democrats."

The second change that he underwent was religious.

Both before and after his conviction, Volkman had described himself as a non-observant Jew. He explained that he had completed a bar mitzvah during his teenage years, and his two children had also participated in the religious ritual symbolizing the passage into adulthood. At one point, in a letter, he told me that he stood by his "cultural and ethnic identity as a Jew," and, though he didn't believe in God, he felt Judaism offered "good moral guidelines by which to live."

During these conversations, he also spoke with open contempt of his daughter's conversion to Messianic Judaism. By adopting this new Christian faith, Jane had "rejected her cultural, ethnic, and family roots" and "embraced a creed historically responsible for the persecution, torture, and murder of Jews for 2000 years," he said in a 2011 letter. After noting that, in Nazi Germany, she would have been treated like any other Jew, he wrote, "Once she realizes that I am a lost cause as a baptism candidate, Jane will, thankfully, be done with me."

But by 2019, something had changed. On May 1, Jane wrote on Facebook that she was "overjoyed" to share that her father had converted to Messianic Judaism. In fact, she said, he was already "testifying" to his fellow inmates. "He is working on his testimony, which I will share in the future," she wrote, before adding, "Hallejulah!!! [sic]"

Sure enough, a couple of weeks later, she shared a nearly four-thousand-word essay that Paul had written. The Facebook post was titled "Conversion Testimony of My Father Paul, From Atheist, Nominal Jew to Messianic Believer."

What followed was an autobiographical narrative with a focus on the religious aspects of Volkman's life. He explained how his maternal grandfather was a rabbi, though he "never heard either parent discuss their belief in God." He said that, as an adult, "I led Passover Seders, and we of course did Hannukah and went to services on the High Holidays. But that was pretty much as far as our Judaism went."

Alongside this spiritual tale, he outlined his life story, with a few trademark flourishes of grandiosity. He noted that the chairman of the pharmacology department at the University of Chicago had "told me that I was the best grad student he had had in 30 years." Later, he mentioned the "groundbreaking, potentially lifesaving treatment regimen" he had (supposedly) discovered during post-med-school research, which his supervisor had refused to publish, prompting Volkman to leave academic medicine in "utter disgust." He described his criminal case as a "horrific injustice imposed on me by the government."

Volkman said that his religious awakening began when he noticed how his daughter had responded to his "coldness" and "anger" with forgiveness, love, and kindness. When he asked her how this was possible, she said that Jesus had helped her, and if he was interested, Jesus could help him, too. "At that realization," he said, "I knew that I had to take a serious look at the faith of Jane and [her husband] Steve." At the time, he said, he was in a state of "deep spiritual turmoil and reorganization."

From there, in a section titled "God Opens My Heart," he described reading books by pastors, professors, two astronomers, and a renowned Finnish biochemist. He also read a fifteen-hundred-page tome called *The Complete Jewish Bible*, which had convinced him that believing in Jesus and identifying as Jewish were not mutually exclusive, because, as he wrote, "Jesus was and is the Messiah for all mankind." He was also impressed by the online testimonial from one of Donald Trump's lawyers, Jay Sekulow, who had written about a spiritual journey that began with secular Judaism ("quite similar to mine," Volkman noted) and eventually led to Messianic Judaism. Volkman said that he was inclined to trust Sekulow, whom he had previously heard on Sean Hannity's radio show and saw as "a brilliant lawyer and a great advocate for my favorite POTUS of all time."

By the end of this journey, he said that he had been "well and properly convinced to believe in God, that Jesus is the Son of God, that Jesus died for all of mankind's sins, and that Jesus was resurrected."

Later, via email, he confirmed to me that he did, indeed, now identify as a Messianic Jew and that he practiced, read, and studied scripture. He also said that he prayed daily for his family, the United States, and "the coming of the Kingdom of Yashua on Earth, which should be soon, considering that the Great Tribulation is upon us right now."

———

I was initially somewhat mystified by these changes in Volkman's life. In the ten years I had known him, he had transformed from a nonpracticing secular Jew who watched MSNBC and admired Bernie Sanders to a Donald-Trump-supporting, right-wing-radio-listening, climate-change-denying Messianic Jew.

But the more I thought about these changes, the more sense they made. These were, after all, not the first times I had seen Paul undergo dramatic shifts in opinion.

In an email written shortly after his arrival in southern Ohio in 2003, he had described Denise Huffman as a "brilliant, tough matriarch" who had started her clinic for honest reasons. But by the time I met him in 2009, he portrayed Denise as an untrustworthy serial gambler who stole pills from the dispensary and who was "crafty" in the ways she hid her true nature and motives. He viewed her with contempt.

Similarly, during our early interviews, he had been extremely disparaging toward his court-appointed defense attorney Wende Cross, whom he described as a "floozy" and a "nasty . . . bitch." But then, following a judge's demand that he work amicably with her, he told me that she had undergone an "amazing transformation" after which she struck him as "earnest" and "bright." After his conviction, though, he reverted to his initial disdain and anger. Cross was (once again, apparently) an "incompetent Benedict Arnold."

I would add myself to this category as well, since, though my own stated goals for this project never wavered, Volkman's actions and comments toward me oscillated wildly. First, in 2009 and 2010, he welcomed my interest in the story. Later, in early 2011, he called me angrily to criticize my reporting and call my approach "incredibly stupid." After his conviction, he told me that a friend had described my refusal of his demands that I become an advocate on his behalf as "perfectly appropriate positions as a budding young journalist," and he resumed speaking to me. At one point in our ensuing correspondence, he wrote, "Could I be the father you didn't have, and you be the son I didn't have? Perhaps." But then, years later, after reading my *Cincinnati* magazine article, I was a "corrupt, brainwashed journalist" who had written a "vicious, biased screed" that showed my "absolutely amazing arrogance and stupidity."

And though his own claims about his general innocence never changed, the exact *reasons* for that innocence did. In 2006, while protesting the DEA's seizure of his bank accounts, Volkman had written, "In approximately ten instances over about three years, patients of mine expired from apparent overdoses," and added that "these deaths were most likely self-inflicted in chronic pain patients well known to have a high risk of suicide." But later, after his trial, he would claim — in many places, but specifically his Doctors of Courage open letter from 2018 — that "none" of his deceased patients "had toxicology results which were consistent with drug overdose deaths" and that they had "died from their chronic conditions," including "severe heart disease."

Throughout these extreme fluctuations in his stated positions, Volkman described himself as a man of principles.

He was, in the words of one letter, a "good, principled, honest, courageous" man, and, in another, a "law abiding, responsible physician and family man." Elsewhere, he described himself as an "empathic physician" and a "careful and conscientious doctor for my patients." In another letter, he said that he had been motivated to work in pain management "out of compassion and concern."

Integral to this portrayal of himself were his descriptions of his scientific training. In a letter to me from the Butler County Jail, when, discussing the University of Chicago, he wrote that he still maintained the "scientific, data-based approach" that he learned there. And in his 2019 narrative describing his conversion to Messianic Judaism, he returned to that idea. "As a physician and medical scientist, I was very much an advocate of scientific evidence," he wrote. "If something could not be seen, heard, felt, weighed, or measured, I did not believe in it."

He was, in other words, asking me — asking you — to believe that virtually everyone but him was wobbly, unreliable, and corrupt. Meanwhile, *he* was the good, principled, and honest man of science.

To believe Paul Volkman, you needed to believe that despite his wild, glaring, and transparently self-interested changes of heart and mind, *he* was the one who was steady and unchanging.

ALL-AMERICA CITY

In August 2018, more than fourteen hundred people gathered in downtown Portsmouth to break the Guinness world record for simultaneous plant-potting. A few months later, more than 1,850 assembled nearby to break the record for most people singing Christmas carols at one place and time, snatching the record from its previous holder, Waukesha, Wisconsin. A year later, in December 2019, the city claimed yet another Christmas-themed record when 1,482 people gathered in Portsmouth to wrap gifts simultaneously.

Each of these events was accompanied by a blast of press releases, which often led to coverage from local news outlets. "Portsmouth, Ohio has been in the national spotlight for over a decade due to the devastating effects from the rise and fall of its 'pill mills,'" read a release promoting the plant-potting record attempt. "Our hope is that an epic one-day downtown transformation and setting a GUINNESS WORLD RECORDS title will encourage outsiders, including businesses, to plant Portsmouth as a destination for business relocation, tourism, and raising a family."

At the bottom of the release was the name and email address of a local attorney, Jeremy Burnside, who had started an organization called Friends of Portsmouth. And because I had written an article about Paul Volkman and his pain clinics in *Cincinnati* magazine in 2017, I later received a personal email from Burnside.

"As you can imagine, you are not the only national reporter to write about our problem," he said. "As you also can imagine, there had to be a breaking point — a rally cry where the whole community got together to say, 'enough.'"

He was writing to inquire if I would consider writing a follow-up story about how, in his words, "the opioid epicenter is now . . . rising from the addiction ashes to rebuild through restoring community pride."

Burnside wasn't the only one who was eager to shift the narrative about Portsmouth. In a *Cincinnati Enquirer* op-ed from 2019, Ryan Ottney, a former *Portsmouth Daily Times* reporter who had become a councilman in the nearby village of New Boston, said that he appreciated the need to tell stories about Portsmouth's opiate-related struggles. "But there's another side to Scioto County that doesn't often make the news," he said. "It's the people who have stayed in town and are working together to help rebuild our community." In the essay, he touted the achievements of local advocates for the homeless, as well as community programs focused on mental health, job training, and GED courses. In a separate *Enquirer* essay from 2019, Brad Wenstrup, the congressman for Ohio's Second District, echoed Ottney's message: "For every negative statistic and damaging headline, there are stories of dedicated Portsmouth citizens pouring their hearts and souls into making a positive difference in their city."

In May 2019, community members in Portsmouth held a pep-rally-style press conference at the city's riverfront to call attention to various projects taking place in and around the city. On hand were the mayor, the county commissioner, the president of Shawnee State University, and a squad of pom-pom-waving cheerleaders. Among the developments mentioned were a new series of mountain-biking trails in the nearby hills, the return of powerboat racing to a local stretch of the Ohio River, and plans to build a new hotel downtown, which would mark the first multistory construction project in the neighborhood in decades.

The momentum continued the following year, when the National Civic League named Portsmouth one of its ten "All-America Cities" for 2020. The distinction, bestowed by the Colorado-based nonprofit to cities and towns annually since the late 1940s, carried no formal reward. But it did offer a morale boost, and, as the league noted, recently named All-America Cities often saw a surge in tourism and interest from businesses and prospective residents.

In its application, Portsmouth had mentioned that at, one point, there were as many as eleven rogue pain clinics in Scioto County that "operated almost exclusively to push opioid painkillers on people who were not aware of how addictive such medication could be." Over time, the application said, "routine and repetitive" negative press coverage had helped to cement the town's reputation as one of the nation's worst-hit places of the opiate epidemic.

The application argued that an All-America City distinction would help to change the city's image. And it would fit nicely alongside the city's beautification and restoration initiatives.

In late October 2022, I made one last reporting trip to Portsmouth.

This trip marked my tenth time visiting the city, though it was my first time back since shortly after Volkman's sentencing, in February 2012. Due to a fortunate bit of timing, I happened to arrive during a photogenic week in mid-autumn, when the hills surrounding the city were splashed with vibrant yellows, oranges, and reds.

At first glance, the city itself didn't look much different from previous visits. I saw plenty of empty storefronts, hollowed-out houses, and abandoned buildings with boarded-up windows. But on closer inspection, there were in fact several new sights. On the drive downtown, I passed a new, three-story, $10 million facility recently built by the local hospital, Southern Ohio Medical Center. Not far away was an upscale coffee shop called the Lofts and a gastro pub called Patties & Pints. Next to city hall was a new dog park; on the other side of town, the city had built a skate park with the help of funding from the foundation of legendary skateboarder Tony Hawk.

Meanwhile, downtown, new banners hung from lamp poles touting notable people who once lived in the area. One was dedicated to Theodore Wilburn Jr., a navy veteran who was the city's first Black police chief in the early 1960s. Another featured the teacher and abolitionist Betsy Mix Cowles, who had served as the president of Ohio's first Women's Rights Commission in 1850.

The city wasn't transformed, by any means. But it did seem to be moving in a good direction.

In late 2022, Scioto County was still one of the poorest counties in Ohio, with higher poverty and unemployment rates than the state and country. And it remained the lowest-ranked county in the state for health indicators like length of life and quality of life.

Opiate-related problems persisted. Between 2015 and 2020, Scioto County was, by far, the Ohio county with the highest rate of unintentional drug overdose deaths. In 2019, the county recorded seventy-nine overdose deaths, which meant that, on average, the epidemic was still claiming at least one life per week. These totals long surpassed the numbers that had prompted County Health Commissioner Aaron Adams to declare a state of emergency in 2010. But here, as in many places around the country, the state of emergency had simply become the status quo.

At the same time, though, rehab facilities had proliferated. The list of Portsmouth-based treatment centers now included Shawnee Counseling Center, BrightView, Hopesource, Sunrise Treatment Center, and ASCEND Counseling and Recovery Services. Rehab or residential facilities had also popped up in the nearby towns of West Portsmouth, Franklin Furnace, and Wheelersburg.

One of these organizations, Pinnacle Treatment Centers, made news when it purchased the sprawling South Shore, Kentucky, mansion that had once belonged to the region's pill mill "godfather," Dr. David Procter. After renovation, the house was repurposed as a thirty-two-bed residential facility. When the center opened in 2016, the *Cincinnati Enquirer* announced: "Karma: Pill Mill Doc's Home Gets New Use." The report noted that, while Procter had pleaded guilty to illegal distribution of pills in 2003 and served eleven years in federal prison, "his former home on 37 acres, complete with pool and 10-acre lake set against the rolling hills of Appalachia, will now help addicts get sober and stay clean."

The largest of all these local rehab facilities was the Counseling Center, which had expanded dramatically in recent years. I had interviewed its CEO Ed Hughes during one of my first visits to town in 2010, and he had told me that the local rehab system couldn't keep up with the demand for services.

But in 2022, the center had a zero-waitlist, zero-wait-time policy for most of its programs. It was serving between six hundred and seven hundred people at a given time, and around three thousand clients per year. The facility boasted more beds than the largest local hospital, and it offered an array of services, including a twenty-four-hour crisis hotline, an opiate-withdrawal treatment program, a program through which mothers could receive treatment without being separated from their children, and a career-oriented "Success Center" that offered classes on money management and workplace etiquette. "We are the Cleveland Clinic of treatment agencies," Hughes told me. "People come from everywhere to get to us for treatment, because we offer things that nobody else offers."

In 2021, the center announced plans to move most of its operations into a former shoe factory on the city's East End. The long-abandoned building would be refurbished and repurposed as a state-of-the-art recovery hub that would allow the center to add a hundred new jobs and dramatically increase its treatment capacity. A video about the project called it "the largest redevelopment project in Southern Ohio in a lifetime." In a press release the Counseling Center's CEO said, "What has previously been viewed as a beacon of despair will now grow to be a beacon of hope for the neighborhood, the city, the region, and beyond."

I spent some of this trip going about now-familiar routines. I drove past Volkman's house on Center Street and the now-empty former clinic on Findlay Street. I visited the public library's local history room to comb through a thick manila folder of news clippings labeled DRUG BUSTS — SCIOTO COUNTY one last time. And one morning I drove to the city health department for a final interview with Lisa Roberts.

Roberts was the person I had spoken with most frequently during my trips to Portsmouth. In the years since we first met, as Portsmouth's profile rose, I had watched her become a kind of mini-celebrity. She had appeared on national television, testified before Congress, and traveled to conferences near and far — in Michigan, South Carolina, Puerto Rico, Las Vegas — to tell the story of what had happened in Scioto County. But in conversation, she was still the same person: earnest, easygoing, generous with her time, and surprisingly cheery for someone who had spent years on the front lines of an overdose epidemic.

Roberts, who was now a few months from retiring, told me that the region had seen some improvement in the decade after Volkman's sentencing. Thanks to new laws on the city and state level, and a concerted campaign of law enforcement, the local pain clinics had all permanently closed. The region also now offered what she described as "the full spectrum" of rehab and recovery services.

But the city's problems were by no means solved. There was still a lot of addiction in Scioto County, she explained, and the *lethality* of the drugs in circulation had gotten worse. Most recently, the region had, like many others around the country, been flooded with the hyper-potent opioid painkiller fentanyl, which had caused local overdose rates to soar even higher. "These people die really fast, like within minutes," she said. "It's not like back when we had the opioid pain pills [and] they tended to be a little bit alive when [paramedics] got there."

Roberts was still incredulous that the opiate crisis had gone under-addressed for so long. She said that if thousands of people had been dying in motorcycle wrecks or skydiving accidents, there would have been a major outcry. She felt the muted response had to do at least in part with the fact that the crisis was initially limited to Appalachia. For whatever reason, decision makers in state and national seats of power weren't as concerned about the people who lived there.

She was also still angry about how the crisis had originated: from pharmaceutical companies, doctors, and others in the medical field. Healthcare isn't supposed to harm or addict or kill you, she said. But that's what happened in Scioto County.

"That's what made me the maddest," she said.

One morning, toward the end of my visit, I drove to the Scioto County Welcome Center. The center is located downtown, in a low brick building next to the floodwall murals. Inside, near a large banquet hall that hosts regular bingo games, are offices for the Portsmouth & Scioto County Visitors Bureau and the Portsmouth Area Chamber of Commerce.

When I entered the building, I passed through a hallway lined with glass display cases featuring Portsmouth-themed mini-exhibits. One case was dedicated to Portsmouth's bygone shoe industry. Another featured VHS tapes of Roy Rogers films, a smattering of Rogers-themed memorabilia (books, mugs, lunchboxes, a wristwatch), and a framed photograph with a handwritten message from Roy that read, "Happy Trails to all the folks in Portsmouth, Ohio."

I visited the center because I wanted to buy some souvenirs at the gift shop. (And I did, indeed, walk away with a Roy Rogers mug.) But I also wanted to see if Lisa Carver was still working.

Carver had been the executive director of the Portsmouth Area Chamber of Commerce during my first trip, in 2010. During my interview with her then, when I asked if there was a problem with prescription drugs in the area, she quickly replied that there was.

Pain clinics were a local nuisance, she had said. "I mean, what doctor has people lined up outside their doors?"

As it turned out, in late 2022, Carver was still in the same job, and she agreed to an impromptu interview on the morning I visited.

Carver, like so many people in Scioto County, had a personal connection to the opiate epidemic. She had adopted and spent years raising the daughter of a cousin due to that cousin's struggles with addiction and accompanying legal troubles. And in 2001, her husband died from an overdose of pain medication prescribed by his family practitioner.

During our interview, she acknowledged that Portsmouth had faced its share of suffering. After most local manufacturing dried up or moved away, the pain clinics had made a bad situation worse. That, in turn, had made it hard to recruit good doctors to the area. Due to Portsmouth's bad press, Shawnee State University had faced hurdles when attracting students.

But these days she was feeling genuinely optimistic. She mentioned some thriving smaller-scale industries in the region, including a shoelace manufacturer and a plastics-recycling facility. And she reported that the town was seeing a surge in historic preservation.

She also pointed to the natural beauty of the place, which she saw every morning as she drove from her home in Kentucky across the river into Portsmouth. By this time I, too, was familiar with this view: a panorama of buildings and church spires set against a backdrop of gently sloping green hills.

She was feeling better about Portsmouth than she had in years. They had faced some hard knocks, she said, "but we knew we were more than that."

AFTERWORD: IN MEMORIAM

Danny Coffee was forty-seven when he died in November 2003. He was a father of three and a grandfather. He was survived by five siblings.

Danny loved baseball, Creedence Clearwater Revival, and the chili that his mother made.

He kept a neat appearance. His hair was always combed and his jeans were carefully pressed with a seam down the front.

His gentle disposition was a recurring theme in conversations about him. His daughter Carley told me that she couldn't remember him ever raising his voice. "I was never sad when I was with him," she said.

People told me that Danny's pleasant nature served as a kind of binding agent for his family. And when he was gone, that cohesiveness disappeared. His daughter Amanda told me that after his passing, his family didn't gather for holidays or reunions the way they used to. "We haven't been a family since," she said. Danny's brother, Lloyd, said, "Once he was gone, when we got together, who was trying to get us to laugh?"

Danny is buried in Greenup, Kentucky. The cemetery is tucked into the rolling, wooded hills, next to a small white church. On the day I visited, his headstone was surrounded by flowers and small keepsakes, including a tiny statue of a bunny. The grave was etched with dates of his birth and death, along with the inscription BELOVED SON, FATHER, DADAW AND BROTHER.

Charles Jordan was forty when he died in November 2003. He was the youngest of six children, "the baby of the family," as one relative described him to me. His family and friends knew him as Hobie, a shortened version of his middle name, Hobart.

Hobie had cofounded a successful home-restoration business, and he would occasionally wear a suit and tie for work-related meetings. But mostly his uniform was boots, jeans, a T-shirt, and a bandanna around his head.

He was an outgoing guy who enjoyed being social. His niece, Sherry, told me, "I can still hear his laughter and his voice as plain as if he was standing beside me."

Hobie is buried in a family cemetery in the small town of Blaine, Kentucky, about seventy miles south of Portsmouth. At the time of his passing, family members shared notes on the website of the funeral home that arranged his burial.

"Hobie was kind and had a big heart. We Loved him very much," one read.

Another said, "I can't believe he is gone."

A third said, "I Loved Hobie more than he will ever know, and I will miss him."

Mary Catherine Carver was thirty-two when she died in January 2004. She was survived by her husband, Stoney, and a daughter, Deanna.

When I spoke on the phone with her aunt, Lori, she told me that Cathy was smart, funny, and opinionated. She was a "wonderful person" who, even at her lowest moments, would help a friend in need. At one point, Lori described how, back when they both played on a co-ed softball team, Cathy was a skilled second baseman who wasn't afraid to stop a fast-moving ball with her shin.

Lori didn't overlook her niece's struggles with addiction in our conversation. But she emphasized that Cathy was "far more than just an addict." And she said that, even if Cathy did struggle with addiction, it didn't make her — or any of Volkman's patients who died — any less important. "They were somebody's mother, somebody's daughter, somebody's niece, somebody's granddaughter . . . somebody's sister," she said.

Cathy is buried in a small cemetery in Lucasville, a rural area about ten miles north of Portsmouth. To get there, you turn off a main road at a faded sign that reads BIG RUN CEMETERY. OPEN DAWN TILL DUSK and drive up a steep dirt road, through a dense forest, to an oval-shaped clearing at the top of a hill. When I visited, it was a breezy autumn day. I could hear branches swishing and the jangle of a wind chime. Leaves drifted slowly to the ground.

Cathy's headstone lies flat in a bed of leaves and pine needles near the edge of the cemetery. It reads:

CATHY JENKINS CARVER

1971–2003

OUR HEARTS STILL ACHE IN SADNESS

AND SECRET TEARS STILL FLOW

WHAT IT MEANT TO LOSE YOU,

NO ONE WILL EVER KNOW

Jeffrey Reed was thirty-seven when he died in 2003. He was survived by his daughter, a stepdaughter, his mother, and six siblings. He and his wife, Cheryl, had been married for thirteen years.

On Facebook in the years after his death, Jeff's family and friends posted frequently about him. In one photo, he looks dapper in a suit and tie. In others, he holds his infant daughter and smiles. In one post, his stepdaughter admits that she was "bratty" when she was younger, but now, as an adult, she cherished his parenting wisdom. In another post, Jeff's sister remarks about how delighted he would have been to meet his grandchildren.

Jeff is buried in a small family cemetery about ten miles due south of Portsmouth, in a rural area outside the town of Greenup. The cemetery is located about two hundred yards from the main road, near an old and dilapidated barn. Visitors have to walk through a cow pasture to get there. On the day I visited, the cemetery was blanketed in dry leaves that crunched underfoot.

The cemetery is perhaps an acre, in total. Jeff's grave marker is carved from shiny black stone. It includes his dates of birth and death, an oval-shaped photograph of him, and the inscription A LOVING HUSBAND AND FATHER, SON AND BROTHER.

Dwight Parsons was forty-seven when he died. He was survived by five siblings and two stepchildren. One of those stepchildren, Brad Nolan, spoke to me at length about the man he knew as his dad.

Brad told me that Dwight was a larger-than-life character, in both the literal and figurative sense. Dwight was six foot two, weighed over 350 pounds, and had a big gray beard. His friends knew him affectionately as Tiny.

Dwight loved hot-rod cars and motorcycles. And he also loved music. He played a variety of instruments, including guitar, drums, and the synthesizer. He sang with what Brad described as a "a huge, wonderful voice."

Dwight is buried in a cemetery outside of Greenup, Kentucky. His grave is marked by a simple stone, set flat into the grass. It reads DWIGHT PARSONS 1957–2004.

Brad told me that, more than fifteen years after his stepfather's passing, he still hadn't visited the site. It was too painful. But he said he carried his stepdad's memory with him in other ways, especially during his own journey into stepfatherhood and, later, adoption of those stepchildren.

He told me that memories of Dwight gave him strength during this process. He had learned so much from his stepdad in such a short amount of time, including the lesson that fatherhood isn't necessarily defined by blood relation. He said his memories of Dwight's love and support made him realize, "Hey, I might be able to do this."

Kristi Ross was thirty-nine when she died in 2004. She had three children.

She is buried in the town of Wheelersburg, a few miles east of Portsmouth on Route 52. Unlike the small, rural burial places for some Volkman patients, her grave is in a large, sprawling cemetery where visitors can hear the distant sound of rumbling engines on a nearby highway.

She is buried on a hill that overlooks the Ohio River and the Kentucky hills. Many of the nearby graves are surrounded by small decorations: American flags, flowers, plastic pinwheels that spin in the wind. Her gravestone reads KRISTI JO JENNINGS OCT. 9, 1964 MAR. 9, 2004, with engravings of flowers on either side of her name.

In a phone interview, Kristi's half brother Jeff told me that he doesn't like to visit graves. But he said he often thinks of Kristi. He sometimes thinks about where she would be now if things had turned out differently.

During that conversation, Jeff said that he had endured health issues related to his legs and feet and had undergone multiple surgeries. But when he was prescribed pain pills, he said he rarely took them all. He preferred to throw them away or flush them down the toilet. He told me that he had nine grandkids, and if he ever found out that a doctor or someone else was peddling drugs to them, "I'd probably have to kill somebody."

James Estep was thirty-two when he died. He was an only child, and he was survived by his wife and a daughter.

James was an outgoing guy. He liked to play cards and shoot pool. He liked cars. He loved to watch *The Sopranos* — though, as his daughter noted, he didn't live to see the show's final seasons. He loved to be outdoors and enjoyed hunting and fishing.

James was a hardworking guy, and he applied the same work ethic to fatherhood. His widow, Angela, told me that he would go out of his way to buy things for his daughter. "He tried to do whatever he could do to make her happy," she said.

James is buried in a large cemetery in the town of Flatwoods, Kentucky, about thirty miles southeast of Portsmouth. The grave is marked by a large, wide stone, with an etching of his name and dates of birth and death on one side and his wife's name on the other. Between their names is an image of interlocking wedding rings and the date of their marriage: Sept.

26, 1992. On the day I visited, stone vases on either side of the stone were filled with flowers. One bouquet had a small decorative baseball glove tucked into it.

When I spoke with Angela, she mentioned how young her husband had been when he died. His daughter, Megan, had mostly grown up without a dad. And James himself had missed out on so much of life.

"He died before he even lived, honestly," she said.

Aaron Gillispie was thirty-three when he died in June 2003. He had three daughters and two stepdaughters.

Aaron's loved ones posted many photos to Facebook in the years after his death. A response to one post reads, "I still miss him and he's in my thoughts so much. I will never get over this loss." Another says, "I miss my brother so so much! It never gets easier."

In my conversation with one of Aaron's daughters, Brittany Adkins, she remembered little details about him: that one of the last movies she and her dad watched together was the Tom Hanks film *Castaway*; that he and her mother used to roller-skate together; that he liked strawberry milk-shakes from the local fast-food joint, Rally's.

Brittany was a mother herself by the time of our interview. She said that her dad had only been a father to girls and had always wanted a boy. So when her son Aiden was born, she was pleased to know that her dad would have been happy. Some folks thought that Aiden bore a striking resemblance to his late grandfather.

Brittany believed Aaron would have relished being a grandparent. "I think he would have loved it," she said.

Ernest Ratcliff was thirty-eight when he died. He was survived by his daughter, two brothers, his parents, and his wife, Melissa.

I spoke with Melissa numerous times over the course of this project. And during those conversations I got a good sense of what Ernest — or at least, the person she referred to as the Old Ernest, before his struggles with addiction — was like.

The Old Ernest was a charismatic, boisterous guy who was quick to make friends wherever he went. "Anyone and everyone loved Ernest," she said.

Ernest loved the outdoors. He loved to fish and hunt. He and Melissa enjoyed going on canoeing trips together, and she showed me photos of the two of them from a trip to the Shenandoah River in 1997, smiling while each of them proudly holds a freshly caught fish.

Ernest loved Christmas. Melissa said that sometimes he went overboard buying gifts and pushed the couple into debt as a result. "Lord, that man loved Christmas," she said.

Melissa told me that although she generally isn't a fan of the term *soulmate*, it accurately described her and Ernest's relationship. From the first instant they met, there was an undeniable chemistry that she hasn't felt since.

Even long after his death, she felt flashes of that connection. In one Facebook post from 2019, more than thirteen years after his passing, she wrote, "I slept hard last night and dreamt about Ernest. I could see him plain as day, after all this time. My heart still skipped a beat when I saw him."

Mark Reeder was thirty-four when he died in 2005. He was survived by an older brother, Matt, who looked so much like Mark that people sometimes mistook them for twins.

Mark was a big guy who, according to one acquaintance, was always laughing. She described him to me as "one of the best-natured, sweetest guys you'd ever meet."

Mark loved to watch Ohio State football. He coached Little League baseball in Portsmouth. He also loved motorcycles, and his gravestone is etched with an insignia of the Harley-Davidson company.

He is buried in the tiny town of Friendship, a few miles west of Portsmouth. The cemetery is in a meadow bordered by trees and a white post-and-rail fence. The morning that I visited was chilly, and the ground was still wet with dew. While I was there, the sun rose higher over the Kentucky hills, and the shadows from the graves moved slowly across the grass.

Bryan Brigner was thirty-nine when he died in October 2005. He had four children.

His daughter told me about how he needed a cigarette and a glass of sweet tea first thing in the morning, or else he would be in a sour mood. She remembered him as a "goofball" who was also fiercely protective of his children.

Bryan's son Tyler described his father as his best friend. Another son, Bryan Jr., described him as a caring man who was always proud of the grades that he brought home from school. He called him a "gentle giant."

Bryan Jr. clearly remembered the sound of his dad's laugh. "He smoked two packs a day resulting in him having a deep, hearty laugh that kind of crackled at the end," he said.

Bryan is buried in Owl Creek Cemetery, about twenty miles northeast of Portsmouth, near the town of Beaver, Ohio. His headstone features his name, his dates of birth and death, and an etching of a fish jumping out of the water.

Steven Hieneman was thirty-three when he died in 2005. He was an only child.

His mother, Paula, was one of a small group of family members of deceased patients to testify at Volkman's trial, and she was the only family member to speak at the sentencing hearings for Volkman, Denise Huffman, and Alice Huffman. She also took the stand in a civil lawsuit against Denise and Paul in Scioto County in 2008. During the closing arguments of that civil case, one of Eastley's lawyers said, "Her life centered around him."

When I spoke with Steven's longtime partner, John, in 2013, he told me how handsome Steven was. He was around six feet tall, with a trim build and salt-and-pepper hair. John told me, with a laugh, that Steven was so attractive that "every girl in town was trying to get a hold of him but obviously he didn't stand on that side of the bus."

John told me that a person has just one true love, and, for him, it had been Steven. He could tell what Steve was thinking just by looking at him. They enjoyed traveling together. They had been to Asheville, North Carolina, and Montreal, among other places, and they were planning a trip to Key West at the time of his death. Their relationship was "perfect," he said.

Steven is buried in a small family cemetery next to a cow pasture in Greenup County, Kentucky. His headstone is made from polished black stone with an accompanying statue of an angel in a mournful posture. A few steps away stands a bench dedicated to Steven's memory. Affixed to the backrest is an oval-shaped photo of Steven in which he is wearing a tuxedo and smiling.

Scottie Lin James was the youngest of the deceased patients listed in Paul Volkman's indictment. She had turned thirty just a few days before her death in 2005. She was a mother of two, and she had two younger sisters, Jakkie and Terrie, for whom she had been a mother figure.

Scottie had long, dark, curly hair and what one friend described as "perfect teeth." Her personality was electric. Jakkie told me, "You could literally stand on any corner in Portsmouth and ask about Scottie and they would tell you how bright and beautiful she was."

Scottie's sisters described her to me as generous and nurturing. "She was just always there for us and always knew how to fix everything," Jakkie said.

Scottie's combination of smarts and charisma made her a natural leader. And one of her friends, Laura Garcia, who was in recovery from addiction herself, told me about the impact Scottie could have had as a mentor in the recovery world. "She would have been fantastic," Laura said.

Scottie is buried in a small plot on the property of a family-owned home in the town of McDermott, Ohio, about ten miles north of Portsmouth.

When I spoke with Jakkie more than fifteen years after her sister's passing, she told me that she thinks about Scottie every day. She said that sometimes she'll be driving through town and see someone who looks or moves in a way that reminds her of Scottie. And for a moment, she'll think, "There she is."

NOTES

"Criminals hate the truth, which is why journalism
is necessary for any fair and just world."
— Sebastian Junger

This is a work of nonfiction.

The people and events described are real. In the rare instance where a name was changed, I have noted that in the text. Wherever possible, I have based my storytelling on testimony, affidavits, or other documents produced under penalty of perjury. Still, there are many places where I rely on the memories of people I interviewed, which comes with inherent limitations. The overwhelming majority of quotations that appear in the text were told directly to me, or come from a transcript or news report.

I reported this book over the span of more than a decade. And I fact-checked the book myself throughout eight weeks in 2023. This involved combing through the text, line by line, to confirm its accuracy and to identify my source for a given fact, quote, or description. I also spoke via phone with numerous sources to confirm the accuracy of what I had written.

None of this means that this book is flawless. As the journalist David Carr wrote at the beginning of his book *The Night of the Gun: A Reporter Investigates the Darkest Story of His Life. His Own,* "All human stories are subject to errors of omission, fact, or interpretation regardless of intent." What Carr promised, instead, was that his book was "as true as I could make it."

This book was written to that same standard: It is as true as I could make it.

Any errors or inaccuracies are mine alone.

Much of the book's sourcing is explained in the text itself. But in the spirit of the Society of Professional Journalists' Code of Ethics — in particular, the principle that "ethical journalism means taking responsibility for one's work and explaining one's decisions to the public" — the following notes offer additional info on each chapter's sourcing.

Without question, the largest single source for this book was the record of Volkman's criminal trial, which began on March 2, 2011, and ended on May 9. Between those dates, jurors heard from eighty witnesses: seventy from the prosecution, and ten from the defense. The transcript of those proceedings, once assembled, was more than four thousand pages. I accessed it through the government-operated website Public Access to Court Electronic Records (PACER; pacer.uscourts.gov).

During that criminal trial, attorneys submitted hundreds of exhibits. They included prescription slips, patients' medical files and records from their visits with Volkman, and other documents from Volkman's tenure in southern Ohio (Tri-State's application to establish an on-site dispensary, Volkman's job-application email to the Cleveland Clinic in which he calls his patients "hillbillies," the signed lease for his office in Chillicothe). This evidence also included photos of the clinics and two videos: a hidden-camera recording of a visit to Tri-State taken by a patient in early 2004 and a walk-through video of the Tri-State building from the DEA's raid in June 2005.

I had difficulty accessing these materials. My initial requests for access — to court clerks, attorneys, and even Judge Beckwith — were denied. My subsequent Freedom of Information Act (FOIA) request to the Department of Justice, filed in February 2012, was delayed for years. It was only after a lawsuit against the DEA, filed with the help of the

Rhode Island ACLU and two pro bono attorneys, Neal McNamara and Jessica Jewell, that
I pried free those videos, photos, and nineteen thousand pages of other material. You can
learn more about this lawsuit, *Eil v. DEA*, at the Rhode Island ACLU's page on the case:
riaclu.org/en/cases/eil-v-dea.

Many chapters of this book, especially those in parts 2 and 4, are based on these transcripts and exhibits.

Prologue: The Arrest

Descriptions of Volkman's Lake Shore Drive apartment are based on interviews with
him, his daughter, his son, and his daughter-in-law. My account of Volkman's arrest
draws from interviews with Volkman and his daughter, Jane, who was in the apartment
on the morning of the arrest. Other details come from court records, including the transcript of Volkman's July 26, 2007, bail hearing in Cincinnati. Volkman's indictment is
accessible on the PACER docket for his criminal case. I accessed his post-arrest letter to
the magistrate judge via a separate PACER docket, with documents related to his arrest,
in the US District Court for the Northern District of Illinois.

The DEA's press release about the indictment from May 23, 2007, "Three Indicted for
Operating Illegal 'Pain Clinics' in Southern Ohio," remains accessible online. The quote
"I honestly thought that one day I would pick up the newspaper and I would see that Paul
had been given the Nobel Prize in Medicine" comes from my June 2010 interview with
Lawrence Cohn, a friend of Volkman's from both the University of Rochester and the
University of Chicago, where Cohn attended business school.

The article I cite about doctors' opiate-epidemic criminal activity is "Characteristics of
Criminal Cases Against Physicians Charged with Opioid-Related Offenses Reported in
the US News Media, 1995–2019," from *Injury Epidemiology* in October 2020. Information
about specific cases comes from media reports and Department of Justice press releases.

Details about Volkman's case come from trial transcripts and evidence, as well as DEA
agent Jerrel Smith Jr.'s twenty-five-page sworn "Declaration" about the agency's investigation, which was filed in support of the asset-forfeiture case against Volkman. The description of Volkman as an "experienced, competent physician working in a rural under-served
area trying to help manage the pain of his patients" comes from attorney Kevin Byers's
motion to dismiss the asset-forfeiture case against Volkman, filed in October 2006.

Volkman's comments in this chapter come from interviews with me in 2009 and 2010,
his sentencing hearing in February 2012, the autobiographical narrative he wrote and
shared from prison in 2014 and 2015, emails he wrote from prison in 2015 and 2016, the
open letter he wrote for the site Doctors of Courage in 2018, and the religious-conversion
essay he published via Facebook in 2019.

PART 1: MALPRACTICE

The Valedictorian

Much of the info in this chapter is based on primary-source documents accessed via
Ancestry.com. Ancestry is where I found draft-registration cards for Volkman's maternal
grandfather, Simon (from World War I), and his father, Murray (from World War II), as
well as documents that describe the immigration journeys of Volkman's grandparents.
Ancestry was also a source of census records from 1910 through 1950, which further
illuminate his family history, and yearbook pages from Volkman's years at Coolidge
High, in Washington, DC. Other information in this chapter comes from interviews
with Volkman; his daughter, Jane; and my father. I also draw from Volkman's 2019 autobiographical essay, which was published by his daughter, Jane, on Facebook under the
title "Conversion Testimony of My Father Paul, from Atheist, Nominal Jew to Messianic
Believer."

MSTP

According to the National Institutes of Health, there are now more than forty-five schools with federally funded Medical Scientist Training Programs (MSTP). A helpful primer on the program's history is the 2017 *Academic Medicine* article "History and Outcomes of Fifty Years of Physician-Scientist Training in Medical Scientist Training Programs." My account of Volkman's specific experiences at the University of Chicago draws on interviews with four MSTP classmates: my dad, Richard Pauli, Jeffrey Kant, and J. Ross Milley. I also interviewed Oliver Cameron (who completed an MD/PhD from the U of C but was not part of the MSTP), Lynda Erinoff (who was one of Volkman's fellow pharmacology PhD students), Paul Nausieda (who overlapped with Volkman in medical school), and Larry Cohn (a friend of Volkman's at both the University of Rochester and the U of C, where he went to business school).

Nancy

My biographical sketch of Nancy Krinn is based on interviews with family members, a draft of her eulogy written by one of her best friends, and high school and college yearbook photos accessed via Ancestry.com. Volkman's accounts of his early relationship with Nancy, his choice of pediatrics as a specialty, and his departure from medical research come from interviews in 2009 and 2010, emails from 2014 and 2016, an autobiographical narrative Volkman shared in 2014 and 2015, and his autobiographical 2019 essay about converting to Messianic Judaism. My conversation with Ronald Albrecht, whom Volkman accused of blocking the publication of his "major" research findings, took place via phone in 2011. After Albrecht's death in 2017, a tribute in the newsletter for the Association of University Anesthesiologists noted, "Dr. Albrecht was passionately involved in the education of medical students and anesthesia residents, influencing their academic advancement and professional future . . . He was tireless in mentoring his academic anesthesiologists to achieve their highest goals."

The Pediatrician

Volkman boasted at one point that "many" of his pediatric patients and their families had "stuck with [me] for 25 years." But when I asked for names of folks I could interview, he declined, writing, "In light of the govt's smear campaign against me it would be an imposition and burden and painful for good people I do not wish to hurt."

Later, by coincidence, two of them found me. Ellen Leahy first contacted me on Facebook after reading my 2017 *Vice* interview ("The Blurry Line Between Healing and Dealing") with the director of a documentary about convicted pain doctor William Hurwitz. Jean Martinez's daughter, Sara, found me via my website after "doing a random late-night search on updates in Paul Volkman's case." Volkman was her former pediatrician, and her mother had worked for him. She later arranged my interview with her mom.

Malpractice, Part I: The Child in the Waiting Room

The bulk of this chapter draws on six posttrial legal filings from the Frey case. Those documents are:

- A fifty-eight-page "Brief and Appendix of Defendant-Appellee" filed by the Corporation Counsel of the City of Chicago in 1994 with the Appellate Court of Illinois, First District, Fifth Division.
- An eighteen-page "Brief of Defendants-Appellee" filed by attorneys for Paul Volkman in 1994 in the same appellate court district and division listed above.
- A fifty-five-page "Brief and Argument of Plaintiff-Appellant/Separate Appellee" filed by attorneys for George Frey (the special administrator of

the estate of Amanda Frey), filed on January 6, 1995, in the same appellate court district and division.

- A fifteen-page "Brief of Defendants-Separate Appellants" filed by attorneys for Volkman on May 8, 1995, in the same appellate court district and division.
- A five-page "Brief of Defendants-Separate Appellants" filed by attorneys for Volkman on June 4, 1996, in the same appellate court district and division.
- A four-page "Petition for Rehearing" filed by attorneys for George Frey, on July 9, 1997, in the same appellate court district and division.

Additional sources for this chapter include a *Chicago Sun-Times* article of the lawsuit ("Suit Charges Paramedic Fault in Girl's Death"), as well as thirteen pages of disciplinary records from the Illinois Department of Professional Regulation, released in response to my Illinois Freedom of Information Act request. Volkman's account of the case is drawn from in-person interviews in December 2009, as well as emails from prison in 2014 and 2021.

Locum Tenens
My understanding of the places Volkman worked as a locum tenens physician comes from his CV, info from state medical boards, a deposition he gave as an expert witness in 2001, and his testimony in the Williamson civil trial in 2002.

Helpful sources for my writing about the history of locum tenens medicine included:

> *Deseret News*, "S.L. Firm Fills in When Physicians Need a Break," February 8, 1990.
> *Tooele [Utah] Transcript-Bulletin*, "Temporary Physicians Come to Tooele," July 15, 1993.
> *The Courier* [Waterloo, Iowa], "Country Doctor in an RV: Have Stethoscope, Will Travel," June 13, 1994.
> *Salt Lake Tribune*, "Local Company Leads in Physician-Staffing Services," October 1997.
> *New York Times*, "Roving Doctors Paying House Calls to Towns," April 16, 2002.
> *Orlando Sentinel*, "Physician, Heal Thyself of Aches and Pains," November 12, 2003.

All except the *New York Times* article were accessed via Newspapers.com.

Malpractice, Parts II–III: Emergency Rooms
In addition to my interview with Mary Cooper's daughter Dale, my writing about the Cooper case draws from more than eleven hundred pages of documents accessed through the Lake County, Illinois, clerk's office. Those documents include the initial complaint and subsequent amended complaints, motions, transcripts, affidavits, medical records, and court orders.

In addition to several interviews with Todd and Roger Kirchhoff's attorney, Steve Jambois, my writing about the Kirchhoff cases draws from more than a hundred pages of documents accessed via the Macon County, Illinois, clerk's office. Those documents include the initial complaint, affidavits, motions and memoranda in support of those motions, and other records, including a locum tenens contract signed by Volkman for his work in Decatur, beginning in December 1994.

Volkman's comments on the Cooper and Kirchhoff cases come from in-person interviews in 2009 and emails from 2014.

Malpractice, Part IV: Bankrupt

I accessed Volkman's twenty-seven-page bankruptcy filing via PACER. The portion of the chapter about the De Masi lawsuit is based on interviews with Volkman; Nicole De Masi; Nicole's mother, Joanne De Masi; and their attorney in the case, Margaret O'Leary.

The Expert Witness

Volkman's estimate that he gave "two to three hundred" depositions as an expert witness comes from his testimony during the *Williamson v. Volkman* trial in 2002. His answers about the number of depositions he gave annually, the number of times he had testified in court, and his fees for those appearances come from a deposition he gave as an expert witness in 2001 for the lawsuit *Robertson v. University Hospitals of Cleveland*. The *New York Times* articles I quote about the growth of the expert-witness industry in the 1980s are "Rush to Judgement Among Expert Witnesses" (February 6, 1983) and "Expert Witnesses: Booming Business for the Specialists" (July 5, 1987).

Malpractice, Part V: Angie and the G-Tube

The *Williamson v. Volkman* malpractice trial took place over five days in Marion, Illinois, in December 2002. The 1,096-page trial transcript was my main source for this chapter. I also interviewed the plaintiff's attorney, John Womick, as well as Angie Williamson's granddaughter Sarah Olson.

Uninsurable

The research I cite about the malpractice-claim risks of different medical specialties comes from the 2019 *International Review of Law and Economics* article "Physicians with Multiple Paid Medical Malpractice Claims: Are They Outliers or Just Unlucky?" The 2000 interview with two malpractice attorneys from *Medical Economics* is titled "How Plaintiffs' Lawyers Pick Their Targets." I accessed it through the Internet Archive's "Wayback Machine" at archive.org. In addition to Tom Baker's 2005 book, *The Medical Malpractice Myth*, I also consulted a 2009 article from *Clinical Orthaepedics and Related Research*, "Juries and Medical Malpractice Claims: Empirical Facts Versus Myths." In the article's abstract, author Neil Vidmar wrote: "Juries in medical malpractice trials are viewed as incompetent, antidoctor, irresponsible in awarding damages to patients, and casting a threatening shadow over the settlement process. Several decades of systematic empirical research yields little support for these claims."

Milwaukee

This chapter draws from an in-person interview with Dr. Paul Nausieda in Milwaukee in August 2011. The Winter 2002 magazine from St. Luke's hospital, *The Spirit of St. Luke's*, which contains a feature about Nausieda and his career, is accessible online. Volkman's comments in this chapter come from letters and emails he wrote to me in 2011 and 2021, as well as a lengthy autobiographical narrative he wrote from prison and shared with various people in December 2014 and January 2015.

PART 2: CRIME SCENES

Boomtown

During my many visits to Portsmouth, I spent hours in the local history room at the Portsmouth Public Library, combing through filing cabinets filled with archival articles and newspaper clippings. Much of my knowledge of the local history, from Roy Rogers to the steel mills to the community's struggles with poverty and drug addiction, traces back to this research. I also benefited tremendously from the PPL's online collections (yourppl.org/history/), which include thousands of scanned photos and documents from Portsmouth's past. For this chapter, I also consulted Elmer Sword's 1965 book *The Story of Portsmouth* and the Scioto Historical website (sciotohistorical.org), a project by Shawnee

State University professor Drew Feight. Professor Feight was also generous with his time and expertise during my years of research.

"The Oxycontin Capital of the World"

For my writing on Drs. Procter, Cohn, Snyder, Santos, and Lilly, I drew on the work of reporters at the *Louisville Courier Journal*, *Lexington Herald-Leader*, *Columbus Dispatch*, and Associated Press. My vignettes about these corrupt doctors also draw on court records, documents from the Kentucky Bureau of Medical Licensure, and, in the case of Lilly, coverage in the *Portsmouth Daily Times*, *U.S. News & World Report*, and the ABC News show *20/20*.

Tri-State Healthcare

The most useful document I had for understanding Denise Huffman's life was a 177-page transcript of a deposition she gave in 2006 as part of a wrongful-death lawsuit filed by the mother of Steve Hieneman, Paula Eastley. It's an extraordinary document, less for what she revealed than for just how uncooperative she was. When the plaintiff's attorney, Stanley Bender, asked her what she did after she quit high school, she claimed that she didn't really remember. "You're going back a long time," she said. "I mean I'm 53 years old." She was similarly foggy about whether she got a job after receiving her GED in the late 1970s ("I'm not sure"), about the nature of a medical course she once took at Shawnee State ("I'm at a loss right at this moment as to . . . what the actual course [was]"), and about when her husband stopped working and began receiving disability benefits ("I am not sure, to give you an actual date"). At other points, when Bender asked if she knew what a limited liability corporation was, she said that she was "not positive." When he asked if she knew what it meant when a physician was "board certified," she said she was "not sure at the moment."

Other sources for this chapter include the trial testimonies of Denise and Alice Huffman and online message-board comments by Denise that were included in the Portsmouth police's sixty-two-page search warrant for 1310 Center Street.

The second half of the chapter draws on documents from the Kentucky Bureau of Medical Licensure (KBML) about pre-Volkman Tri-State doctors Richard Gritzmacher and Richard Ruhling. Those KBML records, and records discussing doctors in the previous chapter, were all accessed at the bureau's "Physician Profile/Verification of License" database, at kbml.ky.gov. My writing about the early days of Tri-State Healthcare also draws on articles from 2003 and 2004 in the *Lexington Herald-Leader*. My interview with Richard Ruhling took place via phone in October 2021.

First Impressions

In addition to trial transcripts and evidence, this chapter draws on online message-board comments by Denise Huffman that were included in the Portsmouth police's search warrant for 1310 Center Street and letters to me from Alice Huffman in July 2012.

Volkman's comments come from in-person interviews in 2009 and 2010; letters to me from Butler County Jail in 2011; his handwritten presentencing memo from February 2012; his autobiographical narrative shared from prison in 2014 and 2015; emails to me from prison in 2015, 2016, and 2021; and his sworn testimony at his DEA-registration hearing, which was included in DEA deputy administrator Michele Leonhart's lengthy 2008 opinion denying his appeal.

My writing about state-level intractable pain laws draws on multiple sources, including the 1995 article "Intractable Pain Treatment Laws and Regulations" from the *American Pain Society Bulletin* and the 2011 article "State Pain Laws: A Case for Intractable Pain Centers Part III" in *Practical Pain Management*. My writing about Ohio's intractable pain law draws on press coverage from the time, including the Associated Press's "Legislature

Considering Morphine" and *Akron Beacon Journal*'s "Powerful Pain Relief a Bitter Pill for Doctors" (both from 1997), as well of the text of the bill itself.

The Decade of Pain Control and Research

The list of sources I draw on in this chapter includes:

> World Health Organization, "Cancer Pain Relief," 1986.
>
> *Pain*, "Chronic Use of Opioid Analgesics in Non-Malignant Pain: Report of 38 Cases," May 1986, Russell Portenoy and Kathleen Foley.
>
> *Advances in Alcohol and Substance Abuse*, "American Opiophobia: Customary Underutilization of Opioid Analgesics," 1985.
>
> *Pain*, "Opioid Pseudoaddiction — An Iatrogenic Syndrome," March 1989.
>
> *Current Addiction Reports*, "Pseudoaddiction: Fact or Fiction? An Investigation of the Medical Literature," 2015.
>
> US General Accounting Office [GAO], report to congressional requesters, "Prescription Drugs: OxyContin Abuse and Diversion and Efforts to Address the Problem," December 2003.
>
> *American Journal of Public Health*, "The Promotion and Marketing of OxyContin: Commercial Triumph, Public Health Tragedy," February 2009.
>
> *New York Times Magazine*, "The Alchemy of OxyContin," July 29, 2001.
>
> *American Pain Society (APS) Bulletin* 13, no. 3, "The Decade of Pain Control and Research," 2003 ("Transcript of the Decade of Pain Control and Research Special Lecture presented by Dr. [John] Loeser at the APS Annual Meeting on March 20, 2003").

I also benefited immensely from the work of other journalists and writers about the broader opiate epidemic. For those interested in learning more, any one of these texts is a good place to start:

> Barry Meier, *Pain Killer: A "Wonder" Drug's Trail of Addiction and Death*, 2003.
>
> Sam Quinones, *Dreamland: The True Tale of America's Opiate Epidemic*, 2015.
>
> Anna Lembke, *Drug Dealer, MD: How Doctors Were Duped, Patients Got Hooked, and Why It's So Hard to Stop*, 2016.
>
> Beth Macy, *Dopesick: Dealers, Doctors and the Drug Company That Addicted America*, 2018.
>
> Patrick Radden Keefe, *Empire of Pain: The Secret History of the Sackler Dynasty*, 2021.
>
> Alex Gibney, *The Crime of the Century* (two-part HBO documentary), 2021.

Aaron

The *Columbus Dispatch* article with a timeline of eighteen deaths of Volkman's patients was headlined "More Died as 3-Year Probe Unfolded." It was published on June 3, 2007. In 2012, following Volkman's sentencing, the *Lexington Herald-Leader* ran an article, "Pill-Mill Doctor Sentenced to Four Life Terms in Prison," which reported, "The U.S. Drug Enforcement Administration looked into 34 overdose deaths among Volkman's patients, 19 of them from Kentucky, said James Geldhof, DEA diversion program manager for the region that includes Kentucky." In September 2020, DEA investigator Chris Kresnak, one of the lead agents on the Volkman investigation, delivered a presentation to the Kentucky Medical Association called "Rising Drug Trends in the US and KY," which was later uploaded to YouTube. During this presentation, Kresnak described Volkman as a "murderous drug dealer" and referred to thirty-nine deaths associated with him. In a subsequent interview with me, Kresnak confirmed that this was the number of deaths with possible ties to Volkman that the agency investigated.

The section of the chapter about Aaron Gillispie draws from trial transcripts and evidence, as well as a March 2022 interview with Gillispie's daughter, Brittany Adkins.

DEA

There seems to be no authoritative, independently written book about DEA history. So I drew on multiple sources in this chapter. The agency has published its own detailed history, *A Tradition of Excellence: The History of the DEA from 1973 to 1998*, which it updated in subsequent years, through 2013. That (conspicuously pro-DEA) narrative is still available on the agency's website, on a page called "Our History" (dea.gov/about/history). When writing about DEA history, I also used the Internet Archive to access speeches, congressional testimony, press releases, and other info from the early years of the agency's crackdown on prescription drug diversion and abuse that was once published on dea.gov.

For an independent perspective, I also dug into the archives of the *New York Times*, *Washington Post*, and other sources. These archives detail the agency's not-so-rare issues with corruption (like the *New York Times* report from 1989, "Agents Accused: The Drug Fight's Dark Side — A Special Report: Corruption in Drug Agency Called Crippler of Inquiries and Morale") as well as debates in the 1970s, '80s, and '90s about whether to fold the agency into the FBI. One *Washington Post* article from 1977 reported, "DEA's first administrator, John R. Bartel[s] Jr., admitted that the public seemed to regard its agents 'as corrupt Nazis who don't know how to open the door except with the heel of their right foot.'"

The section about critics of the DEA draws on various sources. Two examples are the 2018 *New York Times* op-ed by Leo Beletsky and Jeremiah Goulka, "The Federal Agency That Fuels the Opioid Crisis," and the 2020 *Vice* article "The Defund the Police Movement Is Coming for the DEA." In 2020, the American Civil Liberties Union (ACLU) described the DEA in a tweet as "the scandal-ridden federal law enforcement agency powering America's racist drug war." The *New York Times* op-ed that I cite for its criticism of the DEA's crackdown on pain doctors is called "Handcuffs and Stethoscopes," from July 23, 2005.

The details of the DEA's early investigation into Paul Volkman come from a twenty-five-page sworn "Declaration" by Special Agent Jerrel Smith Jr. that was filed in support of the DEA's asset-forfeiture case against Volkman. That document, which I also draw on in the chapters "The Raid" and "Chillicothe," offers a detailed chronological narrative of the agency's work on this case. I accessed it via PACER.

Danny and Jeff

The Danny Coffee portion of this chapter is based on trial exhibits and testimony, as well as interviews with Danny's sister, Diana Coffee McCabe; his brother, Lloyd; and two daughters, Carley and Amanda. The quotes from Danny's mother, Lena, come from two articles published after Volkman's indictment: "Indictment: Doctor Moved Millions of Pills," from the Associated Press on May 29, 2007; and "More Died as 3-Year Probe Unfolded," from the *Columbus Dispatch* on June 3, 2007. The portion of the chapter about Jeff Reed is based largely on trial exhibits and testimony, particularly the testimony of Reed's widow, Cheryl.

1219 Findlay Street

In addition to trial transcripts and testimony, this chapter draws on DEA deputy administrator Michele Leonhart's eighteen-thousand-word opinion denying Volkman's appeal of the agency's suspension of his registration to prescribe controlled substances. The DEA's estimates about Tri-State's revenues come from a January 2012 filing in Denise Huffman's case, "Motion of the United States for a Preliminary Order of Forfeiture," and its accompanying documents, which I accessed via PACER. My writing about the deaths of Volkman's patients was largely based on court transcripts and exhibits. But it was also informed by interviews with Charles Jordan's niece Machelle Stratton; James Estep's widow, Angela, and daughter, Megan; Mary Carver's aunt Lori Dickens; and Kristi Ross's brother, Jeff Swick.

Gambling

Volkman's comments in this chapter come from emails he sent in 2010, the autobiographical narrative he shared from prison in 2014 and 2015, and emails to me from prison in 2021. Other portions of the chapter draw on Facebook messages from Denise Huffman, plus the transcript of her sentencing hearing on February 14, 2012.

Dwight

In addition to criminal trial transcript and evidence, this chapter draws on two lengthy interviews with Dwight's stepson, Brad Nolan, in 2022.

The Cleveland Clinic

The Cleveland Clinic declined to comment for this book when I reached out in 2022. In addition to criminal transcripts and evidence, this chapter also draws on Volkman's comments at his sentencing hearing on February 14, 2012.

Steven

In addition to criminal trial transcript and evidence, this chapter draws on evidence and testimony from a separate civil trial in Portsmouth in 2008, stemming from a lawsuit against Huffman and Volkman in Scioto County's Court of Common Pleas. Steven's mother, Paula Eastley, testified in both the civil and criminal proceedings. I also interviewed Steven's partner, John Kiser, in 2013.

The Raid

The June 2005 raid of Tri-State Healthcare was discussed in detail by witnesses at the Volkman trial. Additionally, photos and video from the raid were presented at trial, and later released to me. Details of the day were also included in DEA agent Jerrel Smith's twenty-five-page "Declaration" about the investigation of Volkman, as well as DEA deputy administrator Michele Leonhart's eighteen-thousand-word opinion denying Volkman's appeal of the suspension of his registration, "Drug Enforcement Administration. Paul H. Volkman; Denial of Application." Volkman also discusses the raid (a "ransacking," in his words) in his 2014 autobiographical narrative emailed from prison.

The End of the Partnership

In addition to criminal trial transcripts and testimony, this chapter draws on letters Alice Huffman sent me from prison in July 2012, as well as Denise Huffman's 2006 deposition from the *Eastley v. Volkman/Huffman* civil lawsuit. Volkman's comments in this chapter draw from in-person interviews with him in 2009 and 2010, a January 2012 letter from Butler County Jail, and his 2014 autobiographical narrative written and sent from prison. My interview with the owner and operator of the website Moe's Forum, Joe Ferguson, took place in Portsmouth in December 2010.

Scottie

In addition to trial transcript and evidence, this chapter draws on the Portsmouth police's sixty-two-page search warrant for 1310 Center Street, as well as interviews with Jakkie Layne, in 2021 and 2022, and a friend of Scottie, Laura Garcia, in 2022.

The House on Center Street
This chapter draws on notes and photographs from my personal visits to Center Street; the October 5, 2005, *Portsmouth Daily Times* article "Dr. Volkman Again Target of Police Raid"; a sixty-two-page search warrant for 1310 Center Street prepared by the Portsmouth police; and May 2010 interviews with Volkman's next-door neighbor in Portsmouth, Sammie Ishmael, and WSAZ reporter Randy Yohe. The section on Bryan Brigner draws on interviews with his sons, Tyler and Bryan, and daughter, Sanyll. Volkman's comments in this chapter come from the autobiographical narrative that he wrote and shared from prison in 2014 and 2015, as well as other emails from 2014. The sourcing for the section on Harold Eugene Fletcher is discussed in my note for the part 3 chapter "The Pharmacist."

Naked Truths
This chapter is based on a series of *Portsmouth Daily Times* articles, "Naked Truths: The Story Behind Portsmouth's Prostitution Culture," from early October 2005. All were written by reporter Phyllis Noah. The articles are:

- "Part 1: Process Starts with Addiction," October 2.
- "Part 2: "Prostitution's Effects Far-Reaching," October 3.
- "Part 3: More Drugs, More Prostitution," October 4.
- "Part 4: Program Shows How to Get Out," October 5.

Ernest
In addition to trial transcripts and evidence, this chapter draws on lengthy interviews with Melissa Ratcliff in 2017, 2021, and 2022. Volkman's commentary comes from his handwritten presentencing memo from February 2012.

Chillicothe
In addition to trial transcripts and evidence, this chapter draws on Volkman's autobiographical narrative from 2014 and 2015. The section on the DEA's investigation draws on the twenty-five-page sworn "Declaration" of DEA agent Jerrel Smith. The section on Mark Reeder draws on an interview with Reeder's sister-in-law, Kimberly Swords Reeder.

Order to Show Cause
Volkman's descriptions of his Chillicothe research plans come from interviews in 2009 and 2010, as well as a lengthy autobiographical narrative he shared with various people, including me, in 2014. The quote, "The long-term view was to publish the eventual findings in the most widely-read and prestigious American medical journal, *The New England Journal of Medicine*," comes from a motion to dismiss the criminal indictment filed on Volkman's behalf by attorney Kevin Byers in early 2009. I accessed Volkman's DEA "Order to Show Cause and Immediate Suspension of Registration" via the Ohio Medical Board's website, where it was included among other documents related to the suspension and, later, revocation of Volkman's license. That site is elicense.ohio.gov.

Losing Battles
Volkman's former attorney Kevin Byers described some of his conversations with Volkman during a 2011 interview. Other documents from Volkman's fight against the DEA's seizure of his assets are accessible via PACER.

Some details of Volkman's (unsuccessful) fight to retain his DEA registration are included in the Sixth Circuit US Court of Appeals's June 2009 decision denying his appeal. A much more detailed account is the DEA deputy administrator's eighteen-thousand-word decision in the case, "Paul H. Volkman; Denial of Application," published in May 2008 in the federal register. This opinion describes the multiday hearing in great detail and quotes directly from various witnesses, including Volkman. It also includes voluminous details about Volkman's tenure in southern Ohio and the response of various authorities, including the DEA and Ohio Pharmacy Board.

Indicted

Volkman's indictment is accessible via the PACER docket page for his criminal case. This chapter also draws on in-person interviews with him from 2009 and 2010. Prosecutor Timothy Oakley's remark that Tri-State Healthcare's locations were "in essence . . . a crack house dealing OxyContin and oxycodone" comes from Alice Huffman's sentencing hearing on November 8, 2011.

PART 3: FACE-TO-FACE

The Phone Call

My account of my father's career draws from numerous interviews with him as well as his CV. I also interviewed his longtime medical partner, Dr. Howard Lilienfeld, in Florida in 2011. My descriptions of Nancy Volkman's funeral and shiva are based on her *Chicago Tribune* death notice and a draft of a eulogy shared with me by her friend Natalie Cohen, as well as interviews with my parents and Oliver and Susan Cameron.

The Query Letter

I still have many of the documents mentioned in this chapter, in either hard copy or digital form. This includes my application essay to the Columbia MFA program from 2008, my diary entry about learning about Paul Volkman and his case from 2009, and my first query letter to Paul Volkman in 2009. Reporter Randy Ludlow's *Columbus Dispatch* article about Volkman's case, "More Died as 3-Year Probe Unfolded," published shortly after his indictment in 2007, was a tremendous help to me during the early stages of my reporting. The book *America's Dumbest Doctors: Ever Wonder About Yours?*, which briefly features Volkman, was published in 2009 by Dog Ear Publishing. Dr. Alex DeLuca's "War on Doctors/Pain Crisis" website, Doctordeluca.com, was an invaluable resource of materials about various accused and convicted pain doctors' cases. The website is accessible through the Internet Archive's "Wayback Machine."

Remarried

This chapter draws on interviews and correspondence with Paul Volkman; an in-person interview with his second wife, Clara (not her real name), in 2011; and correspondence with Jane Volkman. The date of Paul and Clara's October 2008 marriage in Las Vegas was confirmed with online marriage records from the Clark County, Nevada, clerk's office.

Chicago

My first interviews with Paul Volkman took place on December 23 and Christmas Day, 2009, in Chicago. These conversations were recorded with his permission. We spent most of that time in his apartment, though we also went to lunch at a nearby restaurant, drove around the University of Chicago campus, and sat in a Starbucks. The total length of those first recorded sessions was 10.5 hours. I returned to Chicago for three more days of in-person interviews in August 2010, which added 5.5 hours of recorded conversation. Our final in-person interview took place over dinner in Newport, Kentucky, following a pretrial hearing in Cincinnati in 2010. This conversation, which was also recorded with permission, brought the total amount of in-person interviews to around 17.5 hours. At one point, years after his trial, when we were discussing my book project via email, he wrote: "There is nothing which I have said or written to you which would be a problem for me if it is published. Go for it."

A State of Emergency

I made ten reporting trips to Portsmouth over the course of this project. This chapter is based on the first two of those visits: a seven-day trip in May 2010 and a four-day trip in July and August 2010. I spent those trips soaking up as much of the place as I could. I took photos, walked through museums and parks, collected printed materials (pamphlets, newspapers), and jotted lots of notes. I also conducted interviews with professors, pastors, prosecutors, police officers, shop and restaurant owners, elected officials, public health workers, journalists, leaders in the recovery community, and various other people around town. Some of those interviews are mentioned or quoted in the chapter; many are not. I also attended numerous events, including meetings for the recently assembled prescription drug action team.

The Facebook group Fix the Scioto County Problem of Drug Abuse, Misuse, and Overdose remained active until 2022, when it was deactivated by one of its administrators. However, posts from the group going back to 2010 are still accessible on the group's page, which made it a valuable resource in my reporting on Portsmouth's fight against prescription drug abuse.

My writing on the Wheelersburg pain clinic of Margie Temponeras draws from court records, documents from the Ohio Medical Board and DEA, as well as an excellent report by John Caniglia of the *Cleveland Plain Dealer*, "'Unfathomable': How 1.6 Million Pills from a Small-Town Doctor Helped Fuel the Opioid Crisis in Ohio," from September 2019. Other resources cited in the chapter include the Ohio Prescription Drug Task Force's "Initial Report: Progress & Recommendations" from May 2010 and the May 17, 2010, *Chillicothe Gazette* article "Eyes Turn to Pain Clinics in Prescription Drug Abuse," which I accessed via Newspapers.com.

Adam and Elizabeth

I spoke at length with Adam Volkman many times over the course of this project. His wife, Liz, joined us for many of those conversations. This chapter is based on interviews with the couple at their home on the evenings of August 15 and 16, 2010. The first interview was around two hours long and the second lasted nearly three and a half hours. All of these interviews were recorded, with their permission. This chapter also draws from Adam's testimony at his father's July 26, 2007, bail hearing in Cincinnati. Adam shared family photos with me, as well as numerous letters he had received from his father in prison. He had not responded to those letters.

The Pharmacist

My reporting on Harold Eugene Fletcher in this and other chapters ("The House on Center Street," "Chillicothe," "Co-Conspirators") draws mainly from court records. These include Fletcher's 2010 lawsuit against the DEA, his criminal indictments from September and December 2010, and transcripts of his change-of-plea and sentencing hearings in 2011 and 2012, respectively. I also accessed records from the Ohio Board of Pharmacy, which included disciplinary proceedings that predated his involvement in the Volkman case. Perhaps the most detailed and helpful document about Fletcher's case was DEA deputy administrator Michele Leonhart's opinion, published in the Federal Register in October 2010, affirming the suspension of East Main Street Pharmacy's registration. Like Volkman, Fletcher had contested the DEA's suspension of his registration to distribute controlled substances, which had led to an administrative hearing. And just as Volkman's failed fight for his DEA registration had eventually produced an eighteen-thousand-word opinion from Leonhart packed with details from the case and hearing, Fletcher's fight produced a similarly detailed, twenty-one-thousand-word opinion, "East Main Street Pharmacy; Affirmance of Suspension Order," published in the Federal Register in October 2010.

Jane

Jane Volkman and I corresponded regularly from mid-2010 through to this book's final fact-checking process in 2023. Most of that correspondence took place via Facebook message. The second half of this chapter draws, with her permission, from our corre-

spondence between 2010 and January 2011. The biographical sketch at the beginning
of the chapter is based on numerous sources, including my correspondence with Jane,
her public Facebook posts, press coverage of Paul's indictment by the AP and *Chicago
Tribune*, documents on Ancestry.com, her testimony at her father's July 2007 bail hearing
in Cincinnati, and an essay she posted on Facebook in 2019 titled "My Conversion from
Nominal Jew to Messianic Follower of Yeshua (Jesus)."

PART 4: "A TRULY DANGEROUS MAN"

The Judge
Two particularly helpful resources for my biographical sketch of Judge Sandra Beckwith were
a profile in the Federal Bar Association's magazine from 2000 ("Hon. Sandra S. Beckwith,
Judge, Southern District of Ohio") and a six-minute YouTube mini-documentary released
in 2011 to accompany her Great Living Cincinnatian award ("Hon. Sandra Beckwith, 2011
Great Living Cincinnatian").

The archives of the *Cincinnati Enquirer*, which I accessed through Newspapers.com,
were hugely helpful for my reporting on Judge Beckwith's pre-Volkman-trial years on
the bench, and, in particular, the University of Cincinnati radiation case. Other helpful
sources about the radiation case included the *New York Times* article "Cold War Radiation
Test on Humans to Undergo a Congressional Review," from April 1994, and *Case Western
Law Review*'s "The 'Kingdom of Ends': In Re Cincinnati Radiation Litigation and the
Right to Bodily Integrity," from 1995.

I also conducted an hour-long phone interview with Judge Beckwith in August 2022,
after her retirement. During that conversation, I remarked on the visibility and contro-
versy surrounding the radiation case and asked if she viewed it as the most important
of her career. She replied that it was probably the second most important case she had
handled. This, naturally, led me to ask which one she felt was the most important.

"Oh, I think Volkman," she said.

Courtroom Chapters*
My main sources for these six courtroom-based chapters were the trial transcripts and
the trial exhibits. The transcripts are available for anyone to read and download via
PACER. The exhibits were mostly accessed through my FOIA lawsuit. I attended the first
few days of the trial, including jury selection, opening statements, and the testimony of a
handful of witnesses. I also attended the sentencing hearing. Thus, some of my descriptions of the courtroom and its characters are based on firsthand observation.

Press coverage of the Volkman case consisted mainly of short articles announcing
the start and end of the trial and the sentencing. As far as I know, no trial coverage went
into much detail about the witnesses, their testimony, or the evidence presented. The
nickname "Pill Mill Killer" comes from one of those news reports. The first and only time
I heard that name used was in a story about the trial verdict by Chuck Goudie, of ABC7
Eyewitness News in Chicago.

The Devil in Scioto County
Many of the sources mentioned in this article remain available to read or watch online.

Ohio governor John Kasich's 2011 State of the State address is viewable at ohiochannel
.org. The city of Portsmouth's pain-clinic ordinance, passed in March 2011, is available via
American Legal Publishing (codelibrary.amlegal.com), under "Codified Ordinances of
the City of Portsmouth, Ohio." The articles I mention about Scioto County's prescription
drug problem are:

---

*The Prosecution's Case, Part I: The Clinics, The Prosecution's Case, Part II: The Deaths, The
Defense's Case, Closing Arguments, Verdict, Sentenced

Andrew Welsh-Huggins, "Ohio County Fights Extreme Pill Addiction
     Abuse," Associated Press, December 22, 2010.
Melody Petersen, "Pain Killers," *Men's Health*, January 2011.
Sabrina Tavernise, "Ohio County Losing Its Young to Painkillers' Grip,"
     New York Times, April 19, 2011.

Inside the Jury Room

This chapter is based on four interviews with jurors from the Volkman trial. One of those interviews took place in Newport, Kentucky, on February 17, 2012. Another took place via email in May 2017. Two further interviews took place, via phone, in October and December 2021. I accessed Volkman's late-trial order not to contact witnesses via PACER.

Inside His Mind

My portrait of Paul's brother, Alan, is based largely on lengthy interviews with Alan's only child, David, in 2011 and 2023. I found other info and documents, including college yearbook photos and a marriage license from the state of Virginia, via Ancestry.com. The section involving Jane Volkman draws from more than a decade of Facebook-message correspondence with Jane, starting in August 2010 and continuing through 2023.

Butler County Jail

Between July 2011 and January 2012, in response to my letters, Volkman sent me thirteen handwritten letters from the Butler County Jail, totaling more than seventy pages. I have the original hard copies of those letters, as well as scanned PDF versions.

Dr. Drew's May 2011 segment about Portsmouth's drug problem remains on YouTube under the title "Prescription Pill Use Destroying Whole Town." Video of then governor John Kasich signing the so-called Pill Mill Bill is available via the Ohio Channel website under the title "Governor John Kasich: Signing H.B. 93, Preventing Prescription Drug Abuse." Coverage of that bill is accessible from the *Columbus Dispatch* ("'Pill Mill' Bill Awaits Kasich's Signature") and *Cleveland Plain Dealer* ("Ohio Gov. John Kasich Signs Bill Cracking Down on Dangerous Pill Mills"). My description of the closure of the last pill mill in Scioto County comes from coverage by the Associated Press ("Documents: Ohio 'Pill Mill' Was Corrupt Drug Den") and the *Columbus Dispatch* ("Prayers Answered: Scioto County's Last Pill Mill Shut"). The *Dispatch*'s December 28, 2011, editorial applauding this milestone was headlined "Healthy Progress."

PART 5: AFTERMATH

Crime Wave

My reporting on post-Volkman pill mill cases from southern Ohio is based on various court documents (indictments, transcripts, presentencing memoranda, appellate-court opinions), as well as media coverage and press releases from federal and state prosecutors. While it was rare to find news coverage that conveyed the scope of the crime wave, one 2019 article from the *Cleveland Plain Dealer*'s John Caniglia succeeds. Caniglia's report, "The End of an Era: Pill Mills Are Gone at Ohio's Opioid Epicenter, but Crisis Continues," was prompted by the sentencing of former Wheelersburg pain-clinic doctor Margaret Temponeras. Caniglia wrote that it "mark[ed] the end of a deadly era," during which, "for more than 15 years, rogue doctors preyed on patients in the southern Ohio county." The article reported that, during that time, "nearly 20 doctors and business owners" in Scioto County went to prison. One of them was Paul Volkman.

Other reports from Scioto County that I mention at the end of this chapter are:

The Guardian, "'The Pill Mill of America': Where Drugs Mean There Are
     No Good Choices, Only Less Awful Ones," May 17, 2017.

CBC News, "Why Portsmouth, Ohio Became the Epicentre of America's
Opioid Crisis," uploaded to YouTube on June 20, 2017.
New York Times, "'Become My Mom Again': What It's Like to Grow Up
Amid the Opioid Crisis," May 31, 2019.

My review of Sam Quinones's *Dreamland* for *The Millions*, "The Corporate Drug
Cartel: On Sam Quinones's 'Dreamland,'" remains available to read online.

Terre Haute
Both Sixth Circuit US Court of Appeals rulings on Volkman's case, from 2013 and 2015,
are accessible online, as is the US Supreme Court's short opinion from 2014. I accessed
other legal filings mentioned in this chapter through PACER. Volkman's descriptions
from Terre Haute come from our written and emailed correspondence. My summary
of his oft-repeated tale of his own innocence is stitched together from various sources:
handwritten letters from Butler County Jail; emails from his time at Terre Haute and
subsequent prisons; emails to other journalists and appeals for crowdfunding websites,
which he shared with me; a lengthy autobiographical narrative that Volkman wrote
and shared with various people in 2014 and 2015. Perhaps the clearest distillation of his
post-sentencing stance is his open letter published on the Doctors of Courage site in
2018. "I thought I was smart enough to practice medicine in a snake pit," he wrote. "But
the government snakes followed no Rule of Law."

Defenders
Siobhan Reynolds's documentary *The Chilling Effect — Pain Patients in the War on Drugs*
remains available on YouTube. Linda Cheek's website is doctorsofcourage.org. The organization stopthedrugwar.org is also still active and regularly publishes its newsletter,
Drug War Chronicle.

Loved Ones
There is one additional moment from my conversations that bears mentioning. During
my last visit to southern Ohio in 2022, I interviewed one of Scottie Lin James's friends,
Laura Garcia. She had not attended the trial and before our meeting was not aware that
Volkman defense expert Hal Blatman had described Scottie from the stand as "a drug
addict" and "a liar" who had "probably been manipulating people since she was a child."

When I offered Garcia a chance to respond, she called Blatman's remarks "highly
disrespectful" and said it was unprofessional of him to describe someone whom he had
never met in such a way. She added that Scottie wasn't manipulative; she was direct and
"said what was on her mind."

Garcia was a recovering addict herself, and she told me that being in the throes of
addiction "feels like your skin is going to fall off or your insides are going to explode or
your brain is doing laps in your head." She felt that Volkman had taken advantage of this.

Mainly, though, she wanted people to know that Scottie was a human being, who was
"loved by many."

The Magazine Article
In print, my 2017 article in *Cincinnati Magazine* was given the headline "Post Script: How
a Small-Time Chicago Doctor Came to the Southeastern Ohio Town of Portsmouth and
Helped Spur an Epidemic." Online, where it is still accessible, it was called "The Pill Mill
That Ravaged Portsmouth." This chapter also draws on letters and emails between me
and Paul Volkman, in 2018 and 2021.

Co-Conspirators
The sourcing of this final section on Harold Eugene Fletcher is described in my note
for the chapter "The Pharmacist." Obituaries for Alice Huffman (whose name was Alice

Dawn Leffingwell at the time of her death) are viewable online. Documents from Denise's criminal case, including the transcript of her sentencing hearing, are accessible through PACER. Info about the prison releases of Fletcher and the Huffmans came from the Bureau of Prison's "Federal Inmate Locator" site: bop.gov/inmateloc.

Adam and Jane

The details of Volkman's assaults and injuries in prison come from letters he wrote to his son (which were shared with me), emails to me from 2016 and 2021, as well as Facebook posts by Jane in 2018, 2019, and 2020. Jane Volkman and her husband's July 2020 GoFundMe campaign page, "Compassionate Release for Paul Volkman," is still live at gofundme.com/f/compassionate-release-for-paul-volkman. (After Volkman had a falling-out with the attorney he hired, Jane Volkman says she returned the money that was raised to the fundraiser's donors.) Their affidavits were included in Volkman's unsuccessful filings for compassionate release, which were uploaded to PACER. The details of Jane's shift in opinion about her father come from Facebook messages and calls in July and August 2023. My final interviews with Adam Volkman and his wife, Liz, took place in October 2022.

A Man of Principle

As with much of my reporting on Volkman, this chapter draws on the entirety of our communication, including our in-person interviews in 2009 and 2010 and our posttrial correspondence from 2011 to 2021. It also draws on other Volkman writings, including emails he wrote in 2003 that were submitted as evidence during his trial; a letter that he wrote in 2006 in opposition to the DEA's asset-forfeiture case against him; online comments that he wrote in response to an April 2007 post on the *New York Times* TierneyLab blog, "Judge Dismisses the Most Serious Charges Against Dr. Hurwitz"; a letter he handwrote from jail to a magistrate judge in June 2007 after his initial arrest; his 2018 open letter published on the Doctors of Courage blog; and his 2019 religious narrative, which was published by his daughter, Jane, on Facebook.

All-America City

This chapter draws on my last trip to Portsmouth: an eight-day visit in late October and early November 2022. Portsmouth's "All-America City" application was shared with me by Mayor Sean Dunne. A video of the May 2019 Friends of Portsmouth pep rally / press conference is on YouTube, with the title "Why Portsmouth, Ohio Is Leading the Nation in Recovery and Small Town Resurgence." More info about the organization is available at friendsofportsmouth.com. And more info on the Counseling Center is available at thecounselingcenter.org.

The two *Cincinnati Enquirer* op-eds I mention are "There's Another Side of the Portsmouth Community That Doesn't Make the News" by Ryan Ottney, on March 25, 2019, and "Drugs Only Part of Portsmouth Story" by US representative Brad Wenstrup, on August 15, 2019. Lisa Roberts and her work on southern Ohio's opiate epidemic has been discussed on various TV reports, podcasts, and print articles. Her 2018 testimony in Washington, DC, before a subcommittee of the House Oversight and Accountability Committee, "Local Responses and Resources to Curtail the Opioid Epidemic," is also available online.

Afterword: In Memoriam

These vignettes draw upon multiple sources, including interviews, obituaries, Facebook posts, trial transcripts and evidence, and information from Ancestry.com. Physical descriptions of grave sites are based on my own visits, which took place during my October 2022 trip to Portsmouth.

READING GROUP GUIDE

1. Do you believe justice was served in the criminal case of Paul Volkman? Why or why not?

2. What emotions did you feel while reading this story?

3. Decades of public polling data have shown that doctors are among America's most trusted professionals. Do you trust your doctors? What is that trust based on? Did this story affect that trust, or change the way you view the medical field?

4. Who or what do you feel is to blame for the decline of towns like Portsmouth, Ohio? Do you have hope for the future of these towns? Why or why not?

5. Chronic pain and drug addiction are two public health issues at the heart of this book. Did your proximity or personal history with either of those issues affect your reading experience?

6. We hear extensively from Volkman in this book. What were your impressions of him as a person? And as a doctor?

7. The book also includes perspectives from people in Volkman's personal life, including his adult children. How did their thoughts shape your opinion of him?

8. One of the issues at play in Volkman's criminal case — and, in particular, at his trial — is the question of responsibility in the doctor-patient relationship. How much responsibility do patients have for being honest with their doctors and taking medications as prescribed? And how does this compare to a doctor's responsibility to be skeptical of patients' stories and to exercise discretion when prescribing medications?

9. The book includes a chapter titled "Defenders" in which various people express partial or total sympathy for Volkman. Did you find any of their arguments persuasive?

10. This book tells the story of one particular doctor during the opiate epidemic. But the overall responsibility for the crisis has been placed

on a variety of actors, including pharmaceutical companies, medical distributors, pharmacies, federal regulators, and others. Who or what do you hold most responsible for causing this man-made crisis? Why?

11. This book is categorized as "true crime." How does it compare to other stories from that genre that you have read, watched, or listened to? Were there ways this was an unusual or unique true crime story?

12. Do you think the story of Paul Volkman points to systematic issues in US healthcare? Or did you view it more as the story of one "bad apple"?